Scholarly, comprehensive, but also beautifully written and readable, Bethany L. Brand has truly given us the landmark book on the important but often overlooked topic of dissociation. A must-read for all clinicians working with trauma.

—**Janina Fisher, PhD,** author of *Healing the Fragmented Selves of Trauma Survivors* and *Transforming the Living Legacy of Trauma*

Dr. Bethany L. Brand has provided a wealth of contemporary information about dissociation and its assessment and treatment in a concise format. She is known for her deep expertise on these topics and her ability to communicate complicated information in a straightforward and accessible way. I highly recommend it as a must-have reference for all mental health professionals.

—**Christine A. Courtois, PhD, ABPP,** author of *Healing the Incest Wound: Adult Survivors in Therapy* and coeditor of *Sexual Boundary Violations in Psychotherapy*

In this state-of-the art book, Bethany L. Brand eloquently guides the reader through the assessment and treatment of trauma-related dissociation in children and adults, as well as its critical importance in forensic settings. A must-read for all clinicians working with clients who experience dissociation and trauma-related disorders!

—**Ruth Lanius, MD, PhD,** Professor of Psychiatry, University of Western Ontario, London, Ontario, Canada

The Concise Guide to the Assessment and Treatment of Trauma-Related Dissociation

Concise Guides on Trauma Care Series

The Concise Guide to the Assessment and Treatment of Trauma-Related Dissociation

Bethany L. Brand

 AMERICAN PSYCHOLOGICAL ASSOCIATION

Published by
American Psychological Association
750 First Street, NE
Washington, DC 20002
https://www.apa.org

Order Department
https://www.apa.org/pubs/books
order@apa.org

Typeset in Charter and Interstate by Circle Graphics, Inc., Reisterstown, MD

Printer: Sheridan Books, Chelsea, MI
Cover Designer: Beth Schlenoff Design, Bethesda, MD

Library of Congress Cataloging-in-Publication Data

Names: Brand, Bethany L., author.
Title: The concise guide to the assessment and treatment of trauma-related
    dissociation / Bethany L. Brand.
Description: Washington, DC : American Psychological Association, [2024] |
    Series: Concise guides on trauma care series | Includes bibliographical
    references and index.
Identifiers: LCCN 2023023513 (print) | LCCN 2023023514 (ebook) |
    ISBN 9781433837715 (paperback) | ISBN 9781433837722 (ebook)
Subjects: LCSH: Dissociative disorders. | Dissociation (Psychology) |
    Dissociative disorders--Treatment. | Psychic trauma--Complications. |
    Psychic trauma--Complications--Treatment. | Post-traumatic stress
    disorder--Complications. | Post-traumatic stress
    disorder--Complications--Treatment. | BISAC: PSYCHOLOGY /
    Psychopathology / Dissociative Identity Disorder | PSYCHOLOGY /
    Psychotherapy / General
Classification: LCC RC553.D5 B73 2023 (print) | LCC RC553.D5 (ebook) |
    DDC 616.85/23--dc23/eng/20230817
LC record available at https://lccn.loc.gov/2023023513
LC ebook record available at https://lccn.loc.gov/2023023514

https://doi.org/10.1037/0000386-000

Printed in the United States of America

10 9 8 7 6 5 4 3 2

This book is dedicated to my mentors and colleagues who helped me learn to listen, watch, and understand what I observed and to the trauma survivors who trusted me to bear witness to their stories and understand their struggles. I am humbled and inspired by your resilience, courage, and perseverance.

Contents

Series Foreword

Exposure to traumatic events is all too common, increasing the risk for a range of significant consequences affecting health and well-being. In recent years, new reports of incidents of mass trauma—from gun violence and combat to intimate partner abuse and child maltreatment—have propelled trauma into a brighter public spotlight. Public awareness ad education campaigns, such as #metoo and Start by Believing, have coincided with an increasing number of trauma survivors seeking services for mental health consequences of traumatic stress.

Despite the far-ranging consequences of trauma and the high rates of exposure, relatively little emphasis has been placed on trauma education in undergraduate and graduate training programs for mental health service providers in the United States. This book series, Concise Guides on Trauma Care, addresses that gap by providing truly translational books that bring the best of trauma psychology science to mental health professionals working in diverse settings. To do so, the series focuses on what we know (and do not know) about specific trauma topics, with attention to how trauma psychology science translates to diverse populations (diversity broadly defined, in terms of developmental stage, ethnicity, socioeconomic status, sexual orientation, and so forth).

This series represents one of many efforts undertaken by Division 56 (Trauma Psychology) of the American Psychological Association to advance trauma training and education (e.g., see https://www.apatraumadivision.org/68/teaching-training.html). We are pleased to work with Division 56 and a volunteer editorial board to create this series, which continues to move forward with the publication of this important guide to the assessment of trauma-related dissociation by Bethany Brand. As clinicians, researchers, policy makers, and system leaders seek to better engage children, youth, and adults in the assessment process, this monograph offers a practical and accessible guide to the assessment process using a trauma-informed framework. The information provided in this guide will be of great use to mental health professionals in understanding the etiology of dissociation, methodology for assessing dissociation, and considerations with assessing for dissociation with specific populations such as children and adolescents or within a forensic context. This knowledge will be helpful when working with individuals who have been exposed to traumatic events and there are questions of dissociative symptoms impacting presentation and functioning. Future books in the series will continue to address a range of assessment, treatment, and developmental issues in trauma-informed care.

—*Anne P. DePrince*
Ann T. Chu
Series Editors

Foreword

The History and Complexity of Trauma-Related Dissociation

Although first formally described in the late 19th century (van der Hart & Horst, 1989), dissociation has only recently received detailed scientific and clinical scrutiny, and it continues to be controversial for some. Reasons likely include (a) the seemingly bizarre nature of some dissociative symptoms, engendering disbelief and dismissal in some and overexcitement in others; (b) its relationship to trauma, which itself has been subject to cycles of professional rejection and acceptance; (c) its early linkage to "hysteria," a construct that was freighted and ultimately devalued by its inherent sexism and fading relevance to modern psychology; and (d) the lingering effects of the "False Memory" debates of the 1990s and early 2000s, which challenged and derided the notion of amnesia for past traumatic events.

Another reason may be its complexity. Dissociative symptoms can range from depersonalization and derealization to psychogenic amnesia, cognitive disengagement, emotional constriction, somatic disturbance, fugue states, identity confusion, discrete "personalities" that recurrently take control in the same person, and, in some cultures, dissociative trance and possession states. It can present with a range of comorbidities, including somatization, depression, anxiety, self-injury, conversion disorder, eating disorders, substance abuse, personality disturbance, and posttraumatic stress.

These aspects of dissociation continue to feed active and sometimes heated professional debates, including whether dissociation inevitably arises from trauma exposure or, especially in the case of amnesia or dissociative identity disorder, whether it can be dismissed as feigned or fantasy based. There are even questions about whether dissociation exists as an independent entity. Nevertheless, recent research and clinical investigations have tended to settle on a set of probable facts, although even these are currently debated or disputed by some and are likely to be revised based on future research. In general, the following can be said of dissociation:

- It arises from traumatic experiences, especially in childhood (Dalenberg et al., 2012), as well as, in some cases, early relational deprivation and attachment insecurity (Liotti, 2009).

- It is probably best understood as an avoidance strategy (as detailed in this volume), often marshaled in the context of underdeveloped emotional regulation capacities (Cavicchioli et al., 2021). It can also represent an idiom of distress or spiritual disruption in some cultures (e.g., Lewis-Fernández et al., 2010).

- It is multidimensional in nature, involving a range of only moderately correlated symptom clusters (Briere et al., 2005).

- It frequently presents with other psychological problems and symptoms that share a common etiology in childhood adversity (Lyssenko et al., 2018).

- It is often treatable, despite sometimes complicated clinical trajectories (Brand et al., 2022).

Given these various issues, it is important to assess dissociation accurately before attempting to treat it. This is, of course, also true for other clinical presentations. But dissociation is especially noteworthy for its etiologic intricacies and diverse presentations, as well as its sometimes shape-shifting qualities that make it hard to identify and quantify. When successful, for example, the avoidant aspect of dissociation can serve as a self-cloaking device that conceals the severity of the client's distress and impairment and, ironically, may interfere with its own clinical resolution.

As described in this book, evidence-based assessment is critical in determining the specific forms of dissociation that are present in any given clinical scenario and their level of clinical acuity; the role of trauma- and attachment-based responses; the emotional dysregulation often underlying dissociation and the client's response to therapy; the functions that dissociation serves, including numbing, self-protection, or distress reduction; and safety issues such as suicidality, self-harm, and diminished environmental vigilance. It also informs treatment by identifying specific targets and determining appropriate treatment approaches. For example, assessment data can bear on the correct pace and intensity of interventions for a given client, help determine whether safety, stabilization, emotional dysregulation, and major comorbidities require attention before the treatment of "dissociation" per se, and help evaluate the appropriateness of emotional processing methodologies (i.e., prolonged exposure and eye movement desensitization and reprocessing) at any given point in therapy. Assessment may also reduce undue skepticism or countertransference regarding the validity of specific dissociative presentations as the clinician becomes more familiar with the client's history and phenomenology.

Unfortunately, there are a limited number of resources available to clinicians on the modern assessment and treatment of clinical dissociation. Fortunately, we now have Dr. Brand and colleagues' groundbreaking book, *The Concise Guide to the Assessment and Treatment of Trauma-Related Dissociation*. It addresses almost all conceivable questions about dissociation and how to assess it and does so in a way that is both accessible and authoritative. The extensive review and description of psychometric instruments would be enough to merit its inclusion in any clinician's bookshelf, let alone the detailed coverage of the etiology and theory of dissociation, how it can inform intervention, and its forensic implications. Dr. Brand and colleagues' work, here and in other recent books (e.g., Brand et al., 2022), reflects a signal moment in our field, demarcating a growing shift toward empiricism and science, leavened with compassion, as we seek to improve the lives of those struggling with dissociative symptoms and disorders.

—*John Briere, PhD*
Professor Emeritus of Psychiatry & the Behavioral Sciences,
Keck School of Medicine, University of Southern California

REFERENCES

Brand, B. L., Schielke, H. J., Schiavone, F., & Lanius, R. A. (2022). *Finding solid ground: Overcoming obstacles in trauma treatment*. Oxford University Press. https://doi.org/10.1093/med-psych/9780190636081.001.0001

Briere, J., Weathers, F. W., & Runtz, M. (2005). Is dissociation a multidimensional construct? Data from the Multiscale Dissociation Inventory. *Journal of Traumatic Stress*, *18*(3), 221–231. https://doi.org/10.1002/jts.20024

Cavicchioli, M., Scalabrini, A., Northoff, G., Mucci, C., Ogliari, A., & Maffei, C. (2021). Dissociation and emotion regulation strategies: A meta-analytic review. *Journal of Psychiatric Research*, *143*, 370–387. https://doi.org/10.1016/j.jpsychires.2021.09.011

Dalenberg, C. J., Brand, B. L., Gleaves, D. H., Dorahy, M. J., Loewenstein, R. J., Cardeña, E., Frewen, P. A., Carlson, E. B., & Spiegel, D. (2012). Evaluation of the evidence for the trauma and fantasy models of dissociation. *Psychological Bulletin*, *138*(3), 550–588. https://doi.org/10.1037/a0027447

Lewis-Fernández, R., Gorritz, M., Raggio, G. A., Peláez, C., Chen, H., & Guarnaccia, P. J. (2010). Association of trauma-related disorders and dissociation with four idioms of distress among Latino psychiatric outpatients. *Culture, Medicine and Psychiatry, 34*(2), 219–243. https://doi.org/10.1007/s11013-010-9177-8

Liotti, G. (2009). Attachment and dissociation. In P. F. Dell & J. A. O'Neil (Eds.), *Dissociation and the dissociative disorders: DSM-V and beyond* (pp. 53–65). Routledge/Taylor & Francis Group.

Lyssenko, L., Schmahl, C., Bockhacker, L., Vonderlin, R., Bohus, M., & Kleindienst, N. (2018). Dissociation in psychiatric disorders: A meta-analysis of studies using the Dissociative Experiences Scale. *The American Journal of Psychiatry, 175*(1), 37–46. https://doi.org/10.1176/appi.ajp.2017.17010025

van der Hart, O., & Horst, R. (1989). The dissociation theory of Pierre Janet. *Journal of Traumatic Stress, 2*(4), 397–412. https://doi.org/10.1002/jts.2490020405

Foreword

An Overview of The Concise Guide to the Assessment and Treatment of Trauma-Related Dissociation

I have known Dr. Bethany Brand since 1988, when she worked on the Female Growth and Development Study, our 35-plus year, prospective, longitudinal study of the effects of sexual abuse on young girls. From that time forward, it was clear that Bethany was to become an outstanding trauma clinician and researcher. Over the following decades, we have collaborated on multiple research projects related to trauma-related dissociation (TRD), most of which were initiated by Dr. Brand. I have followed her career closely, and she is a well-regarded international leader in the field of dissociative and trauma-related disorders across many domains: treatment, prevention, research, political, and public education. Her work, both clinical and nonclinical, is characterized by innovation, sensitivity, and a dogged persistence, often in the face of egregious pushback by trauma deniers. She brings an enormous depth and breadth of expertise to *The Concise Guide to the Assessment and Treatment of Trauma-Related Dissociation.*

In many respects, this book is more of a "complete" than a "concise" guide, as it covers virtually everything that is important for the typical clinician to know about trauma-related dissociation. Having consulted with innumerable patients, Dr. Brand is alert to the myriad clinical presentations of TRD across gender, age, and diagnostic categories. She is sensitive to the concerns and cautions that both clients and clinicians feel as they begin to unpack the complicated contributions of TRD to their lives and problems. Having conducted multiyear longitudinal studies of the treatment of TRD by community clinicians,

Dr. Brand appreciates the ups and downs in the usual course of treatment as well as common pitfalls.

This guide contains a comprehensive review of assessment measures and methodology, including forensic evaluation and assessing children and adolescents. Amply illustrated with case studies and tables comparing the strengths and limitations of the numerous assessment and diagnostic measures, this guide should help even neophyte clinicians feel confident that they are pursuing state-of-the-art approaches to assessing their clients.

For more than 30 years, we have had reliable and valid measures to screen for pathological dissociation and structured diagnostic interviews for formal diagnosis of the *Diagnostic and Statistical Manual of Mental Disorders* (*DSM*) dissociative disorders. Research with these instruments has repeatedly found that high levels of dissociation are strongly linked to antecedent trauma and associated with clinically significant morbidity and comorbidity including suicide attempts, depression, posttraumatic stress disorder (PTSD), self-mutilation, and substance abuse. In addition to the *DSM* dissociative disorders, patients with borderline personality disorder and PTSD may manifest high levels of dissociation. Research finds that "non–dissociative disorder" patients with high levels of dissociation are significantly more resistant to the standard treatments for their conditions than are patients with the same diagnoses but with low levels of dissociation. A growing number of treatment studies indicate that irrespective of the *DSM* diagnosis, directly addressing high levels of dissociation is associated with significant clinical improvement but is of little to no benefit in low dissociative patients with the same diagnoses.

What is surprising is that when faced with complicated, treatment-refractory patients, many clinicians do not consider the possibility that dissociation may be making a major contribution to their patient or client's clinical picture. As we gain a better understanding of how to treat pathological dissociation, failure to assess complex, treatment-nonresponsive patients appropriately for pathological dissociation becomes increasingly indefensible.

There are a variety of reasons why many clinicians fail to include pathological dissociation in their differential diagnosis. These range from an unfamiliarity with dissociation as a clinical process to an active rejection of dissociation as a legitimate psychopathological construct. Indeed, dissociation and the dissociative disorders have faced literally centuries of professional ignorance, skepticism, and aggressive denial.

The Concise Guide to the Assessment and Treatment of Trauma-Related Dissociation summarizes the current state of empirical knowledge about pathological and normal dissociation. The *Guide* also addresses common misunderstandings as well as the misguided denials of dissociation as a major clinical process. The *Guide* wisely focuses on "trauma-related dissociation" (TRD) because this is the basis of most clinically significant dissociative symptoms.

The *Guide* approaches dissociation from a number of perspectives, including the *DSM* dissociative disorders as well as cardinal dissociative symptoms such as dissociative amnesias, fugues, identity alterations, depersonalization and derealization, and deep absorption. It details the pros and cons of the continuum versus dichotomous and normative versus pathological characterizations of dissociation.

Most important, the *Guide* stresses the transdiagnostic, but often covert, nature of TRD. The astute clinician should be alert to the possibility of pathological dissociation in every patient reporting a significant trauma history, especially childhood trauma. An extensive table aids in differentiating the dissociative disorders from borderline personality disorder, bipolar disorder, and schizophrenia, for which they are most often mistaken.

The *Guide* summarizes the wide range of psychological and biological mechanisms and historical models advanced to explain the nature and psychobiological functions of dissociation. Ranging from TRD as a classic psychoanalytic defense mechanism to TRD as a third alternative (i.e., "freeze") to W. B. Cannon's classic "fight-or-flight" response to life threats, the *Guide* considers all the major (and many minor) theories advanced to account for TRD. In particular, it excels in contrasting the trauma versus fantasy models of dissociation, the focus of a long-running, passionate debate in which Dr. Brand is a major participant. The *Guide* also updates the seminal neurobiological findings of Ruth Lanius and others that distinguish TRD from "classic" PTSD. Further, it summarizes the equally important, but often overlooked, longitudinal developmental research linking disrupted early attachment with later elevations of dissociation in adulthood.

Building on this empirical and historical foundation, readers are introduced to the importance of a "collaborative" and "therapeutic" approach to assessment, especially respecting an individual's trauma history and life experiences. Particularly salient in this regard are discussions of clinically observable signs of dissociation, grounding techniques to help patients with overwhelming dissociative experiences, and approaches to building a therapeutic relationship with these complex, often mercurial, patients. A detailed mental status exam is included.

Richly illustrated with case studies, the *Guide* includes the author's emotional reactions and intellectual responses to the complex clinical and challenging forensic case studies that she offers as heuristic examples. Important, but seldom acknowledged, confounds such as cultural issues, transference and countertransference, and clinical complexity are amply covered. Starting with the Dissociative Experiences Scale, the domains and psychometrics of the leading self-report dissociation measures are reviewed in detail. Similarly, the major structured *DSM* diagnostic interviews are covered. Projective testing, such as the Rorschach and Thematic Apperception Test, can be diagnostically helpful, particularly because they provide an opportunity to observe the client exhibiting traumatic and dissociative reactions in response to projective stimuli. Of critical importance is a comprehensive section devoted to differentiation of genuine pathological dissociation from factitious or malingered symptoms.

Dr. Brand has extensive experience in the assessment of pathological dissociation in forensic settings including death row cases. Understanding the manifestation of dissociation in forensic contexts, especially its effects on a victim's recall of events and demeanor in court, is critical in conducting an informed and objective forensic evaluation.

A chapter by Amie Myrick, MS, LCPC, and Joyanna Silberg, PhD, on assessing child and adolescent dissociation covers this extremely important area. Many dissociative disorders begin in childhood or early adolescence and initially present as serious behavioral problems. Normal childhood developmental processes (e.g., imaginary companionship and adolescent identity crises) are common and must be distinguished from pathological dissociation. This has become increasingly important in an era of "TikTok and YouTube multiples"—adolescents who post Internet videos exaggerating different facets of their personality. Of particular importance is the discussion of differentiating normative childhood identity alterations, such as imaginary companionship, from more pathological manifestations. The leading self-report and parent/observer-report measures of dissociation in youth are detailed and compared, together with informative case studies.

The final chapter is a comprehensive survey of state-of-the-art approaches to the treatment of TRD, to which Dr. Brand has made significant contributions. Stressing the need for individualizing treatment depending on a client's needs, she outlines a three-phase treatment model along the lines of the therapeutic approach first articulated by Dr. Judith Herman for rape and incest victims with complex PTSD. Specific symptom and behavior treatment targets, issues raised by working with self-states, techniques for clinical stabilization, and approaches to assessing efficacy are detailed. Dr. Brand addresses the nuances of working with dissociative identity states, something that many clinicians find uncomfortable and confusing. In addition, she includes therapist- and client-report measures of treatment progress with which to help gauge progress. The references section is extraordinarily complete. Lessons learned from the seminal Treatment of Patients With Dissociative Disorders (TOP DD) studies directed by Dr. Brand complete the *Guide*.

Author and coauthor of many peer-reviewed publications and the winner of numerous professional awards for her work, Dr. Brand is the ideal author for this guide. Throughout her career, she has been deeply involved in research, clinical practice, and forensic evaluations—all of which require extensive knowledge of the tools and techniques required to assess dissociation and the dissociative disorders empirically. The information contained in *The Concise Guide to the Assessment and Treatment of Trauma-Related Dissociation* will be invaluable for clinicians working with trauma victims for years to come.

—*Frank W. Putnam, MD*
Professor, Department of Psychiatry,
University of North Carolina at Chapel Hill

Preface

Most individuals seeking mental health treatment have experienced trauma, and their symptoms and struggles are often directly or indirectly related to, or exacerbated by, trauma. Clinically significant dissociative symptoms are one of the impacts of trauma. Trauma-related dissociation (TRD) is more common and is associated with greater risk and symptom severity than most clinicians realize. The prevalence of dissociation in population studies ranges from 3.4% to 6.4% (Maaranen et al., 2005, 2008; Mulder et al., 1998; C. A. Ross et al., 1990). Dissociation is associated with reduced ability to work; unemployment; younger age; and poor finances, social support, and physical health (Maaranen et al., 2005). One in 20 veterans in a U.S. nationally representative sample experienced dissociative symptoms; dissociation was associated with a fivefold greater likelihood of suicidal ideation and fourfold greater likelihood of lifetime suicide attempt (Herzog et al., 2020). Hospitalized veterans who were diagnosed with somatoform or dissociative disorders had 3.6 greater odds of completing suicide after being discharged (Kessler et al., 2015). Dissociation conferred more risk for completed suicide than did depression, psychosis, and past suicide attempts. Clearly, dissociation urgently needs to be assessed and adequately treated.

Unfortunately, most clinicians receive little to no training about assessing and treating dissociation. This book is an attempt to remedy this concerning gap. It is my hope that this book facilitates accurate diagnosis and appropriate treatment for individuals who experience TRD.

Dissociation is associated with longer treatment, higher dropout rates, and poorer response to treatment. If chronic TRD is not attended to in treatment, symptoms of TRD, particularly those related to complex dissociative symptoms, do not significantly improve (Brand, Sar, et al., 2016; Jepsen et al., 2014). Research shows that when the complex dissociative disorders as well as milder forms of dissociation are targeted in treatment, patients show a wide range of improvements including stabilization of nonsuicidal self-injury and suicidal ideation, decreased rates of hospitalization and treatment costs, improved functioning and emotion regulation, and reduced symptoms of PTSD, dissociation, depression, and substance misuse (e.g., Brand, Schielke, et al., 2019; Jepsen et al., 2014). Said differently, if TRD is targeted in treatment, trauma survivors can greatly benefit.

AN OVERVIEW OF THE BOOK

Chapter 1 provides definitions of dissociation and the disorders in which TRD occurs. The prevalence, impairment, comorbidity, chronicity, and mortality associated with dissociation are reviewed. The reasons and costs of dissociation being underrecognized and undertreated are discussed. I present information about differentiating dissociative disorders from other disorders, including schizophrenia, bipolar disorder, and borderline personality disorder.

Chapter 2 reviews the debate about the etiology of dissociation from the perspectives of the trauma model of dissociation and the fantasy model of dissociation. I review the impact of this debate on individuals living with TRD and the impact on the training and knowledge of mental health professionals.

In Chapter 3, I describe practices that foster developing a collaborative working relationship with traumatized clients so that they feel sufficiently supported and safe to share and reflect on their life experiences, symptoms, and resiliencies. The impact of circumscribed incidents of trauma are compared with those from exposure to complex trauma. I suggest adaptations that need to be made depending on the type of trauma experienced, the individual's level of resources, and the severity of TRD. I argue that a careful assessment for trauma and its impact should be part of the standard intake assessment process for all individuals seeking mental health treatment, regardless of their presenting problems, and should precede and inform the choice of psychotherapeutic interventions including psychotherapy and psychiatric medications.

Chapter 4 presents the validated measures of TRD, including self-report measures, clinician-report measures, semistandardized diagnostic interviews, performance measures, and less formal assessment procedures that can be used in clinical practice. I provide descriptions of a battery of tests and interviews that may be useful for formal psychological testing when TRD is a concern. A summary of research-based methods for differentiating exaggerated, factitious, or malingered dissociation is presented, along with two cases of individuals presenting for assessment of possible TRD.

Chapter 5 addresses the assessment of TRD in forensic contexts. It reviews the measures that are useful in differentiating response styles among individuals who may have been exposed to trauma and may have TRD, as well as measures that have low utility scores in forensic research with individuals with TRD. A forensic case in which TRD was assessed is presented.

Chapter 6 guides clinicians in recognizing dissociation in children and adolescents and discusses methods for differentiating between dissociation and other symptoms and disorders, including attention-deficit, psychotic, mood, and anxiety disorders. Developmentally sensitive and appropriate interviewing techniques and youth symptom screens for TRD are reviewed. The authors, Joyanna Silberg and Amie Myrick, describe the presentation and treatment of a young girl whose TRD was initially not recognized or treated, as well as the symptoms that signaled TRD, which, when addressed in treatment, resulted in substantial improvement.

In Chapter 7, I describe the importance of assessment results being used to conceptualize and individualize treatment for TRD. I discuss measures that can be used to assess treatment progress. I review treatment studies with TRD samples and discuss the debate about whether treatment needs to be adapted for dissociative individuals. I address the strengths and weaknesses of randomized controlled trial studies and the clinical guidelines that have relied on this research design. Research indicates that treatment focusing on improving emotion regulation, stabilizing safety, and educating TRD patients about symptom management techniques is associated with a wide range of improvements in symptoms, reductions in nonsuicidal self-injury and treatment costs, and increased engagement in social and vocational activities.

THE NATURE OF BEING A CONCISE GUIDE

This book is part of the American Psychological Association's Concise Guide series, with related page limitations. Therefore, there are limited citations of research and theoretical material. I prioritize recent over older research, meta-analytic studies and reviews over original studies, and tables that present findings in summary format rather than discussing each study in the text. Other sources offer excellent, thorough reviews of the theory and clinical wisdom related to complex trauma, complex PTSD, and dissociation.

Here, the focus remains resolutely on TRD. I limit the discussion of assessment measures strictly to measures that are validated and widely used measures of TRD, rather than measures of complex PTSD or PTSD. I emphasize practical application over theoretic discussions. Inevitably the need to be concise and practical means I am not citing the brilliant work of many scholars, clinicians, and researchers, upon whose work my clinical, forensic, and scientific work rests. I humbly acknowledge that what I share here is a compilation and distillation of wisdom and practices developed and generously shared by dozens of mentors, authors, and colleagues; I attempt to acknowledge many of these people in the Acknowledgments and list some of the foundational work in Appendix C.

MY BACKGROUND

I matriculated from the University of Michigan, then earned my master's and PhD from the Clinical/Community Psychology program at the University of Maryland, College Park. I completed an externship in psychological testing at Johns Hopkins Hospital and a clinical internship at George Washington University. I have worked in inpatient units at several psychiatric hospitals as well as in a variety of outpatient settings. I continue to assess and treat patients and serve as a forensic expert in my private practice.

This book is informed by more than 30 years of clinical and research experience with trauma survivors, including a 2-year postdoctoral fellowship in severe trauma disorders at Sheppard Pratt Health Services followed by several years as an attending and supervising psychologist. I supervised the psychological testing performed by trauma disorders postdoctoral fellows for more than 20 years at Sheppard Pratt. I have taught courses in diagnostic interviewing and differential diagnosis, as well as other clinical courses, for 25 years at Towson University. I have served as an expert in a variety of forensic contexts, most often on criminal cases in which the defendant was facing capital punishment or had already received a sentence of capital punishment and was residing on death row. I conduct research in five primary areas: the assessment and differentiation of clinical dissociation from malingered dissociation, the treatment of dissociation, training clinicians in the assessment and treatment of complex trauma, assessing the accuracy and adequacy of textbooks' coverage of trauma and dissociation, and the debate between the proponents of the trauma and fantasy models of dissociation. I have been a coauthor on national and international task forces that have developed guidelines about the assessment and treatment of trauma and TRD.

A NOTE ABOUT TERMINOLOGY

I use the terms *client*, *patient*, and *trauma survivor* interchangeably and synonymously throughout this book.[1]

ACKNOWLEDGMENTS

I want to acknowledge and thank the incredible group of the Treatment of Patients With Dissociative Disorders (TOP DD) consultants who are gifted researchers, clinicians, trainers, and writers, and unfailing supporters and friends: Suzette Boon, Catherine Classen, Paul A. Frewen., Ellen K.K. Jepsen, Willemien Langeland, Ruth A. Lanius, Richard J. Loewenstein, Amie Myrick, Clare Pain, Frank W. Putnam, Karen Putnam, Hugo J. Schielke, and Kathy Steele. I am also indebted to the colleagues and mentors who have profoundly influenced my work through their inspiration, insights, supervision, and support, notably Pamela Alexander, Judith Armstrong, John Briere, Richard Chefetz, Christine Courtois, Constance Dalenberg, Nel Draijer, Barton Evans, Catherine Fine, Richard Kluft, Richard Loewenstein, Frank Putnam, Joyanna Silberg, and Kathy Steele.

My understanding of the assessment and treatment of trauma survivors has been strongly influenced by many brilliant colleagues. Some of these individuals include, but are not limited to, Su Baker, Peter Barach, Ruth Blizard, Lisa Butler, Dan Brown, Laura Brown, Eve Carlson, Etzel Cardena, James Chu, Martin Dorahy, Paul Dell, Janina Fisher, Brad Foote, Julian Ford, Steve Frankel, Jennifer Freyd, David Gleaves, Steve Gold, Naomi Halpern, Judith Herman, Ingunn Holbæk, Elizabeth Howell, Phil Kinsler, Ulrich Lanius, Peter Levine, Roberto Lewis-Fernandez, Giovanni Liotti, Karlen Lyons-Ruth, Alfonso Martínez-Taboas, Warwick Middleton, Andrew Moskowitz, Ellert Nijenhuis, John O'Neil, Simone Reinders, Colin Ross, Vedat Sar, Alan Schore, Daniel Siegel, Daphne Simeon, Eli Somer, David Spiegel, Joan Turkus, Onno van der Hart, and Eric Vermetten. I also want to thank Sebastian McNary, Thom Lieb, Richard Loewenstein, and Barton Evans for their outstanding editing and useful guidance on early versions of this book. You are fabulous thinkers and writers!

---

[1]Throughout this book, case study information is fictional, uses composites, or has been altered by changing names and removing identifying information to preserve client confidentiality.

I have learned a great deal from individuals who have lived with trauma-related dissociation and other sequalae of trauma. Their perseverance, resilience, and courage in the face of horror and violence inspire and motivate me. I deeply thank them for sharing their experiences and struggles with me. It is an honor to have the opportunity to work with and guide them on their healing journeys.

On a more personal level, I want to acknowledge and thank my close friends, my two dear sons (who inspire me with their work for social justice), and my loving partner, Denzil. You have listened and cared when I was full of enthusiasm as well as when I hit obstacles while writing. You supported and encouraged me and had faith in me and this book. Thank you for accompanying me.

The Concise Guide to the Assessment and Treatment of Trauma-Related Dissociation

1 AN INTRODUCTION TO TRAUMA-RELATED DISSOCIATION

Dissociation is an intriguing, complex phenomenon. It has become so popularized that it is frequently featured in movies, TV series, news reports, and social media, yet it is often misunderstood, even by mental health professionals. Clinicians, researchers, forensic experts, and attorneys have become interested because of growing awareness about the importance of trauma, its potential impact, and the need to address trauma in mental health treatment. As this chapter will show, trauma-related dissociation (TRD) is underrecognized, inadequately treated, associated with disability and impairment, as well as high financial costs to the individual patients and society. Mental health professionals are rarely trained to assess for dissociative symptoms, although all patients should be assessed for TRD so individualized treatment plans can address its impacts. Earlier recognition and treatment of TRD could result in reduced levels of disability, considerable economic savings, and improved quality of life for individuals with TRD. It is time to stop making traumatized individuals and their loved ones pay for the lack of training about trauma and TRD among mental health professionals. Systemic trauma education needs to become ubiquitous in training programs so that the enduring

https://doi.org/10.1037/0000386-001
The Concise Guide to the Assessment and Treatment of Trauma-Related Dissociation,
by B. L. Brand

impact of childhood abuse, neglect, and adult traumatization are no longer overlooked, misdiagnosed, and mistreated.

The *Diagnostic and Statistical Manual of Mental Disorders, Fifth Edition– Text Revision* (*DSM-5-TR*; American Psychiatric Association, 2022) defines *dissociation* as "disruption of and/or discontinuity in the normal integration of consciousness, memory, identity, emotion, perception, body representation, motor control, and behavior" (p. 291). Dissociation includes a wide range of phenomena that extend from common, nonpathological experiences (e.g., being so completely absorbed by a book that one does not hear a conversation) to severe symptoms (e.g., feeling one's body does not belong to oneself). If dissociation occurs frequently and is disruptive to functioning or causes distress, it may indicate the presence of a dissociative disorder.

Dissociation is increasingly studied in assessment, experimental, psychological, clinical, neurobiological, and treatment research because researchers have recognized dissociation is common and yet often disruptive to psychological functioning (American Psychiatric Association, 2022; World Health Organization, 2021). The focus of this book centers on pathological TRD— that is, dissociation occurring during or after trauma or overwhelming stress that causes dysfunction or distress (Brand & Frewen, 2017; Brand, Schielke, & Brams, 2017; Lanius et al., 2018; Lebois et al., 2021). TRD impacts a wide range of higher level integrative and regulative capacities, thereby interfering with emotion regulation, thinking, memory, perception, emotional learning, and other psychological processes (Cavicchioli et al., 2021). Alterations in the neural pathways that process sensations between the inner, psychological and outer social, physical worlds have been hypothesized to have cascading effects on higher order cognitive functions including social cognition, emotion regulation, and goal-oriented behavior, thus shaping dissociative individuals' perception of and engagement with the world (Harricharan et al., 2021). Indeed, the *DSM-5-TR* notes that "dissociative symptoms can potentially disrupt every area of psychological functioning" (American Psychiatric Association, 2022, p. 329). This widespread disruption can contribute to the development of intrusive fragmented traumatic memories and a fragmented sense of self. Dissociation can be so disruptive to emotional and cognitive functioning that individuals with TRD have difficulty being fully present and able to benefit from psychotherapy, making recognizing and treating dissociation of central importance.

There are many types of dissociative symptoms. *Depersonalization* involves feeling disconnected or estranged from one's body, thoughts, or emotions. *Derealization* is perceiving one's environment as unreal, foggy, distorted, or unfamiliar. *Dissociative amnesia* is characterized by an inability to recall important autobiographical information that is inconsistent with normal forgetting. Some people who experience amnesia also travel away from home with amnesia for one's name and other aspects of identity; this is *dissociative fugue* (American Psychiatric Association, 2013). *Identity confusion* is the feeling of uncertainty, puzzlement, conflict, or struggle regarding one's identity (e.g., a conflict about one's values and beliefs). *Identity alteration* refers to the observable behaviors associated with shifts in dissociative self-states; note that "self-states" have also been referred to as alters, parts, personalities, and identities. *Absorption* occurs when a person loses track of background events (e.g., does not hear their name being called while reading a book or misses their exit while driving on a highway). There is debate about whether absorption should be included as a pathological versus normal form of dissociation. Because the extreme form of absorption is linked to pathologies (Allen et al., 1996), it is included here as a dissociative symptom. Dissociative symptoms serve as "building blocks," which the *DSM-5-TR* categorizes into disorders based on particular clusters and patterns.

The *DSM-5-TR* identifies five categories of dissociative disorders (DDs). These DDs are further explained in the section Disorders With High Levels of Trauma-Related Dissociative Symptoms. The disorder of *dissociative amnesia* is an inability to recall important autobiographical information, usually of a stressful or traumatic nature, that is inconsistent with normal forgetting. The *DSM-5-TR* identifies that *depersonalization/derealization disorder* is characterized by persistent or recurrent depersonalization and/or derealization (American Psychiatric Association, 2022). *Dissociative identity disorder* (DID) is diagnosed when an individual experiences a disruption of identity characterized by two or more distinct personality states (in some cultures this may be experienced as possession) and "recurrent gaps in the recall of everyday events, important personal information, and/or traumatic events that are inconsistent with ordinary forgetting" (American Psychiatric Association, 2022, p. 330). The *DSM-5-TR* further delineates that individuals with DID experience (a) recurrent intrusions into consciousness and sense of self (e.g., voices; intrusive thoughts, emotions, impulses; actions including speech that are perceived as disconnected from one's control); (b) alterations in the sense of self (e.g., emotions, thoughts, preferences that are experienced as "not mine"); (c) depersonalization or derealization; and (d) intermittent neurological symptoms (e.g., amnesia that patients often report as "blackouts" or "time loss," nonepileptic seizures, paralyses, sensory loss) that are psychogenic in nature, meaning that they are not caused by substance use, head trauma, or other medical conditions.

The fourth DD, *other specified dissociative disorder* (OSDD), involves dissociative symptoms that cause distress or impairment but that do not meet the full criteria for another DD. There are four specified types of OSDD: (1) chronic, recurrent dissociative symptoms (i.e., identity disturbance suggestive of DID but without dissociative amnesia, referred to as OSDD-1); (2) identity disturbance due to prolonged, coercive persuasion (e.g., brainwashing); (3) acute dissociative reactions due to stressful events; and (4) dissociative trance (i.e., profound unresponsiveness to environmental stimuli). Individuals with DID or OSDD-1 are considered "complex DDs" (Mueller-Pfeiffer et al., 2012). They are often grouped together due to their similarities, so they are often considered together in this book. *Unspecified dissociative disorder* applies to conditions in which dissociation is causing impairment, but the criteria are not fully met for a specified DD or there is insufficient information to make a specific DD diagnosis.

DEFINITIONS AND CONCEPTUALIZATIONS

Dissociation has been conceptualized in a multitude of ways: as existing along a continuum versus a dichotomous, taxon group; as a state versus a trait; as positive versus negative symptoms; and as a mechanism versus an outcome.

Continuum Versus Taxon and Normative Versus Pathological

Dissociation is often discussed as existing along a continuum from normative to moderate to severe, with absorption exemplifying the normative end of the continuum and identity alteration exemplifying the most severe form. In contrast to a continuum, the results of taxometric analyses have been used to suggest that a pathological group or "taxon" exists. A dissociative taxon would consist of individuals with the most severe of DDs. The dissociative taxon has often been measured by the scores on eight items known as the Dissociative Experiences Scale (DES) taxon, often written as DES-T (Bernstein & Putnam, 1986; Waller et al., 1996). Sometimes the dissociative subtype of posttraumatic stress disorder (DPTSD) is also categorized as belonging to the dissociative taxon (Lanius, Wolf, et al., 2014).

The ideas of a continuum and taxon are not necessarily antithetical (Brand & Frewen, 2017). From the perspective of a continuum, dissociation ranges from mild detachment that may occur during peak athletic performance and some religious experiences (Butler et al., 1996), to more significant derealization or depersonalization that can occur briefly with stress, to the DPTSD and some DDs. The conceptualization of a continuum is applicable to individuals who do not fall into the dissociative taxon. The dissociative taxon includes those individuals with DID and OSDD-1.

State Versus Trait

Some authors refer to dissociation as a state that is transient and nonrecurrent, with trait-like, recurring dissociative experiences that endure after the trauma has ended. Peritraumatic dissociation is dissociation that occurs during or immediately after trauma exposure; it is usually a transient state that does not persist for more than a few weeks. However, for a subgroup of individuals, it endures, becoming a chronic symptom that can eventually be diagnosed as DPTSD or a DD (Carlson et al., 2012). Some individuals who are terribly frightened and hyperaroused during or after trauma may experience depersonalization and derealization due to hyperventilating. This state does not necessarily become chronic or lead to the development of PTSD (e.g., Briere, Scott, et al., 2005; Cardeña & Carlson, 2011; Tichenor et al., 1996).

Positive Versus Negative

The unbidden intrusions into awareness and behavior are considered *positive symptoms*, whereas the inability to access information or to control mental functions that are normally under one's control (e.g., amnesia or inability to access knowledge of well-learned facts or skills) are considered *negative symptoms* (American Psychiatric Association, 2022). Positive and negative, in this context, do not refer to an individual's perception of symptoms as positive or negative. Rather, symptoms are classified as positive when they cause newly presenting experiences or behavior and are termed negative when they cause an absence of typical functioning.

Mechanism Versus Outcome

Dissociation can also be discussed as a mechanism versus an outcome. When referred to as a mechanism, dissociation is viewed as psychological process of voluntarily or involuntarily narrowing the field of consciousness such that an individual appears to be in a trance. Dissociation is used in the mechanistic way here: "He dissociated while thinking about being trapped in his car when it caught fire." In contrast, research often refers to dissociation as a symptomatic outcome such as, "The group who had experienced more forms of childhood abuse had higher dissociation."

Detachment Versus Compartmentalization

Within the conceptualization of mechanism versus outcome, scholars have also conceptualized dissociation as detachment—that is, as being estranged from oneself, people, and/or the environment, versus compartmentalization, which is a lack of integration between psychological processes including identity, behavior, and memory (Holmes et al., 2005). This conceptualization addresses how different aspects of dissociation can contribute to the most severe presentation of DDs—that is, DID. Viewed through this lens, detachment can contribute to compartmentalization in some individuals. For example, during episodes of chronic abuse, a child may have responded with neurobiologically driven detachment from their emotions, body, and surroundings. Over time, this could contribute to the child developing compartmentalized, nonintegrated states. In some states, the child may be able to access and feel the emotions, physical pain, and betrayal they experienced by the caretaker. In other states, the child may not be able to recall these episodes or might be able to do so only with confusion at the intrusive images that may depict the abuse, without first-person recollection of having experienced it themselves.

Two prominent theories about compartmentalization and TRD are mentioned here. The *structural theory of dissociation* discusses various features of compartmentalization as the core feature of DID and OSDD-1 (van der Hart et al., 2006). The *discrete behavioral states theory* of dissociation subsumes the structural theory of dissociation and other trauma-based theories of dissociation (Loewenstein & Putnam, 2023; Putnam, 1984, 1994, 1997, 2016). Putnam (2016) argued that developmental and neurobiological studies indicate that many psychiatric disorders are state-change disorders, including mood disorders, panic disorder, and DID. From the perspective of this theory, DID is understood to be a posttraumatic developmental disorder involving extreme traumatic states and attachment pathology interfering with development of a continuous sense of self across states and contexts (Loewenstein & Putnam, 2023). Neurobiological studies indicate that the dissociative phenomena seen in DID are posttraumatic state-dependent, trauma-based nonintegrated states. Loewenstein and Putnam (2023) characterized DID as a "state of multiple simultaneous, overlapping states" (p. 294). On the basis of this trauma, attachment, and neurobiologically informed perspective, the term *self-states* is used throughout this book to refer to trauma-based, dissociative self-states that are found in DID and OSDD-1, as well as other DDs.

DISSOCIATION IS TRANSDIAGNOSTIC

Determining what exactly "counts" as a traumatic event has been debated for decades (Dalenberg, Straus, & Carlson, 2017). As currently defined by the *DSM-5-TR*, trauma includes exposure to actual or threatened death, serious injury, or sexual violence and can include directly experiencing the event, witnessing it in person, learning about it having occurred to a close loved one, or being repeatedly exposed to aversive details of traumatic events (e.g., first responders being exposed to dead bodies). Evidence suggests that events that cause severe emotional loss, such as abandonment by a parent or sudden loss of one's home or loved one, contribute additional variance to the prediction of PTSD symptoms and dissociation, so such events should be included as potential traumas (Carlson et al., 2013).

TRD provides containment and physical analgesia, as well as detachment from stressful, threatening situations (Nijenhuis et al., 2002; Steele et al., 2017). TRD is common among individuals with DDs, who often have experienced trauma, traumatic losses, and attachment difficulties (D. P. Brown & Elliott, 2016; Dalenberg et al., 2012; Ogawa et al., 1997; Şar, Koyuncu, et al., 2007; Trickett et al., 2011). The *DSM-5-TR* placed the DDs in the chapter following trauma- and stressor-related disorders to signify the close relationship between DDs and trauma. However, it is crucial to understand that dissociative symptoms are transdiagnostic, and not all dissociation is trauma- or stress-related or pathological. As discussed in Chapter 2, dissociation can occur in nontraumatic situations.

Research consistently finds that dissociative symptoms are present in many psychological disorders, including ones that are not strongly associated with trauma exposure (Ellickson-Larew, Stasik-O'Brien, et al., 2020; Lyssenko et al., 2018). Two large meta-analyses show that dissociative symptoms are found in a wide range of disorders, although the more severe dissociative symptoms are consistently found in trauma-related disorders (Lyssenko et al., 2018; van IJzendoorn & Schuengel, 1996). The most recent meta-analysis included 216 studies of 15,219 individuals and found dissociative symptoms in 19 diagnostic categories (Lyssenko et al., 2018). Despite the passage of time and differences in methodologies, the findings were strikingly similar. Both found a continuum of dissociation with the most severe symptoms occurring in DID, followed by general DDs, followed by somewhat lower levels of dissociation in PTSD and borderline personality disorder (BPD). The level of dissociation in depersonalization/derealization disorder was somewhat lower than in BPD. Figure 1.1 depicts Lyssenko et al.'s average dissociation scores, as assessed by the DES (Bernstein & Putnam, 1986).

The recent interest in dissociation has led to important new insights about dissociation, including cross-culturally. For example, in the World Mental Health Surveys, Stein et al. (2013) found dissociative symptoms among 14.4% of individuals with PTSD from among 25,018 respondents from 16 countries. Compelling evidence such as that from Stein et al.'s international study documenting high levels of dissociation among a subgroup of traumatized individuals across cultures with PTSD led to the addition of the

FIGURE 1.1. Average Dissociation Scores Assessed With the Dissociative Experiences Scale From a Meta-Analysis of 216 Studies Comprising 15,219 Individuals From 19 Diagnostic Categories

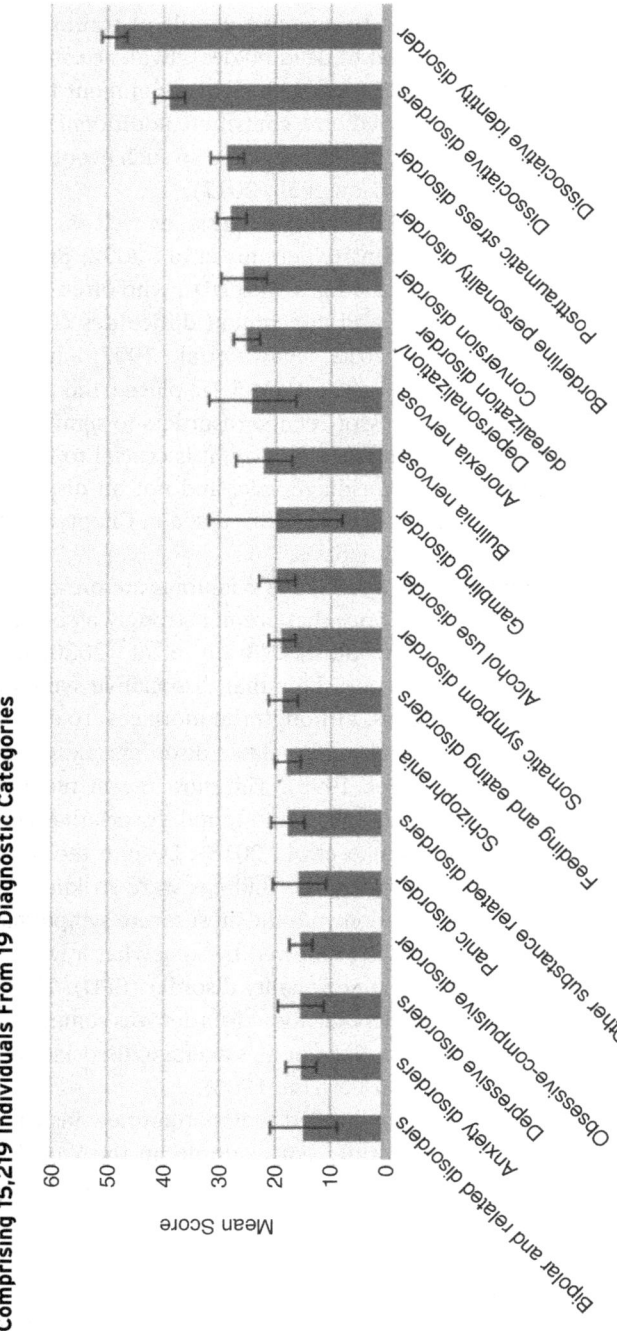

Note. Error bars indicate 95% confidence interval. From "Dissociation in Psychiatric Disorders: A Meta-Analysis of Studies Using the Dissociative Experiences Scale," by L. Lyssenko, C. Schmahl, L. Bockhacker, R. Vonderlin, M. Bohus, and N. Kleindienst, 2018, *The American Journal of Psychiatry, 175*(1), p. 40 (https://doi.org/10.1176/appi.ajp.2017.17010025). Copyright 2018 by the American Psychiatric Association. Reprinted with permission.

DPTSD in the *DSM-5-TR*. Similarly, one mild form of dissociation, specifically referred to as "numbing," is included as a symptom in the *International Classification of Diseases–11* (*ICD-11*; World Health Organization, 2021) diagnosis of complex PTSD (CPTSD).

DISSOCIATION AS A DEFENSE AGAINST TRAUMA

The connection between trauma and dissociation appears to be related to the defensive protection provided by dissociation. Schauer and Elbert (2010) described the *defense cascade*, a progression of neurologically driven self-protective strategies that occur in response to threat. When faced with danger, people typically respond with an "orienting freeze" associated with a decrease in heart rate while they look and listen to gather information. Next, people use a series of strategies to survive the danger. These defenses are not consciously chosen; rather, they are influenced by an individual's prior exposure to trauma (if any). If they have not experienced repeated trauma exposure, they will typically respond actively to protect themselves, through "flight," if possible, or "fight" if flight does not seem possible. (Note that in their common usage the words "fight or flight" are in the incorrect order in terms of actual response to life threat.)

If neither is possible, or if those strategies have not worked with past threats, they are likely to become immobile. This *tonic immobility* involves high physiological arousal, increased autonomic reactivity, and increased muscle tone, yet the person cannot move all or part of their body (Nijenhuis, Vanderlinden, & Spinhoven, 1998; Schauer & Elbert, 2010). (Although tonic immobility is sometimes called "freezing," this heightened muscle tone along with immobility is not the same physiological state as that which occurs during the initial orienting freeze, so the term tonic immobility is preferred.) This stage is sometimes referred to as "death feigning." When an animal feigns death, predators might lose interest, sometimes allowing the animal to escape. However, if the danger is inescapable, the individual or animal may shift to the next stage, emotional collapse or shutdown, which involves further parasympathetic activation, loss of motor tone, anesthesia, and even apnea (Schauer & Elbert, 2010). As Putnam noted 30 years ago, "Dissociation is a very primitive biological response that kicks in when all is lost" (p. 104) (Putnam, 1992).

The psychological defense of tonic immobility has been likened to the experience of dissociative states (Kluft, 1985; Nijenhuis et al., 1998; Spiegel, 1984). When someone has no ability to defend against attacker(s), "dissociation is the escape when there is no escape" (Putnam, 1992, p. 104). Dissociation provides some buffer from the emotional and physical pain caused by trauma, which is especially adaptive when the trauma involves interpersonal betrayal, particularly of a child by their caregivers (Freyd, 1996).

Child Abuse and TRD

Research supports the idea that dissociation may be frequently used if the trauma is chronic and begins early in childhood when the child is more vulnerable and cannot run away or fight. In a meta-analysis of 65 studies that examined the predictors of dissociation among 7,352 adults who had been abused or neglected in childhood, higher dissociation was found in those with an earlier age of onset of abuse, a longer duration of abuse, and abuse perpetrated by a parent (Vonderlin et al., 2018).

Approximately one in 58 children in the United States are maltreated by a parent or caretaker in a given year (Sedlak et al., 2010). Children who are abused by parents are often raised in "high-risk families" with frequent aggression, high conflict, neglect, and lack of support (Repetti et al., 2002). Additional contributing factors include poor family mental health, substance abuse problems, unresolved trauma in the parent(s), and perhaps fewer opportunities for positive, safe interactions within the family. When abuse is perpetrated by a parent, the child is also more likely to develop insecure or disorganized attachment, both of which are associated with risk for dissociation and other negative outcomes (Byun et al., 2016; Granqvist et al., 2017; Lyons-Ruth, 2008; Ogawa et al., 1997).

As is reviewed later in the chapter, adverse childhood experiences (ACEs) such as these are strongly linked to a wide range of negative outcomes, including deficits with autobiographical memory (D. W. Brown et al., 2007), which may be due to dissociation. Sibling relationships may also be disturbed. The child may witness the abuse of other family members or perhaps experience a tremendously stressed parent(s) working long hours to support the family, so caregivers may not be often physically present, or if present, they may be too exhausted to provide consistent, loving interactions. A traumatized child who is not protected by caregivers or is not comforted after experiencing harrowing experiences is left to endure and make sense of overwhelming emotions and painful or shame-inducing body sensations. The child often receives the direct or indirect message not to show or talk about any reaction to the devastating, shocking events that have occurred. They may be told that such things did not occur, which leaves the child bewildered, uncertain, and confused about what is real, depending on their age, cognitive ability, and developmental level.

Long-Term Impacts of Childhood TRD

Almost invariably, children feel that they are at fault for their neglect or abuse. Sometimes they are manipulated with statements such as "If you weren't so bad, I wouldn't do this" or are mocked or abused if they show feelings. Over time, emotions and body sensations can become associated with danger and the possibility of being harmed again. In this context, disconnecting from one's emotions and body, as well as the knowledge that such horrible events occurred, allows the child to go on about daily life. The child may think that by hiding trauma-related distress, they are hiding how "bad" they are and preventing further danger. It may feel unsafe to show feelings anywhere because if anyone notices the child's distress, further questioning about "what's wrong" could prompt disclosure of abuse, prompting possible retaliation, loss of parents' love, or the family being torn apart.

Even after the trauma has ended, perhaps even years or decades later, when the individual remembers the traumatic experience, it is often in fragmented snippets or snapshot images, or other confusing sensory intrusions (Andrews et al., 2000; Halligan et al., 2003; Peltonen et al., 2017). Traumatic experiences can reoccur in "real time" in the person's current life, or in "trauma time," that is, in the psyche as an intrusive emotion, image, body sensation, or other fragment of the memory (Steele et al., 2017). Intrusive recollections can trigger panic or flashbacks, which seem like the trauma is happening *now*. No escape or comfort is possible, so the individual dissociates, which lessens the overwhelm.

Although dissociation is initially automatic and biologically driven, it may become a habitual response to stress and uncomfortable emotions. Danger may later be perceived when there is little to no present-day danger due to PTSD hyperarousal and believing the world is "always dangerous." A person may consciously choose to dissociate sometimes to escape states of overwhelm or in response to recalling traumatic experiences. For example, a client may intentionally watch violent movies to stop intrusive images related to their experience of trauma; in response to violent movie scenes, they may shift from feeling ashamed, helpless, and terrified to being in a dissociated, numb state. Nonsuicidal self-injury (NSSI) and other high-risk behaviors are common methods of inducing dissociative states. Thus, dissociation can serve as a method of emotion regulation even long after there is no direct danger.

TRD may be experienced so frequently, and yet subtly, that it is difficult for traumatized individuals and clinicians to recognize it. It may occur in response to seemingly benign situations. For example, an individual may begin to feel detached from their body as if they are floating when they hear a loud voice because the person who abused them frequently screamed in rage. Due to trauma-based shame, patients may avoid mentioning dissociation to therapists. They may prefer to feel numb rather than experiencing emotions such as shame, likewise preferring to disconnect from their bodies rather than risk having a trauma-related bodily sensation. They may prefer to feel out of touch with reality rather than be aware that someone they depended on and loved (and perhaps even still depend on) has harmed them.

These moments of dissociation can become frequent yet go unnoticed, and the connection to the earlier trauma can be disrupted through repeated reexposure to dissociative states. Individuals with TRD often have "phobia of inner experience," which may include avoidance of emotions, physical sensations and movement, impulses, behaviors, thoughts, wishes, fantasies, needs, and dissociative self-states (Steele et al., 2017). Over time, the individual may have difficulty identifying, experiencing, labeling, and tolerating emotions and body sensations, even when they are not directly linked to trauma.

The inability to identify and describe emotions is called *alexithymia*. Alexithymia and an inability to use emotion regulation strategies predict dissociation (Powers et al., 2015). Treatment of TRD that emphasizes teaching emotion regulation and grounding has been linked with decreased dissociation, PTSD symptoms, and NSSI, as well as improvements in adaptive capacities (e.g., Brand, Schielke, et al., 2019; Cloitre et al., 2011; see also Chapter 7, this volume).

DISSOCIATION: ADAPTATION, PATHOLOGY, OR BOTH?

Calling dissociation pathological can be offensive to individuals because dissociation was an *adaptive* state that fostered survival in the face of awful events, rather than being a state of disease. Many persons with TRD experience decades of being flooded by emotion and bodily sensations ("feeling too much") as well as shutdown experiences of dissociation ("feeling too little"). Individuals with TRD often engage in unhealthy, risky, or unsafe behaviors to manage ongoing feelings of danger and traumatic intrusions (Calati et al., 2017; Nester, Boi, et al., 2022). NSSI is often an attempt to regulate one's emotions, including sometimes as a method for inducing dissociation (more common in DDs) or ending dissociation (more common in BPD; Brand, 2001). NSSI may also be an attempt to manage relationships, such as a way to convey distress and to indirectly seek care. As such, dissociation, NSSI, and other risky or unhealthy behaviors are *adaptations* to trauma. What clinicians and researchers, myself included, refer to as "symptoms" and "pathology" must also be recognized as attempts to survive what may have been otherwise beyond survival. Thus, dissociation can be seen as an essential adaptation and a survival mechanism—yet, over time, it becomes a symptom that interferes with functioning.

Emerging neurobiological research provides support for this notion. Different types of maltreatment appear to impact different brain regions and pathways (Korgaonkar et al., 2023; Teicher & Samson, 2016). For example, verbal abuse and sexual abuse by parents, as well as witnessing parental domestic violence, appear to affect the auditory, visual, and somatosensory cortex and brain pathways related to processing aversive experiences. As Teicher and Samson (2016) stated, "Maltreatment is associated with reliable morphological alterations in anterior cingulate, dorsal lateral prefrontal and orbitofrontal cortex, corpus callosum and adult hippocampus, and with enhanced amygdala response to emotional faces and diminished striatal response to anticipated rewards" (p. 241). Individuals who experienced abuse in childhood, but not adolescence, have altered brain functional connectivity, suggesting altered functioning of systems related to perceptual processing and attention (Korgaonkar et al., 2023). These results indicate that abuse during the brain's sensitive developmental periods is particularly likely to have an impact on perceptual processing and attention. Dissociation was not assessed by Korgaonkar et al. (2023), but early-onset, severe abuse is linked to DID; future whole brain connectivity studies need to include dissociation, given dissociation's impact on perceptual processing and attention.

These and other researchers have hypothesized that certain neurobiological alterations may be adaptations that allow the child to cope with growing up in a harmful environment, yet later contribute to difficulties in nontraumatizing environments, thus serving as a "latent vulnerability" for the development of psychopathology (reviewed in Cassiers et al., 2018). Emotional abuse is correlated with changes in the frontolimbic socioemotional networks responsible for processing emotions. Trauma-related abnormalities in these networks might contribute to vulnerability to depression, anxiety, DDs, and other disorders, as well as indirectly increasing the risk for NSSI, suicide attempts, and interpersonal difficulties.

Another way that dissociation could initially be adaptive, yet later associated with difficulties, could involve its impact on memory. Dissociation might indirectly contribute to traumatic memories being encoded in disorganized, sensory fragments that return as haunting, intrusive symptoms of PTSD (Brewin et al., 1996; Ehlers & Clark, 2000). Prospective research has found evidence that memory fragmentation and dissociation contribute to the development of chronic PTSD in children living in war zones (Peltonen et al., 2017) and adults following motor vehicle accidents (Murray et al., 2002).

Additionally, dissociation that occurs during therapy sessions impedes treatment progress. Patients may not be able to encode, recall, and later use the skills, new beliefs, and other types of learning if they dissociate during sessions. In one study, patients presenting with acute injury to an emergency department were randomly assigned to early intervention (i.e., three sessions of exposure therapy) to prevent the development of PTSD or assessment only (i.e., no therapy outside of routine medical assessment; Price et al., 2014). Dissociation in the first session was the sole significant predictor of treatment response out of many variables assessed, predicting a substantial 51% of the variance in PTSD symptoms. Similarly, individuals with PTSD resulting from child sexual abuse were more likely to improve significantly from trauma treatment involving dialectical behavior therapy and exposure or cognitive restructuring if their state level of dissociation at therapy sessions was low (Kleindienst et al., 2016). Patients also may be unable to acquire inhibitory learning if they are dissociated (Lanius et al., 2012; Price et al., 2014). Inhibitory learning is the acquisition of nonfearful learning and is the presumed mechanism for the efficacy of exposure therapy (Craske et al., 2008). As elaborated in Chapter 7, it is crucial for effective treatment that patients are "grounded" in their bodies and are oriented in present reality.

HIDDEN IN PLAIN SIGHT AT GREAT COST

Dissociative symptoms are not usually the presenting complaint when patients seek treatment. Rather, they typically request treatment for depression, anxiety, or other comorbid conditions. The impact of trauma in general is often unrecognized and untreated (Lanius, Wolf, et al., 2014). Despite being at least as prevalent as other types of mental illness, TRD (particularly DDs) is underrecognized, so these individuals often do not receive treatment specifically targeting dissociation. As a result, their core dissociative symptoms often persist despite receiving treatment for comorbid conditions (Jepsen et al., 2014). A nationally representative study of German youth found that only 16% of the young people with dissociative disorder not otherwise specified had received mental health treatment despite being highly impaired (Tanner et al., 2019). Adults with DDs also tend to be highly impaired. For example, among a representative sample of adults in New York State, those with DDs were 50% more impaired than adults with other psychiatric disorders, even after controlling for gender, age, and co-occurring disorders (Johnson et al., 2006). Swiss researchers concluded DDs should be considered a serious mental illness due to the high levels of impairment beyond the impact of comorbid psychiatric disorders (Mueller-Pfeiffer et al., 2012).

Dissociation is a risk factor for suicidality and NSSI (Brand, Schielke, et al., 2019; Foote et al., 2008). For example, one fifth of the veterans in a U.S. nationally representative sample experienced dissociative symptoms; dissociation was associated with a fivefold greater likelihood of suicidal ideation and fourfold greater likelihood of lifetime suicide attempt (Herzog et al., 2020). A review of completed suicides among 53,769 U.S. soldiers found that inpatients who had been diagnosed with a DD or somatoform disorder during the hospitalization had an alarming suicide risk after discharge (Kessler et al., 2015); specifically, their odds ratio for suicide was 3.6 versus 0.4 for PTSD and 2.9 for psychosis. Dissociation conferred more risk for suicide than did depression, psychosis, and past suicide attempts. The more severe the level of dissociation, the greater the risk for NSSI and suicide attempts among those with DDs (Webermann et al., 2016).

Dissociation is associated with reduced ability to work, unemployment, financial difficulties, and poor social support and physical health (Maaranen et al., 2005). The high level of impairment causes suffering for individuals with TRD and negatively affects their families. Many individuals with TRD are so impaired that they cannot work, and their quality of life greatly suffers (Langeland et al., 2020; Mueller et al., 2007; Mueller-Pfeiffer et al., 2012). They are at high risk for being retraumatized in adulthood (Webermann et al., 2014, 2021). Their children may be at risk for emotional problems, neglect, and abuse (Narang & Contreras, 2005; Noll et al., 2009; Yeager & Lewis, 1996).

Despite these risks, treatment that targets dissociation and emphasizes safety, symptom stabilization, and emotion regulation in individuals with DDs is associated with decreased NSSI and hospitalization and other signs of stabilization (Brand, Classen, Lanius, et al., 2009; Brand, Classen, McNary, et al., 2009; Brand, Schielke, et al., 2019). Once TRD is recognized and directly treated, even previously "chronic" patients may begin to make progress in treatment (Quimby et al., 1993), and treatment costs may decline (Lloyd, 2016; Myrick, Webermann, Langeland, et al., 2017).

In summary, TRD is often hidden in plain sight, leaving these individuals underserved, highly impaired, often disabled, and at risk for NSSI and suicide. Clearly, the mental health field needs to improve the recognition and diagnosis of TRD so that these individuals can obtain proper treatment and improve their stabilization and quality of life. Traumatized, dissociative patients deserve to be seen, heard, and responded to with evidence-supported treatment.

THE IMPACT OF LACK OF TRAINING IN DISSOCIATION AMONG CLINICIANS

The lack of systematic training for mental health professionals in trauma and dissociation is alarming. Only 8% of students graduating from doctoral programs in psychology had been required to take a course in trauma (Foltz et al., 2023). Despite dissociation being a common response to stress and trauma, education about trauma and dissociation is lacking in most mental health training programs (Cook et al., 2011; Henning et al., 2022). Many clinicians report having little or no training in how to inquire about a history of child abuse, or they do not feel prepared to follow up disclosures of trauma with appropriate referrals or treatment (e.g., Hepworth & McGowan, 2013; Lab et al., 2000; C. L. Xiao et al., 2016). Many patients are not assessed for trauma (Rossiter et al., 2015). Given the link between trauma exposure and the development of psychopathology, the lack of consistently inquiring about trauma exposure is unacceptable. This is analogous to physicians failing to ask patients about smoking; smoking is causally linked to so many medical disorders that failing to ask about it might be considered providing treatment below the standard of care.

Without proper training, it is understandable that many clinicians feel anxious about assessing and treating dissociation. Seventy-five percent of clinicians attending workshops about complex trauma in the United States and Australia felt inadequately prepared to treat individuals with complex trauma histories (Kumar et al., 2022). Only 25% of the clinicians attending the workshops had received formal training in trauma during their academic education. At the conclusion of the workshops, many clinicians indicated that learning about the assessment and treatment of TRD was the most helpful part of the workshop.

Many clinicians have difficulty accurately diagnosing DDs, even when a client presents with obvious and classic symptoms of a DD. Almost half of the clinicians who read a vignette clearly describing symptoms of DID did not accurately diagnose the disorder (Dorahy et al., 2017). Clinicians often feel confident about the accuracy of their diagnoses in a client who presents with dissociation, despite overlooking dissociation or misattributing dissociative symptoms to other disorders (Perniciaro, 2014). Individuals with DDs are often misdiagnosed as suffering from attention-deficit disorder, bipolar disorder, psychotic disorders, and personality disorders rather than DDs (Putnam et al., 1986; Vielleux, 2015). Research suggests that there is a consistent tendency to underdiagnose TRD (Mueller-Pfeiffer et al., 2012; Putnam et al., 1986; Şar et al., 2000). However, when a DD diagnosis is given, research shows that clinicians have usually accurately diagnosed the DD based on dissociative symptoms (Nester et al., 2021).

Misdiagnosis of psychological disorders can contribute to an individual receiving ineffective or even potentially harmful treatment. For example, if a client reports hearing voices and these hallucinations have a dissociative rather than a psychotic origin, they may be misdiagnosed with schizophrenia or bipolar disorder and treated for those disorders. Published cases describe patients who were misdiagnosed and treated for years in state psychiatric hospitals or clinics without benefit until the DD was recognized and properly treated, leading to substantial improvement and cost savings (Lloyd, 2016; Quimby et al., 1993).

Misconceptualization and misdiagnosis of TRD can also lead to trauma processing occurring too early or too much. If the severity of trauma exposure and resultant dissociation is overlooked, clinicians may inadvertently overwhelm patients by providing exposure-based treatments too early or too intensively, even though such approaches are considered frontline approaches for "classic" PTSD (Cloitre, Courtois, et al., 2012; Kezelman & Stavropoulos, 2012). To avoid inadvertently causing an escalation in suicidal ideation, NSSI, dissociation, or PTSD symptoms, it is critical that clinicians accurately assess the level of trauma exposure and TRD when conceptualizing treatment plans (see Chapters 4 and 7).

Another consequence of the lack of training is a shortage of clinicians who can appropriately assess and provide treatment of TRD. In a survey assessing treatment barriers among individuals with dissociative symptoms, 36% of the participants reported having had difficulty finding a treatment provider who was trained in treating trauma and dissociation (Nester, Hawkins, et al., 2022). More than a fourth (27.5%) reported that they discontinued treatment after a poor response from a clinician. Others described having felt mocked when they discussed dissociation and trauma or being told they were "faking" dissociative symptoms. One provider reportedly ended therapy sessions if the patient was dissociating. It would be unthinkable to end a therapy session if a depressed person was crying or a psychotic person was hallucinating. Although it is possible that trauma-based traumatic transference (i.e., misperception of others' words or behavior based on one's trauma history; Chefetz, 1997b; Loewenstein, 1993) may have influenced these individuals' experiences of their therapists, there is compelling evidence that sometimes traumatized patients, particularly those with TRD, are mistreated by some clinicians (Dalenberg, 2000, 2004; Leonard et al., 2005).

In conclusion, the lack of systematic training about TRD contributes to enormous social, psychological, and financial costs paid by individuals living with TRD, their families, and the health care system. Clinicians who misunderstand dissociation may sometimes add to patients' suffering through misdiagnosis, misconceived treatment, or hurtful responses. Training in trauma and dissociation are urgently needed so that mental health practitioners and researchers do not add to the burden of individuals who have already been unprotected, neglected, and harmed by those who are supposed to care for them.

TRAUMA AND TRD CONTRIBUTE TO COMPLEXITY AND COMORBIDITY

Trauma contributes to many more negative impacts beyond TRD and PTSD. In the 1990s, the landmark Adverse Childhood Experiences study was conducted by the Centers for Disease Control and Prevention and Kaiser Permanente. It documented extensive and enduring negative effects of ACEs (see https://www.cdc.gov/violenceprevention/aces/index.html). The original study's ACEs included child abuse (emotional, physical, sexual) and neglect (emotional and physical) as well as other adversities (e.g., household member who experienced mental illness, substance misuse, or incarceration; maternal domestic violence; parental divorce or separation). As the number of ACE exposures increases, the risk for negative outcomes increases in step with dramatically higher rates of depression, substance abuse, suicidality, self-destructiveness, interpersonal difficulties, revictimization, number of psychiatric diagnoses, work impairment, hearing voices, and memory problems for early life experiences (i.e., possible dissociation), among others (Felitti & Anda, 2010). Similarly, risky behaviors and medical problems increase in stepwise fashion with increasing exposure to ACEs, including risk of sexually transmitted diseases, early pregnancy, morbid obesity, autoimmune disorders, and serious cardiac, hepatic, and pulmonary problems (Anda et al., 1999).

The alarming findings from the original ACE study have been replicated by dozens of international teams. For example, the enduring impact of 12 childhood adversities were replicated in analyses with more than 9,000 adults in the National Comorbidity Survey Replication (Green et al., 2010). Childhood adversities were associated with 44.6% of all childhood-onset psychiatric disorders and with 25.9% to 32.0% of later onset psychiatric disorders. Trauma-related pathologies have also been found internationally. Researchers from 21 countries assessed 12 childhood adversities with first onset of psychiatric disorders, using data from more than 51,000 adults who participated in the World Mental Health Surveys (Kessler et al., 2010).

The adversities that were associated with problematic family functioning (e.g., child abuse/neglect, parental mental illness) were the strongest predictors of later mental illness. Childhood adversities were found to account for an alarming onset of 29.8% of the 20 psychiatric disorders they studied. Together these and similar studies show that childhood trauma and adversity is strongly associated with lifelong psychiatric and medical illnesses and behavioral difficulties (Ortiz et al., 2022).

As a result of their multiple disorders, chronic NSSI, and frequent suicidality, many patients with TRD require high usage of medical and psychiatric care, often with little recognition or treatment of the underlying primary TRD and antecedent childhood trauma. As a result, TRD, especially DDs, is extremely costly to the health care system (Brand, Myrick, et al., 2012; Langeland et al., 2020).

Chronic and multiple types of interpersonal trauma are called *complex trauma*. Examples include childhood sexual and physical abuse; sex trafficking; being a victim of interpersonal relationship violence; being a child soldier; or being a refugee or civilian war victim who experienced torture, genocide, or other types of organized violence (Herman, 1992b). Complex trauma, particularly when it occurs throughout childhood, is associated with a wide range of clinical problems including the following:

- affective dysregulation (e.g., dissociation alternating with hyperarousal and emotional flooding; problems with anger, anxiety, shame),

- behavioral dysregulation (e.g., impulsive, self-destructive and aggressive behavior; substance abuse; high-risk behaviors),

- identity disturbance (e.g., compartmentalization of self and/or self-fragmentation, difficulties with body image and eating disorders),

- disruption in meaning (e.g., seeing others and the world as traumatizing and untrustworthy and the self as damaged and blameworthy for trauma),

- interpersonal problems (e.g., avoidance of relationships; chaotic, violent, abusive relationships; enmeshed relationships), and

- somatization and medical problems (e.g., gastroesophageal reflux disease, irritable bowel syndrome, chronic fatigue, headaches, heart disease, and autoimmune disorders).

This pattern of widespread deficits has been recognized as CPTSD, disorders of extreme stress not otherwise specified, and developmental trauma disorder (Herman, 1992a, 1992b; Stolbach et al., 2013; van der Kolk et al., 2005). Complex trauma theorists describe slightly different conceptualizations and groupings of trauma-related reactions, although there are generally recognized core problems that require treatment: affect and somatic dysregulation, dissociation, impaired self-concept, and insecure patterns of attachment that manifest in relationship difficulties (Briere & Scott, 2015; Cloitre et al., 2011; Ford & Courtois, 2020a).

These trauma-related deficits underlie the psychiatric comorbidities reviewed here. Assessing for these deficits and patterns of comorbidity, along with adaptations and strengths, is crucial to understanding and successfully treating traumatized individuals. A trauma-informed conceptualization of treatment is built on understanding the impact these trauma-related deficits have on an individual and supporting them in developing secure attachment, self-regulation capacities, and supporting their development of a cohesive identity and stable, healthy relationships.

Dissociation Is Associated With Greater Impairment

Dissociation is of considerable clinical significance because it can be related to functional impairment, regardless of whether it occurs in a trauma-related or a non–trauma-related disorder. Dissociative symptoms are associated with greater symptom severity including poorer neuropsychological performance in BPD and depression, more binges in eating disorders, and greater depression in obsessive–compulsive disorder (reviewed in Lyssenko et al., 2018). Dissociative symptoms confer a higher risk of having a personality disorder among individuals with CPTSD (Dorrepaal et al., 2012). A meta-analysis showed that dissociation is linked to higher suicidality and NSSI across disorders (Calati et al., 2017). Dissociative symptoms were among the strongest predictors of functional impairment in a longitudinal study of patients with mood, substance use, anxiety, somatoform, dissociative, and personality disorder symptoms (Tanner et al., 2019). Dissociation mediated the relationship between PTSD symptoms and functional impairment in a sample of veterans, military members, and first responders (Boyd et al., 2018). A survey of individuals from 16 countries found that dissociative symptoms were linked with more severe role impairment (Stein et al., 2013). Furthermore, the impairment related to trauma typically endures for decades, as shown in the ACE studies.

After finding that dissociation occurs transdiagnostically and is associated with serious impairment, the authors of a meta-analysis of dissociation concluded, "An evaluation of dissociation should therefore be part of every careful psychopathological assessment, and future studies should engage a transdiagnostic perspective to enhance the development of treatment modules to deal with dissociative symptoms" (Lyssenko et al., 2018, p. 8).

Dissociation Must Be Considered in Treatment Planning

Research shows that dissociation often interferes with treatment progress or may necessitate longer or more intensive mental health treatment (Ellickson-Larew, Stasik-O'Brien, et al., 2020; Lyssenko et al., 2018). Dissociative symptoms predict nonresponse or slower response to treatment in PTSD (Bae et al., 2016; Kleindienst et al., 2016), BPD (Kleindienst et al., 2011), panic disorder (Kamaradova et al., 2013), agoraphobia (Michelson et al., 1998), and obsessive-compulsive disorder (OCD; Rufer et al., 2006). A study published in *The New England Journal of Medicine* demonstrated that among treatment-seeking spouses of military personnel, those with DDs utilized the most therapy sessions, compared with 17 other psychiatric disorders (Mansfield et al., 2010).

A prospective study found dissociative memory disturbance was moderately to strongly associated with almost all forms of psychopathology (Ellickson-Larew, Stasik-O'Brien, et al., 2020). Depersonalization/derealization was moderately associated with self-reports of a range of symptoms and diagnoses as well as the strongest predictor of increases in suicidality and internalizing symptoms over time. The authors concluded, "Given the interfering effects of dissociation, assessment and treatment of dissociative symptoms may be needed before treating other symptoms of psychopathology" (Ellickson-Larew, Stasik-O'Brien, et al., 2020, p. 145).

These studies suggest that highly dissociative individuals are likely to require treatment adapted to address dissociation and possibly intensive services. There have been repeated calls for the assessment of dissociation in all clients seeking mental health treatment as well as for considering dissociation when planning treatment (Ellickson-Larew, Stasik-O'Brien, et al., 2020; Lyssenko et al., 2018; Vonderlin et al., 2018; see also Chapter 7, this volume).

Dissociation Is a Complex Construct

Dissociation is a complicated phenomenon composed of a wide range of experiences. Unfortunately, it is often studied as a single construct (Bryant, 2007; Lanius et al., 2012). Many measures aiming to assess dissociation, CPTSD, and DPTSD evaluate only one or two types of dissociation such as numbing or depersonalization, thereby overlooking many types of dissociation. This is problematic because individuals who have experienced complex trauma often experience many types of dissociation (e.g., Briere, Weathers, et al., 2005; Dell & Lawson, 2009). If assessed for only one type of dissociation, it is likely that many highly dissociative individuals with complex TRD will be overlooked, and their treatments will not be adequately individualized.

Similarly, research may miss key relationships among variables and may not generalize to the range of individuals with TRD. Calls to assess dissociation as a complex construct include carefully assessing the timing and type of dissociation that occurs (Bryant, 2007; Lanius et al., 2012).

Different types of dissociation are associated with different patterns of trauma history, clinical status, demographic variables, and longitudinal outcomes, all of which may have considerable clinical relevance (Briere, Dietrich, et al., 2016; Ellickson-Larew, Stasik-O'Brien, et al., 2020). Using the Multiscale Dissociation Inventory, Briere identified various types of dissociation in the traumatized subsample drawn from a nationally representative U.S. sample (Briere, Weathers, et al., 2005). These factors include disengagement (from one's surroundings, such as being in a "trance"), depersonalization/derealization, emotional constriction (i.e., numbing), identity dissociation, and memory disturbance (Briere, Dietrich, et al., 2016). If a clinician assesses only for a type of dissociation the client does not experience, the clinician may incorrectly believe that the patient is able to begin trauma exposure work immediately without first developing the patient's awareness and acceptance of emotions, and their ability to stay grounded in present reality. This could lead to the client becoming overwhelmed and destabilized.

Over a range of populations, trauma experts have shown that these factors have clinical relevance for diagnosis and treatment planning. For example, Briere, Dietrich, et al. (2016) evaluated dissociation as a complex construct using a general population sample and also a sample with incarcerated individuals. They found evidence for what they labeled *dissociative complexity*, meaning the individual experienced several types of dissociative symptoms. Dissociative complexity was higher among women and incarcerated individuals, those with high cumulative trauma, and those with serious comorbidities including suicidality and substance use, even after removing the influence of the general level of dissociation. Assessing for the complexity of dissociation often helps identify individuals who have complex trauma histories and related complex dissociative symptoms. Clinicians need to be aware of and consider dissociative complexity when planning and assessing progress in treatment.

DISORDERS WITH HIGH LEVELS OF TRAUMA-RELATED DISSOCIATIVE SYMPTOMS

Dissociative symptoms are ubiquitous across many psychiatric disorders. As described earlier, a meta-analysis of 216 studies found dissociative symptoms in 19 psychiatric disorders, and it was associated with higher burden of illness and poorer treatment response (Lyssenko et al., 2018).

Figure 1.1 illustrates that DID individuals have the most severe level of dissociation ($M = 48.7$), followed by other DDs ($M = 38.9$), then PTSD ($M = 28.6$), BPD ($M = 27.9$), conversion disorder ($M = 25.6$), and depersonalization/derealization disorder ($M = 25.1$). The figure shows that although dissociation is transdiagnostic, more severe symptoms occur in the trauma-related disorders. This illustrates that a continuum of dissociation with DID being the disorder with the most severe TRD.

The following represent the most prevalent "primary" *DSM-5-TR* diagnoses that people with complex trauma histories may experience, presented in order from lower to higher levels of average dissociation.

Borderline Personality Disorder

Patients with BPD often report childhood adversity, trauma, and attachment problems, all of which put them at risk for experiencing dissociation. They are more than 13 times more likely to report childhood adversity than non-clinical controls in a meta-analysis (Porter et al., 2020). Emotional abuse and neglect were particularly elevated in the BPD group relative to controls. Between 35% and 79% of individuals with BPD have comorbid PTSD (Sack et al., 2013; Zanarini et al., 1998; Zimmerman & Mattia, 1999; Zlotnick et al., 2003). This level of PTSD is considerably higher than that found in individuals with other personality disorders (e.g., Golier et al., 2003).

There is considerable comorbidity between BPD and DDs. In one study (Korzekwa et al., 2009), 76% of the borderline sample had a DD, with almost equal prevalence between dissociative amnesia (29%), depersonalization disorder (29%), DID (24%), and dissociative disorder not otherwise specified (DDNOS; 24%). Correspondingly, individuals with DID also often meet criteria for BPD (30%–70%; e.g., Boon & Draijer, 1991; Dell, 1998; Korzekwa et al., 2009).

DSM-5-TR BPD symptom criteria include "dissociative states under stress," "impairments in identity," and "unstable self-image." These symptoms suggest that dissociative processes may be present and contributing to the comorbidity between BPD and DDs. Although high comorbidity rates between BPD and DDs may be partially due to symptom overlap and misdiagnosis, individuals diagnosed with both BPD and DID are more impaired and symptomatic and have more severe trauma histories, compared with individuals with either diagnosis alone (Ross et al., 2014).

Complex PTSD and Related Concepts

As reviewed earlier, myriad symptoms and difficulties can develop when an individual has been exposed to complex trauma. The range of these difficulties, including TRD, often goes well beyond classic PTSD, which has led theorists to develop conceptualizations including "complex PTSD" and "disorders of extreme stress" (Courtois & Ford, 2009; Herman, 1992a, 1992b; Luxenberg et al., 2001) that encompass these broad, complex reactions. Scholars have shown that dissociation is a common response to complex, chronic trauma, and therefore they include it in their conceptualizations of complex PTSD and disorders of extreme stress (e.g., Courtois & Ford, 2009; Herman, 1992a, 1992b). Many individuals with DPTSD and DDs struggle with these trauma-related reactions and so would fit the conceptualization of complex PTSD. However, the *DSM-5-TR* does not include complex PTSD; instead, it includes DPTSD, although the *ICD-11* includes complex PTSD. The *ICD-11* conceptualization of complex PTSD puts considerably less emphasis on dissociation, only listing "numbing" as a type of emotion dysregulation. Accordingly, the measures created to assess for *ICD-11* complex PTSD inquire only about numbing, rather than the broader range of dissociative symptoms (Cloitre et al., 2018).

Acute Stress Disorder

Acute stress disorder (ASD) is characterized by acute stress reactions that may occur in the first month after experiencing a traumatic event. ASD includes symptoms of intrusion, dissociation, negative mood, avoidance, and arousal. If the trauma-induced symptoms endure beyond 1 month, the diagnosis of ASD should be changed to PTSD, if PTSD criteria are met. The *DSM-5-TR* ASD criteria specifically describe flashbacks as a dissociative symptom. Other types of dissociation include an altered sense of oneself (depersonalization) or one's surroundings (derealization) and an inability to remember an important aspect of the trauma (dissociative amnesia). The prevalence of ASD after trauma ranges between 5% and 33% depending on the type and severity of the trauma (reviewed in Bryant, 2022). Individuals with ASD typically present with high levels of anxiety and distress, intrusive symptoms, and avoidance of reminders of the event. Despite these emotional symptoms, individuals with ASD may present with flat affect, although the flatness typically shifts to distress when discussing the traumatic event. Studies show that 40% to 80% of those with ASD develop PTSD (Bryant, 2022).

Traumatic Brain Injury

When an individual has experienced a traumatic brain injury (TBI), differentiating the effects of TBI from ASD may be challenging. *Mild TBI* is defined as "a traumatically induced physiological disruption of brain function" and may include a loss of consciousness, a loss of memory for events immediately before or after the injury, or an alteration in mental state at the time of the accident (R. W. Evans & Whitlow, 2022). Mild TBI can resemble the ASD symptoms of depersonalization, derealization, dissociative amnesia, and reduced awareness of one's surroundings. It is difficult to distinguish reliably between genuine dissociative amnesia and amnesia secondary to mild TBI; therefore, Bryant (2022) advised not interpreting amnesia occurring after mild TBI as a symptom of ASD. Instead, the presence of the other symptoms of ASD should be relied on. Individuals can develop ASD, as well as PTSD, comorbid with mild TBI. Even when the traumatized individual has partial amnesia for aspects of the trauma, they can nevertheless develop PTSD.

PTSD and Its Dissociative Subtype

"Classic" PTSD can include dissociative symptoms, including flashbacks and inability to remember part or all of the trauma. A dissociative subtype of PTSD (DPTSD) was added to the *DSM-5-TR* due to several types of research. High levels of dissociation were found in a subgroup of individuals with PTSD according to the distribution of dissociation scores (Putnam et al., 1996), taxometric analyses (Waelde et al., 2005), latent class analyses (Wolf, Miller, et al., 2012), and signal detection analyses (Ginzburg et al., 2006). Neuroimaging studies distinguished the classic hyperemotional presentation of PTSD from a hypoemotional DPTSD (reviewed in Lanius et al., 2010). Additionally, some studies indicated that high dissociation was related to different risk factors and could affect treatment course (Lanius, Wolf et al., 2014).

A meta-analysis found that DPTSD typically occurs in 42% of clinical samples of adults, 95% confidence interval (CI) [33%, 51%], and 63% of children with PTSD, 95% CI [50%, 75%] (White et al., 2022). In one of the methodologically strongest studies, DPTSD was found in 14.4% of the individuals with PTSD drawn from 16 countries (Stein et al., 2013). Risk factors for DPTSD included exposure to prior traumatic events and childhood adversities, childhood onset of PTSD, prior history of separation anxiety disorder and specific phobias, and male gender. The DPTSD group had more severe role impairment and higher suicidality. Although Stein et al. (2013) found DPTSD to be associated with males in the general population, clinical studies typically find the highest rates in females (Steuwe et al., 2012; Wolf, Lunney, et al., 2012).

Most studies of DPTSD have been based only on symptoms of depersonalization and derealization. A more complex understanding of the role of dissociation in the course and treatment of traumatized individuals requires that dissociation is conceptualized and assessed with greater breadth. Frewen and Lanius (2015) categorized flashbacks, emotional numbing, and voice-hearing as additional dimensions of dissociative experience (or "trauma-related altered states of consciousness"), and they have shown that these experiences frequently occur in PTSD. Voice-hearing in TRD can be a form of traumatic reexperiencing; for example, many people hear the voices of the individual(s) who traumatized them (Anketell et al., 2010). Amnesia is also a frequent symptom of DPTSD and the most strongly associated dissociation factor in one study (Steuwe et al., 2012).

Although individuals in DPTSD samples are often described as "high" in dissociation, these individuals have moderate levels of dissociation. For example, one group (Hagenaars et al., 2010) categorized individuals with scores on the DES (Bernstein & Putnam, 1986) half a standard deviation (i.e., 25.13) above the sample average mean as "high dissociation." However, traditionally, scores of 30 or higher are interpreted as high enough to suggest that further assessment is needed to determine whether the individual has a DD (Carlson & Putnam, 1993). Indeed, the mean DES scores in individuals with complex DDs are much higher (e.g., 35.9, *SD* = 19.9; Brand, Classen, Lanius, et al., 2009).

The *DSM-5-TR* Dissociative Disorders

DDs are more common than most people realize, with DID being approximately as common as schizophrenia and bipolar disorder in most community studies, as seen in Table 1.1. The 1-month prevalence rate of pathological dissociation and likely DD was 4.1% in the National Comorbidity Survey Replication study (Simeon & Putnam, 2022). This study used rigorous methodology including a U.S. representative sample of 6,644 individuals and seven of the eight DES taxon items. The approximate 1-month prevalence of DID was 1.5%, the prevalence of depersonalization/derealization disorder was 1.3%, and the prevalence of dissociative amnesia was .5%.

DDs are even more common in treatment settings. Among Taiwanese patients in a psychiatric hospital, 19.5% met *DSM-IV* criteria for a DD (Chiu et al., 2017). One patient had possession trance disorder, which was included as a type of DID in the *DSM-5*. The DD patients showed patterns consistent with Western clinical profiles, including considerable comorbidity and high levels of childhood and adulthood trauma exposure, leading the authors to conclude that the "cross-cultural manifestations of dissociative pathology in East Asia are similar to those in North America and Europe" (Chiu et al., 2017, p. 285). However, the only report from China indicates the prevalence

TABLE 1.1. Weighted Means and Ranges of the Prevalence Rates (in Percentages) of *DSM-IV* Dissociative Disorders in Clinical and Nonclinical Populations in Western and Eastern Studies

	Inpatient		Outpatient		Community	
	M	Range	M	Range	M	Range
Dissociative amnesia	2.9	0.0–13.4	1.9	0.0–9.8	3.0	0.2–7.3
Depersonalization disorder	1.2	0.0–4.5	2.0	0.0–4.9	0.8	0.2–2.4
Dissociative identity disorder	3.8	0.0–12.0	3.1	0.3–7.5	0.9	0.0–3.1
Dissociative disorder NOS	6.6	0.7–19.4	5.0	2.0–8.5	2.8	0.0–8.3
Any dissociative disorders	16.6	1.7–58.3	12.5	4.9–29.3	7.3	0.3–18.3

Note. DSM-IV = Diagnostic and Statistical Manual of Mental Disorders (4th ed.); NOS = not otherwise specified. See Chiu et al. (2017) for citations of original studies. Adapted from "Dissociative Disorders in Acute Psychiatric Inpatients in Taiwan" by C.-D. Chiu, M.-C. M. Tseng, Y.-L. Chien, S.-C. Liao, C.-M. Liu, Y.-Y. Yeh, H.-G. Hwu, and C. A. Ross, 2017, *Psychiatry Research, 250,* p. 286 (https://doi.org/10.1016/ j.psychres.2017.01.082). Copyright 2017 by Elsevier. Adapted with permission.

of DDs may be somewhat lower (1.7%–4.9%), although replication is needed (Z. Xiao et al., 2006).

DDs vary among cultures, according to the limited data available. Possession types of DID occur in some Eastern cultures and some sections of the United States with the individual presenting as possessed by external identities (e.g., spirits, demons) and with more florid switching than found in nonpossession forms (e.g., American Psychiatric Association, 2013; Ross, 2011; Şar, Alioğlu, & Akyüz, 2014). The individual may recurrently act as if the individual were replaced by the "ghost" of someone in the same community who died years earlier and is still alive (American Psychiatric Association, 2022). These unwanted and distressing possessions contrast with the majority of possession states that are found internationally and are accepted cultural or religious experiences and do not meet criteria for DID.

Consistent with Western cultures, most (i.e., 83%) of the individuals in the Taiwanese inpatient study who were found to have DDs had not been diagnosed as such, despite dissociative-like behavior being noted in their medical records (Chiu et al., 2017). Instead, they had been diagnosed with psychotic and mood disorders, as is also typical in Western cultures. More investigation about the prevalence, presentations, and treatment of DDs across cultures is needed including culturally related disorders such as *amok, ataque de nervios, latah,* and *pibloktoq* (Krüger, 2020; Lewis-Fernández et al., 2007).

Individuals with complex DDs typically report severe histories of chronic early maltreatment (reviewed in Loewenstein et al., 2017; Spiegel et al., 2011). Studies of DID patients indicate that they report higher levels of child abuse and neglect than any other diagnostic group (Spiegel et al., 2011).

Given the ACE studies' findings, it is not surprising that individuals with complex DDs are at risk for extremely high rates of psychiatric, medical, and behavioral comorbidity (Langeland et al., 2020).

Unfortunately, the ACE studies have not yet addressed DDs, nor somatoform symptoms, conversion disorder, and related somatic symptom disorders, all of which are common among DDs (Langeland et al., 2020). Nonetheless, research consistently shows that high levels of comorbidity are ubiquitous among DDs. Depression is often the most frequent comorbid diagnosis in individuals with DDs and is generally treatment resistant (Ellason et al., 1996; Johnson et al., 2006), although PTSD is also sometimes found to be the most prevalent comorbidity (Brand, Classen, Lanius, et al., 2009). As reviewed by Foote (2022), BPD is comorbid in 30% to 70% of persons with DID. Substance abuse, chronic self-destructiveness and suicidality, treatment-resistant anxiety disorders, and eating disorders (Gleaves & Eberenz, 1995; Johnson et al., 2006) are also common in DD patients. Individuals with complex DDs typically have three or more psychiatric disorders. For example, among a clinical sample with DID or OSDD, 89% had PTSD, 83% had a mood disorder, 54% had a personality disorder from the dramatic cluster, 51% had a personality disorder from the anxious cluster, 50% had an anxiety disorder, 30% had an eating disorder, and 22% had a substance use disorder (Brand, Classen, Lanius, et al., 2009).

Individuals with DDs are at risk for adult victimization as well as complex medical problems (Espirito-Santo & Pio-Abreu, 2009; Myrick et al., 2013; Şar, Akyüz, et al., 2007; Saxe et al., 1994; Webermann et al., 2014). Some of their psychiatric symptoms may seem bizarre (e.g., not recognizing themselves in the mirror) or impossible (e.g., not remembering something they said earlier in the session) if clinicians have not been trained in the wide variety of symptoms associated with trauma. Misunderstanding dissociation and the impact of complex trauma, as well as their elevated scores on validity and symptom measures can lead clinicians to suspect these patients of malingering, although research shows that such elevated and supposedly unusual symptoms are typical in complex DDs, as discussed in Chapters 4 and 5.

Individuals with complex DDs experience a wide range of dissociative symptoms. This psychiatric complexity can be confusing for clinicians, who often struggle to make accurate differential diagnoses. The comorbidity also generally necessitates longer treatment. The complexity and acuity of these individuals make planning treatment challenging, as clinicians may be baffled about which disorder(s), symptoms, (or even, at times, which crisis) to focus on first. Chapters 4 and 7 provide guidance on these issues.

Dissociative Identity Disorder
DID is a disruption of identity with two or more self-states along with marked discontinuity in one's sense of self and agency with alterations in "affect, behavior, consciousness, memory, perception, cognition, and/or sensory-motor functioning" (*DSM-5*; American Psychiatric Association, 2013, p. 292). Gaps in memory for everyday events, personal information, or traumatic events are also required. These symptoms can be reported by the patient or others who know the patient, or they may be observed by a clinician. In some cultures, the personality states, which here are referred to as *self-states*, may be experienced as possession. Possession self-states are typically highly overt, although only a small fraction of DID patients present with overt, dramatic shifting of self-states. Instead of presenting with complaints about dissociative symptoms, most individuals seek treatment for comorbid conditions such as unbearable depression, being overwhelmed with current life crises, and unhealthy relationships (sometimes still experiencing ongoing maltreatment in current abusive relationships or from past abusers). They typically have not derived much benefit from numerous past psychotherapies, medications, or psychiatric hospitalizations. This history and presentation should alert clinicians to the possibility of a complex trauma disorder and lead to a thorough assessment for trauma exposure and assessment for trauma-related disorders, including DDs.

In contrast to the dramatic switching of self-states portrayed in movies and social media, the self-states in genuine DID are generally more subtle or hidden. The symptoms related to self-states' intrusions, such as "missing time" in present-day activities, may wax and wane, so they may be noticeable primarily during "windows of diagnosability" (Kluft, 1991). If individuals with DID overtly presented as if they were "different people" as they are portrayed in media, exhibiting behavior such as flamboyantly switching and announcing their different names, the disorder would not be so consistently underdiagnosed. Some individuals with genuine DID do present this way, but it is highly unusual. Dramatic presentations are also found in some cases of malingered DID.

To be clear, individuals with DID do not have different people inside them. Nonetheless, a small subset of DID individuals with profound dissociative amnesia insist that the other states *are* other people. (In such cases, the individual needs to become gradually aware that they are one person with multiple self-states.) The self-states are generally less noticeable to others unless the individual is in acute crisis or motivated to make their self-states observable to others. Rather than an *external* disorder of dramatic switching, the disorder is experienced as *internal* phenomena that are experienced as sudden alterations, intrusions, or discontinuities in one's sense of self (Dell, 2009). Dell (2009) offered this description: "The phenomena of pathological dissociation are recurrent, jarring, involuntary intrusions into executive functioning and sense of self" (p. 226). For example, a person may suddenly have strong feelings, urges, or thoughts that seem not to be coming from oneself, such as finding oneself inexplicably tearful and sad with no sense of being sad. Most individuals with DID experience almost all the known dissociative symptoms, including depersonalization, derealization, identity alternation and confusion, dissociative amnesia, trance states, flashbacks, and dissociative somatoform symptoms (e.g., part or all of the body feels numb without a medical cause).

Foote (2022) summarized studies about trauma among DID as follows. These individuals typically report multiple types of extreme abuse typically starting before age 6 with 76% reporting having experienced four or more types of sexual abuse and half reporting physical abuse by four or more perpetrators. Summarizing 10 studies of 658 DID participants, a median of 83% reported childhood sexual abuse (range 70%–100%) and 81% reported childhood physical abuse (range 60%–95%). When young children are physically and sexually abused, there is almost always some level of emotional abuse as well, and emotional abuse has been shown to have highly negative impacts, such as enduring risk for depression (Teicher et al., 2006). Despite some authors questioning whether DID are reporting "real" versus "fantasized" trauma (see Chapter 2), corroboration of childhood abuse has been found in 26% to 100% of DID cases (median 85%; Foote, 2022). Given this level of early, severe, and chronic profound childhood abuse, often at the hands of trusted caretakers, it is understandable that these individuals experience complex psychological and medical disorders, have heightened mistrust of authority figures including mental health professionals, and require long-term treatment. This level of complex symptomatology is entirely consistent with the sobering findings about the enduring impact of childhood adversities and complex trauma exposure.

DID's Apparent Similarity to Schizophrenia

A group of symptoms referred to as *Schneiderian first-rank symptoms* were originally considered critical diagnostic features indicating that an individual has schizophrenia. However, Richard Kluft (1987a) documented that these symptoms are prevalent in individuals with DID. Kluft noted these first-rank symptoms in DID "made" feelings (i.e., feelings that are experienced yet do not seem to be one's own), impulses, and actions; voices arguing; voices commenting; influences on the body (e.g., feeling genital pain as if one is being raped); thought withdrawal (e.g., a patient's mind goes completely blank in midsentence, and they experience it as if their thoughts were taken from them); and thought insertion (e.g., the thought comes to a patient to curse at the therapist, yet the thought is repugnant and seems inexplicable to the patient; the thought of cursing originates with another self-state for whom the thought is not repugnant). Patients with DID endorse an average of 3.6 first-rank symptoms with the "made" feelings, impulses, and actions being most common. Two first-rank symptoms are not found in DID: thought broadcasting and delusional perception (e.g., "I saw a man with a beard like my father's right after I told my therapist about my father's abuse. This means my father is still after me"). However, these symptoms can occur when patients with DID experience a psychotic episode (Dell, 2006b). More than a dozen studies have found Schneiderian first-rank symptoms in individuals with DID (reviewed in Dell, 2006b). Many clinicians are unaware of these studies and misdiagnose individuals with DID with schizophrenia due to first-rank symptoms.

First-rank symptoms in DID result from intrusions of self-states into the consciousness of individuals with DID. They are assessed in only some measures and interviews of dissociation. Unfortunately, few researchers outside the DD field are aware of the importance of first-rank symptoms in TRD, and so they do not assess them. If they were included, it would likely help identify more cases of DID and OSDD-1 and perhaps clarify inconsistent patterns across studies and illuminate what trauma treatments work for whom and when.

Unfortunately, measures intended to assess psychotic disorders often include items that could be dissociative in nature without acknowledging the possibility of dissociation or how to make the differential diagnosis between the disorders, thereby potentially leading to the misdiagnosis of DDs as psychotic disorders. For example, the Structured Interview for Psychosis-Risk Syndromes (SIPS; Woods et al., 2019) includes potentially dissociative items such as "Have you ever been confused at times whether something you have experienced is real or imaginary? Do familiar people or surroundings ever seem strange? Unreal? Does your experience of time seem to have changed? Unnaturally faster, unnaturally slower?" The inclusion of potentially dissociative items on an interview for psychosis suggests that some researchers and test developers are not yet trained in dissociation.

Depersonalization/Derealization Disorder

Trauma exposure is less common and typically much less severe in depersonalization/derealization disorder than in the complex DDs (Simeon, 2009). Many individuals with depersonalization/derealization disorder report no clear precipitant for the disorder, traumatic or otherwise. In some cases, serious stressors including severe losses (e.g., interpersonal, financial) precede the onset. In some cases, the disorder appears to develop following ingestion of psychoactive substances (e.g., marijuana and hallucinogens; Loewenstein et al., 2017). (Note that in the *DSM-5-TR*, the name of the disorder was changed from "depersonalization disorder" to "depersonalization/derealization disorder.") Individuals with this disorder reported significantly more childhood trauma, particularly emotional abuse, compared with healthy controls, with parents being the primary abusers (Simeon, Guralnik, Schmeidler, et al., 2001). The average age of onset of depersonalization was 16 years. Those with depersonalization/derealization had higher dissociation scores on the DES than did the healthy controls (24.4 vs. 4.6). The possibility that this disorder might be a type of anxiety disorder has been disproven (Sierra et al., 2012).

Dissociative Amnesia

Dissociative amnesia is typically localized or selective for a specific event or series of events, although sometimes there is generalized amnesia for one's identity and entire personal history. Fugue, "apparently purposeful travel or bewildered wandering that is associated with amnesia for identity or other important biographical information" (*DSM-5-TR*; American Psychiatric Association, 2013, p. 338), sometimes occurs with dissociative amnesia, although in many cases, the individual is ultimately determined to have DID, and the fugue state reflected the intrusion of a self-state. Varying rates of dissociative amnesia have been reported for survivors of traumatic events; for example, it was found in as few as 5% of World War II combatants and as many as 61% of tornado survivors (reviewed in Bryant, 2007).

Unfortunately, there are few systematic studies about dissociative amnesia other than case reports or case series. In some cases, dissociative amnesia appears to have a clear traumatic antecedent, such as when an assault later in life was reminiscent of earlier, severe trauma (Kritchevsky et al., 2004). Loewenstein et al. (2017) summarized the literature, noting that depression and suicidal ideation are common, although there is no common personality profile or antecedent history. A personal or family history of dissociative or somatoform symptoms are risk factors for developing acute dissociative amnesia, as is exposure to childhood abuse or adult trauma. Among wartime cases, the intensity of combat is associated with developing dissociative symptoms.

The classic case of dissociative amnesia described in textbooks, often reinforced by media stories, is of an individual who presents without autobiographical memory for their identity or life history. Less extreme cases occur and are more common such as when someone has acute amnesia for a specific highly traumatic event(s) (e.g., sexual assault or combat). A "nonclassic," covert presentation occurs when a patient presents with symptoms other than amnesia, and the amnesia is only discovered when directly assessed (Loewenstein et al., 2017). These individuals are typically uncomfortable when discussing amnesia, often minimizing or rationalizing it (e.g., "That was so long ago, I forgot about it"). Amnesia appears to serve as a means of avoiding or reducing responsibility or high-risk situations (e.g., financial failure; sexual indiscretions; legal consequences; or anticipated, feared involvement in combat).

Unfortunately, existing case studies have not examined amnesia patients for underlying DDs (R. Loewenstein, personal communication, February 8, 2022). The authors of a *Lancet* review of amnestic disorders called for rigor when studying and assessing amnesia, emphasizing the need for memory-testing paradigms (Staniloiu & Markowitsch, 2014). It is important to assess carefully for the full range of dissociative symptoms because some of the cases have been reported to have the severe histories of trauma and some other features (e.g., having taken on a "different personality" after the onset of amnesia) that suggest they may have had undiagnosed DID or OSDD.

Other Specified Dissociative Disorder

As noted earlier, this category of DDs includes four presentations that do not meet the full criteria for any other DD. *OSDD-1* includes identity disturbance that is less marked than in DID or identity alterations similar to DID but without dissociative amnesia. Those diagnosed with OSDD-1 are thought to have similar clinical features, comorbidities, trauma history, and treatment response to individuals with DID (Loewenstein et al., 2017). When data are presented separately for OSDD-1 and DID, typically the OSDD-1 group has lower symptoms of dissociation but with large standard deviations so that the groups do not statistically differ. For example, 76 individuals with DID reported an average Multidimensional Inventory of Dissociation (MID; Dell, 2006a) score of 51.3 ($SD = 18.7$) compared with 40 DDNOS individuals with an average MID score of 39.0 ($SD = 19.4$).

OSDD-2 is identity disturbance due to prolonged and intense coercive persuasion, such as when individuals are held captive, tortured, confined in long-term political prisons, or exposed to brainwashing. *OSDD-3* includes acute dissociative reactions to stressful events that can last several hours or longer and typically resolves in less than 1 month. Individuals may show depersonalization, derealization, perceptual disturbances such as time slowing, constriction of consciousness, stupor, or alterations in sensorimotor behavior such as paralysis (American Psychiatric Association, 2013). *OSDD-4* is dissociative trance, which is characterized by sudden narrowing of consciousness or even a complete lack of awareness of one's surroundings. Individuals may have minor motor stereotypies (e.g., nodding head) that the individual cannot control or is unaware of. Individuals may also have acute, transient paralysis or loss of consciousness.

DIFFERENTIATING TRAUMA-RELATED DISSOCIATION FROM COMMONLY MISDIAGNOSED DISORDERS

Individuals with DDs, particularly DID, are often misdiagnosed with BPD, schizophrenia, and bipolar disorder (Foote, 2022). However, there are important differences that can inform making differential diagnoses. The distinctions between DID and BPD, schizophrenia, and bipolar disorder are summarized in Table 1.2.

Borderline Personality Disorder

Many of the trauma-related symptoms experienced by people who endured complex trauma can contribute to misdiagnosis. For example, due to dysregulated moods, impulses, identity instability, and dissociation, traumatized individuals are at risk for being diagnosed with personality disorders, particularly BPD, even though most of these symptoms improve with trauma-informed stabilization treatment (Ellason & Ross, 1997). As reviewed above, the two conditions can occur together. Judith Herman (1992b) cogently argued that these symptoms are adaptations to trauma and stabilize in trauma treatment. From this perspective, classifying these trauma-based adaptations and symptoms as indicative of a personality disorder can be seen as blaming the victim for showing signs of the impact of trauma. Although some clinicians consider DID to be essentially BPD due to similarities in some symptoms, research shows that individuals with complex DDs can be distinguished from those with BPD.

Schizophrenia

Many clinicians believe that voice-hearing is pathognomonic for psychotic disorders, especially schizophrenia. However, numerous studies including meta-analyses show that auditory hallucinations are common among individuals who have been traumatized, and hearing voices is correlated with dissociation (e.g., Longden et al., 2012, 2020; Moskowitz & Corstens, 2007;

TABLE 1.2. Features That Typically Distinguish DID/DDNOS1/OSDD1 From Borderline Personality Disorder, Bipolar Disorder, and Schizophrenia

Feature	DID, DDNOS1, OSDD1	Schizophrenia-spectrum disorders	Bipolar disorder	BPD
Trauma	• Typically report early onset, severe, chronic childhood trauma (Boon & Draijer, 1993a; Ross et al., 2014; Korzekwa et al., 2009) • High number of traumatic intrusions on Rorschach (Brand, Armstrong, et al., 2009)	• Less likely to have severe, chronic childhood trauma • Fewer traumatic intrusions on Rorschach compared with DID (Brand, Armstrong, et al., 2009)	• Less likely to have severe, chronic childhood trauma	• Although many report a history of childhood trauma, significantly less severe than for DID (Boon, & Draijer, 1993a; Ross et al., 2014) unless comorbid for DD + BPD (Korzekwa et al., 2009) • Very high rates of trauma reported if have comorbid DID + BPD (Korzekwa et al., 2009) • Do not differ significantly from DID on traumatic intrusions on Rorschach (Brand, Armstrong, et al., 2009)

(continues)

TABLE 1.2. Features That Typically Distinguish DID/DDNOS1/OSDD1 From Borderline Personality Disorder, Bipolar Disorder, and Schizophrenia (*Continued*)

Feature	DID, DDNOS1, OSDD1	Schizophrenia-spectrum disorders	Bipolar disorder	BPD
Dissociative symptoms	• Typically endorse high levels (e.g., DES average score 48.7; Lyssenko et al., 2018), high in depersonalization, derealization, and amnesia with intact reality testing • Often prefer to feel numb rather than have feelings; may self-harm to induce a state of dissociation • When dissociating, may be involved in elaborate inner world involving self-states, some of whom may be related to past traumatic experiences • Some signs of dissociation typically occur during assessment if trauma and attachment are queried	• Endorse moderate symptoms (e.g., DES average score 17.8 schizophrenia; Lyssenko et al., 2018) with poor reality testing • Score lower than DID on 13 of 14 MID primary dissociation scales (Laddis & Dell, 2012) • DID lower on rare symptoms, attention-seeking, and factitious (i.e., imitative) behavior validity scales on the MID, but on most other MID scales, DID scored higher than schizophrenic groups (Laddis & Dell, 2012)	• Lower dissociation scores expected with low scores on identity confusion and alteration (e.g., DES average score 14.8; Lyssenko et al., 2018) • No current-day amnesia except possibly during psychotic episodes • No signs of dissociation noted during interviews and psychological testing	• Endorse moderately high symptoms (e.g., DES average 27.91; Lyssenko et al., 2018) due mostly to absorption and depersonalization/ derealization, typically less amnesia (Ross et al., 2014) than DID with intact reality testing • On SCID-D, not significantly different from DID on derealization and depersonalization, but lower on amnesia, identity confusion, identity alteration (Boon & Draijer, 1993a) unless have comorbid DID (Korzekwa et al., 2009) • Do not usually endorse voices, first-rank symptoms (with the exception of "made" emotions), or amnesia on MID unless have comorbid DD • Often find it distressing to feel depersonalized and numb; may self-harm to end an episode of dissociation

Transformations and confusion about identity	• May admit to transformations in identity (e.g., "There's a part of me that is a terrified kid and another part is mean and screams like my abuser did.") • Typically endorse current-day amnesia for some out-of-character behaviors, although not all are aware of this	• May admit to transformations in identity but with magical or delusional beliefs (e.g., "I am Harry Potter and I had to had to fight when Voldemort took over me.") • No current amnesia (except when recalling periods of florid psychosis)	• None	• When dissociating, patients are merely "trancing" or depersonalized. They do not have an inner world of complex self-states, although they may endorse having a "bad" and "good" side to them • May experience identity changes related to polarized mood changes (e.g., "I was dating my last girlfriend, but when she left me, I became enraged and depressed again.") • Little current amnesia outside of drug and alcohol use. If there's time loss, it is when "trancing." May have less detailed recall for behavior in mood states different from the current one, but not frank amnesia • Endorse high levels of identity confusion including struggles about who they are on MID even without comorbid DD (Korzekwa et al., 2009)

(continues)

TABLE 1.2. Features That Typically Distinguish DID/DDNOS1/OSDD1 From Borderline Personality Disorder, Bipolar Disorder, and Schizophrenia (Continued)

Feature	DID, DDNOS1, OSDD1	Schizophrenia-spectrum disorders	Bipolar disorder	BPD
Hallucinatory and other first-rank symptoms	• Most endorse hearing voices (i.e., 92%; Foote, 2022) but are aware of the "as if" quality ("I know they're not real, but I hear a kid whimpering as a man's voice yells at her."); the voices' opinions and values are often in conflict with the patient's typical opinions and values (e.g., "She wants to go out partying, but I don't drink and want to be faithful to my husband"; Boon & Draijer, 1993a) • Hearing "thoughts that aren't mine" or "arguing thoughts" • Most often, voices are experienced inside their head; may have elaborate conversations with voices; sometimes conversations are in writing; sometimes have multiple conversations going on at the same time	• May endorse voices without awareness of the hallucinatory quality ("God talks to me.") • Typically, voices are not involved in elaborate, ongoing interrelated discussions and arguments • Voices are not typically related to past abusers and/or hurt children • May have visual hallucinations without observing ego • Hallucinations are due to psychotic process • MID's Psychosis Screen is highly correlated with dissociation scores for schizophrenia group, but not for DID • Report more delusions than do DID patients on the MID (Laddis & Dell, 2012)	• Experiences hallucinations only during episodes of psychotic mania or depression • In psychotic depression, the voices are typically solely persecutory (do not have child voices or encouraging voices; "The woman tells me I smell bad.") • Voices are not in conflict with one another	• If hallucinatory experiences occur, they are brief and distressing and occur during significant stress ("I see the lines on the wallpaper behind you moving.") • If endorses hearing voices, they are polarized, internalizations of their own thoughts; they do not dramatically differ from patient's typical values and opinions. ("I hear 'No one will ever love you'"; Boon & Draijer, 1993a) • If they endorse voices on the MID, they typically have a comorbid DD (Korzekwa et al., 2009)

(continues)

- May experience brief periods of "seeing" past trauma in flashback or "seeing" parts of self with reality testing intact
- Auditory and visual hallucinations relate to high hypnotizability
- Often hear childlike and/ or persecutory, angry, and arguing voices
- Report hearing voices more frequently than patients with schizophrenia (Laddis & Dell, 2012)
- Report more passive influence experiences (i.e., thoughts, feelings, and behaviors over which they perceive having no control; Dorahy et al., 2009)

- In schizophrenia, MID Voices scale had very high correlation ($r = .84$) with delusions; this pattern not found in DID group (Laddis & Dell, 2012)
- Average MID scores are lower during periods of remission (18.4) than during psychotic episodes (27.0) but lower than DID average (51.1; Laddis & Dell, 2012)
- Not highly hypnotizable

TABLE 1.2. Features That Typically Distinguish DID/DDNOS1/OSDD1 From Borderline Personality Disorder, Bipolar Disorder, and Schizophrenia (*Continued*)

Feature	DID, DDNOS1, OSDD1	Schizophrenia-spectrum disorders	Bipolar disorder	BPD
Affect	• Typically experience a range of inexplicable, rapid mood changes that begin and end abruptly; may be triggered by internal or external precipitants (e.g., sad to angry to helpless and afraid); many mood shifts can occur per day and within seconds • Shifting self-states often mistaken for borderline or rapid cycling bipolar, but these shifts do not resolve with mood stabilizers or antidepressants • Rarely complain of "emptiness"; inner world is "full" of voices, conflict, parts, and struggles • Often avoid affect and are obsessive, intellectualized (Brand, Armstrong, et al., 2006) • Feel ashamed and unworthy, even when not in a severe depression	• Flat, inappropriate affect	• Shifts in mood state occur slowly (even if rapid cycling, require hours to shift mood state and usually much longer than that) • When manic, often have expansive mood with grandiose views of self ("I have a mission to save people from terrorists.") • Mood is typically stabilized with medications	• Affect is significantly less modulated than in DID (Brand, Armstrong, et al., 2009) and shifts according to external precipitants • Often the most frequent affects are emptiness and intense anger • Endorse high levels of "made" intrusive emotions, mood changes without any reason, and not feeling in control of emotions on the MID even when there is no comorbid DD (Korzekwa et al.)

Ability to perceive accurately and think logically	• Perceptions are generally accurate (Brand, Armstrong, et al., 2009) • Thinking is logical and organized, although can become illogical and disorganized following traumatic intrusions or when decompensated or in crisis (Brand, Armstrong, et al., 2009)	• Perception is not significantly less accurate than in DID (Brand, Armstrong, et al., 2009) • Thinking is significantly less logical and organized than in DID (Brand, Armstrong, et al., 2009)	• Disturbed only during mood episodes	• Perception is significantly less accurate than in DID (Brand, Armstrong, et al., 2009) • Thinking is significantly less logical and organized than in DID (Brand, Armstrong, et al., 2009)
Working alliance	Capable of developing a working alliance with therapist due to capacity to experience others as cooperative, interest in others despite fear of being hurt, capable of emotional distancing and self-reflection, at least in some self-states (Brand, Armstrong, et al., 2009)	Less capable of developing a working alliance than DID due to expecting others to be less cooperative than in DID, significantly less interest in others than in DID, less capable of emotional distancing and self-reflection than in DID (Brand, Armstrong, et al., 2009)	Capable of developing a working alliance	Less capable of developing a working alliance than in DID due to expecting others to be less cooperative than do individuals with DID, about the same level of interest in others as in DID, significantly less capable of emotional distancing and self-reflection than in DID (Brand, Armstrong, et al., 2009)

(continues)

TABLE 1.2. Features That Typically Distinguish DID/DDNOS1/OSDD1 From Borderline Personality Disorder, Bipolar Disorder, and Schizophrenia (Continued)

Feature	DID, DDNOS1, OSDD1	Schizophrenia-spectrum disorders	Bipolar disorder	BPD
Comorbidity	• Usually meet criteria for multiple comorbid disorders including treatment resistant life-long depression, PTSD, anxiety disorders, substance disorders, mixed personality disorder traits, somatic symptom disorder as well as multiple medical illnesses. • Usually meet BPD criteria when severely decompensated or having overwhelming PTSD/DD symptoms; many do not meet BPD criteria once stabilized with trauma treatment	• Typically meet criteria for fewer comorbid conditions, although substance use disorders are common	• Typically meet criteria for fewer comorbid conditions	• Often have a variety of comorbid disorders, especially depression and PTSD (Korzekwa et al., 2009), but less likely to have the same degree of somatization; less often have panic disorder and substance use disorder compared with DID (Ross, 2007)

Relationships and sexuality	• Often so mistrustful of others that may isolate although lonely • Vulnerable to revictimization in adulthood • May be avoidant of sexual relationships, or highly sexual, or vacillate between the two • Often vulnerable to becoming terrified and dissociative during sex • Some parts may interfere with relationships due to internal conflicts ("*You married him, not me. He's not my husband!*")	• Typically less emotionally open with others, even in long-term relationships; may be paranoid and intensely afraid of others, which can be exacerbated if individual has experienced interpersonal trauma	• Capable of close relationships, although risky, self-destructive behavior during mood episodes may damage relationships • May be highly sexual, even indiscriminately, during manic episodes • Unlikely to become terrified during sex unless have experienced sexual assault	• Relationships tend to be chaotic and short-lived • Terrified of abandonment; perceives abandonment even when it is not occurring • May become so hurt and angry, or desperately needy, that they drive supportive others away • Their emptiness can be temporarily eased by others, particularly sexual relationships if they feel attractive and valued, but this is typically transient
Other distinguishing variables	Typically have borderline, avoidant, obsessive, and compulsive personality traits, with borderline features more apparent when decompensated (Ross, 2007; Ross et al., 2014)			In addition to borderline traits, often have histrionic traits (Ross, 2007)

Note. BPD = borderline personality disorder; DD = dissociative disorder; DES = Dissociative Experiences Scale; DID = dissociative identity disorder; DDNOS = dissociative disorder not otherwise specified; MID = Multidimensional Inventory of Dissociation; OSDD = other specified dissociative disorder; PTSD = posttraumatic stress disorder; SCID-D = Structured Clinical Interview for *DSM-IV* Dissociative Disorders.

Pilton et al., 2015; Shinn et al., 2020). A meta-analysis found a large ($r = .52$) positive relationship between dissociative experiences and voice-hearing (Pilton et al., 2015). Despite individuals with DID often being misdiagnosed with schizophrenia, the disorders can be distinguished. More than 70% of individuals with DID report hearing voices, while others with DID do not hear voices yet report hearing their own thoughts "arguing" or having multiple, often simultaneous, internal conversations (Dorahy et al., 2009; Putnam et al., 1986). These results illustrate the importance of assessing a wide range of dissociative phenomena using measures developed with an understanding of the impact of complex trauma, as well interpreting assessment results informed by research on complex trauma. Unfortunately, measures developed to assess psychotic illnesses often include items that could reflect dissociation rather than psychosis, likely due to the lack of awareness about TRD. For example, the Structured Interview for Prodromal Syndromes includes the items, "Do familiar people or surroundings ever seem strange?" "Have you ever been confused at times whether something you have experienced is real or imaginary?" and "Have you felt that you are not in control of your own ideas or thoughts?" (Miller et al., 2003). Such measures likely contribute to the misdiagnosis of TRD as psychosis.

Bipolar Disorder

See Table 1.2 for features that can assist in making the differential diagnosis of bipolar versus DID.

GROWING INTEREST IN THE NEUROBIOLOGY OF DISSOCIATION

The surge of interest in dissociation has led to neurobiological discoveries with important implications for assessing and treating TRD (see Brand et al., 2022). Dissociation-based disruptions to integrative and regulative capacities have a neurobiological basis. The brain–body disconnect that trauma causes is the basis for understanding trauma-related disorders (Kearney & Lanius, 2022). Trauma-related symptoms are hypothesized to be related to dysfunction in brainstem-level somatic sensory processing; its cascading influences result in difficulties with physiological arousal modulation, affect regulation, and higher order capacities (Kearney & Lanius, 2022). Neuroimaging studies have found patterns of brain activation that differentiate dissociative "hypoaroused" posttraumatic reactions from "hyperaroused" forms of "classic" PTSD (Lanius et al., 2010). These reactions are referred to as "feeling too much" versus "feeling too little," respectively. These and other studies contributed to awareness of the need to add DPTSD in *DSM-5-TR*, defined as PTSD along with derealization or depersonalization (Lanius et al., 2010).

Neurobiological research is providing support that TRD is not simply fantasized or malingered. For example, numerous studies provide evidence of brain activation patterns that distinguish DID from PTSD, simulated DID, and healthy controls that professional actors cannot successfully imitate (e.g., Lanius et al., 2010; Lebois et al., 2021; Reinders, 2008; Reinders et al., 2003, 2006, 2014; Roydeva & Reinders, 2021; Schlumpf et al., 2014, 2019). Furthermore, researchers reading trauma scripts to DID patients have found different brain activation patterns that distinguish whether a self-state is present that identifies the autobiographical trauma memory as "theirs" versus a self-state that does not experience trauma memories as "theirs" (Reinders et al., 2006, 2014).

A consistent neurobiological pattern found transdiagnostically among dissociative individuals is temporal lobe epilepsy-like symptoms and temporal lobe abnormalities (Schiavone et al., 2018). Clinicians need to be aware of this because temporal lobe epilepsy-like symptoms have been included in some malingering scales (see Chapters 2, 4, and 5). This is unfortunate because it increases the risk of dissociative individuals who are accurately reporting their symptoms being misclassified as malingering. Teicher's (1993) Limbic Symptom Checklist–33 may be useful for assessing temporal lobe epilepsy-like symptoms.

Researchers are searching for an unbiased, brain-based measure of dissociation severity that could augment self-reports of dissociative symptoms. A group from Harvard University studied patterns of network connectivity using functional magnetic resonance imaging scans of 65 women with histories of childhood abuse and PTSD (Lebois et al., 2021). After controlling for childhood trauma and PTSD severity, they had moderate success in estimating dissociation with the default mode and frontoparietal control networks showing the strongest ability to predict dissociation. Similarly, researchers who reviewed 205 studies found consistent biomarkers of pathological dissociation (Roydeva & Reinders, 2021). Unique network connectivity patterns appear to be associated with depersonalization/derealization (i.e., central executive and default networks) and DID (i.e., central executive network; Lebois et al., 2022).

This area of research is evolving rapidly. Perhaps soon biomarkers of dissociation will be sufficiently sensitive and specific to provide guidance in assessing TRD and guiding the treatment of TRD.

FANTASY-BASED PHENOMENA POSSIBLY RELATED TO DISSOCIATION

A phenomenon that is related to dissociative absorption and fantasy is immersive daydreaming. *Immersive daydreaming* is the ability to immerse oneself in vivid fantasy that can be enjoyable. However, if immersive daydreaming becomes compulsive and difficult to control, and if it creates distress or dysfunction, it becomes maladaptive. At that point, it is considered *maladaptive daydreaming* (MD). MD is based on fantasizing and may sometimes be a method of coping with stress, including childhood trauma (Somer, Somer, et al., 2016). MD is "probably [a] pathological form of obsessive fantasizing characterized by intense inner absorption compromising concentration on external tasks" (Somer, Lehrfeld, et al., 2016). However, it is related primarily to absorption, rather than amnesia, depersonalization, or derealization (Somer, Lehrfeld, et al., 2016). MD is assessed by the 16 Item Maladaptive Daydreaming Scale (MDS; see Chapter 4). Some theorists suggest that MD is a DD (Soffer-Dudek & Somer, 2023). Suggestive evidence includes those with MD have DES scores in the range suggestive of a possible DD (i.e., 29); furthermore, shame and dissociation fully mediated the relationship between emotional trauma and MD severity (Ferrante et al., 2022). Almost half of the inpatients on a trauma unit met criteria for MD; those who had MD reported higher symptoms, including dissociation (Ross et al., 2020). Those with DID had very high MDS-16 scores compared with those without a DD (36.4, SD = 24.3 vs. 7.1, SD = 10.3, respectively). One possibility is that severe, early trauma compounded by impaired attachment and MD can contribute to the development of DID, whereas without severe abuse and attachment problems, socially anxious individuals with high stress and the ability to engage in immersive daydreaming may develop MD rather than DID (Soffer-Dudek & Somer, 2023).

Social media and the COVID-19 pandemic seem to have contributed to the development and skyrocketing popularity of some phenomena that may be related to dissociation, including *reality shifting* in which individuals purposefully induce a state of altered consciousness so they can experience alternate, fictional realities that seem very real to them (Somer, Cardeña, et al., 2021). On some platforms, clips where individuals describe the process of reality shifting have been viewed more than 1.7 billion times. Additionally, there are various forms of experiencing oneself as having a plural, rather than a single, identity that are discussed on social media; online forums provide information about these self-experiences and provide support for individuals who experience themselves as plural (Christensen,

2021). The soaring popularity of these forums, as well as recent increased rates of self-diagnosing mental health conditions, including attention-deficit disorder, Tourette's syndrome, and DID, have concerned some clinicians (Rettew, 2022). These phenomena complicate assessing mental health disorders and bring up questions about possible factitious and malingered presentations of TRD and DDs. Little is known about many of these phenomena, including their similarities and differences from DDs and methods for differentiating them from TRD. They need to be researched and better understood, with methods developed for differentiating them from TRD and treating them when associated with distress. See Chapters 4 and 6 for additional discussion.

SUMMARY AND A CALL TO ACTION

TRD is underrecognized, inadequately treated, associated with disability and impairment, and incurs high financial costs to individuals experiencing it and society at large. Mental health professionals should assess for the complex range of dissociative symptoms with every patient and use the assessment results to individualize treatment planning. Clinicians, researchers, policymakers, and the health care industry need to be aware that earlier recognition and treatment of TRD could result in reduced levels of disability, considerable economic savings, and improved quality of life for individuals with TRD and their loved ones.

It is time to stop making traumatized individuals, their loved ones, and health care systems pay for the lack of training about trauma and TRD among mental health professionals. It is crucial to implement ubiquitous and systematic trauma education in training programs so that the enduring impact of childhood abuse, neglect, and adult traumatization are not continually overlooked, misdiagnosed, and mistreated. In psychology, social work, psychiatry, nursing, and allied fields, this training must become standard practice.

2 THE ETIOLOGY OF DISSOCIATION

There has been considerable discussion about the causes of "normal" versus "pathological" dissociation. This book focuses on pathological dissociation because normal forms of dissociation are not generally caused by trauma or stress. Two competing theories of dissociation, the trauma model (TM) and the fantasy model (FM), are discussed in this chapter, and an overview of the debate between the models is provided. Empirical evidence consistently shows that chronic, severe forms of dissociation develop after antecedent trauma. Additional factors, such as genetics and disorganized attachment, are also included in the TM, as they appear to contribute to a vulnerability to dissociate.

NORMAL VERSUS PATHOLOGICAL DISSOCIATION

Not all dissociation is pathological. For example, dissociation may occur during peak moments of spiritual, creative, and athletic experiences and can contribute to a sense of euphoria and accomplishment rather than distress

https://doi.org/10.1037/0000386-002

and impairment. Dalenberg and Paulson (2009) contended that the construct of "normal dissociation" includes dissociation that is not associated with pathology and/or that is common and temporary and that occurs possibly but not necessarily in response to stress. Many scholars regard absorption as a form of normal dissociation. They suggested that "normal," milder dissociation likely has a genetic basis, whereas severe and pathological dissociation is associated with impairment and pathology and is consistently linked with antecedent trauma.

Dalenberg and Paulson (2009) acknowledged that defining pathological dissociation is not simple. A common method for identifying pathological dissociation has been through the use of the DES taxon—that is, eight items on the Dissociative Experiences Scale (DES; Bernstein & Putnam, 1986) that indicate a high likelihood of having a dissociative disorder (DD; Waller et al., 1996). However, the DES taxon has poor short-term stability; furthermore, findings may have been driven by combining a group with DDs with healthy controls (i.e., an artificial noncontinuous distribution of DES scores may have been created; Watson, 2003). Thus, the DES taxon may not be ideal for identifying pathological dissociation.

Further, even though the Absorption factor measured by the DES is often considered nonpathological, it is highly correlated with the more pathological factors on the DES (Amnesia and Depersonalization/Derealization), as well as a wide range of pathology, such as anxiety, reexperiencing symptoms, traumatic avoidance, and dysfunctional sexual behaviors. Dalenberg and Paulson (2009) posited that individuals who are highly absorbed in one aspect of experience are necessarily detached from other aspects, which may interfere with psychological processes such as encoding memories and higher order cognition. Absorption and repeated inattention may create "unformulated experiences" (p. 149), such that experiences may be unrehearsed, resulting in limited neural connections in memory. The narrowing of attention that underlies absorption may reduce the number of associations in memory, thereby creating what the authors referred to as "extreme state-dependence" (p. 151).

Memories that are extremely state dependent may not be as easily accessed as memories that are encoded in normal, nondissociative states. As such, so-called normal dissociation, if engaged in frequently through exposure to chronic stress and trauma, may cause a person to have difficulty accessing memories of negative experiences unless they are in the same state as when the memory was experienced and encoded. Thus, at the most severe level, even "normal" dissociation may not be benign. Theorists have implicated state-dependent learning in the development and maintenance of dissociative self-states (e.g., Silberman et al., 1985). In summary, "normal" dissociation can be nonpathological, but trauma plays a crucial role in the development and possibly the maintenance of pathological dissociation. Dalenberg and Paulson (2009) advised that "normal" as well as "pathological" dissociation should be assessed and considered in treatment planning and research.

THE TRAUMA VERSUS FANTASY MODEL OF DISSOCIATION

The awareness that dissociative reactions to trauma contribute to psychopathology was observed well over a century ago by Janet (1907). For example, a meta-analysis by Ozer and colleagues (2008) of 68 studies found that prior trauma, prior psychological adjustment, family history of psychopathology, perceived life threat during trauma, lack of social support after trauma, peritraumatic emotional reactions, and peritraumatic dissociation (i.e., dissociation that occurs at the time of or shortly after the trauma) significantly predicted the development of posttraumatic stress disorder (PTSD). However, peritraumatic dissociation was the strongest predictor of PTSD (weighted $r = .35$).

Strong support for the causal connection between trauma-related dissociation (TRD) and psychopathology has been found in prospective studies of peritraumatic dissociation and PTSD (J. Murray et al., 2002; Peltonen et al., 2017). For example, one study assessed people immediately and at 1 and 6 months after vehicle accidents (J. Murray et al., 2002). Persistent dissociation 1 month after the accident, traumatic memory fragmentation, and rumination about the accident explained 41% of the variance in chronic PTSD at 6 months. Dissociative symptoms predicted chronic PTSD even more than the PTSD symptom clusters. The authors concluded that although initial dissociation may pose a risk for PTSD, individuals with persisting dissociation and rumination beyond the initial month posttrauma are those most in need of treatment. Similarly, in a study of war-affected children, even after controlling for severity of war exposure, peritraumatic dissociation predicted high PTSD symptoms 6 months later (Peltonen et al., 2017).

Despite findings from prospective studies and meta-analytic data, a debate continues about whether trauma causes dissociation. Two competing theories have been put forth to account for the relationship between trauma and dissociation. Proponents of the TM hold that the relationship is direct: Antecedent trauma causes pathological dissociation, and dissociation acts as a neurobiological defense against the overwhelm caused by trauma. Proponents of the FM, which has also been referred to as the iatrogenic and sociocultural model, hold that suggestible individuals who are prone to fantasy or sociocultural influence experience dissociation and begin to falsely believe they were abused in childhood (e.g., Giesbrecht et al., 2008; Lynn et al., 2012). The FM has historically been associated with the notions that dissociative identity disorder (DID) is an iatrogenic phenomenon and that false traumatic memories may be "implanted" by suggestive therapists. FM proponents further hypothesized that "dissociation is related to self-reported but not objective trauma" (Giesbrecht et al., 2010, p. 10).

A series of papers in *Psychological Bulletin* articulated the perspectives of the TM and FM proponents; this exchange is considered the most thorough examination of the debate between the TM and FM theorists. Dalenberg and colleagues, including the author of this book, reviewed approximately 1,500 studies and conducted a series of meta-analyses to determine which model had the most empirical support. Dalenberg et al. (2012) examined eight hypotheses regarding the relationship between trauma and dissociation. They found that the preponderance of research overwhelmingly supported the TM.

Dalenberg et al.'s (2012) inclusion standards ensured that methodologically strong studies were analyzed (e.g., samples sizes of 50 or more; control groups designs). Meta-analyses of 38 studies yielded moderate effect sizes for the relationship between childhood sexual abuse, childhood physical abuse, and overall trauma and dissociation. Another meta-analysis of studies comparing nontrauma control participants with DD patients found that trauma-exposed individuals were 4 times more likely than nontraumatized individuals to have a DD (effect size of $r = .5$). The moderate relationship between trauma and dissociation was replicated regardless of culture, research design, and sample variations, as hypothesized by the TM.

Results from another meta-analysis contradicted the FM hypothesis that objectively confirmed trauma would have weaker correlations with dissociation than self-reported trauma. Specifically, the effect sizes of studies with objective measures of trauma exposure (e.g., Child Protective Services reports or poor treatment of the child as reported by trained observers) were compared with studies that used self-report measures of abuse. This meta-analysis is critical because it addresses the fundamental difference between the two models. The objective versus self-report studies on sexual abuse had almost identical correlations (i.e., weighted average r of .30 and .32, respectively), as did the objective versus self-report studies on physical abuse (i.e., weighted average r of .30 and .26, respectively). These results refute the most important tenet of the FM: If the trauma–dissociation relationship was caused by fantasy proneness and exaggeration, the relationship should have been considerably weaker or even nonexistent when trauma was measured objectively, but the analyses showed that the relationship remained the same regardless of the assessment method. Furthermore, when fantasy proneness was statistically controlled, trauma history still predicted dissociation.

Dalenberg and colleagues (2012) also reviewed seven controlled and adequately powered PTSD treatment studies and found that dissociation decreased over time in response to trauma therapy, yet dissociation did not decrease for untreated control participants. Similarly, an additional meta-analysis of eight DD treatment studies showed that dissociation decreased significantly with treatment specifically tailored toward treating trauma-related difficulties including dissociative symptoms.

To evaluate the FM theory that DID individuals are particularly fantasy-prone, studies comparing DID to healthy control participants were analyzed. DID patients were found to have similar levels of fantasy-proneness to healthy control participants. Furthermore, a meta-analysis of 34 studies that assessed the link between suggestibility and dissociation found that suggestibility accounted for only a fraction (1%–3%) of the variability in dissociation. However, individuals with DDs are more responsive than controls to direct verbal posthypnotic suggestions, according to a meta-analysis; the authors note that no study to date indicates that hypnotic suggestibility *causes* DDs (Wieder et al., 2022; Wieder et al., 2023). See below for more information on hypnotizability.

Dalenberg and colleagues (2012) challenged the FM notion that recovered trauma memories are inaccurate. Research data do not support this FM prediction. On the contrary, research shows that recovered trauma memories have similar rates of accuracy as continuously recalled trauma memories (reviewed in Dalenberg, 2006). This finding has significant clinical and forensic implications. It is crucial that evaluators and forensic experts are familiar with evidence-based findings and practices, rather than believing unsubstantiated myths about the unreliability of trauma memories.

Finally, Dalenberg et al. (2012) reviewed the neurobiological research on dissociation, and found that it, too, supported the TM. In summary, considerable neurobiological research indicates that dissociation is a response to fear and other extreme emotions caused by trauma with measurable biological correlates (Harricharan et al., 2021; Lanius et al., 2010).

After realizing how little research supports the FM conjectures, readers may wonder about the basis for the FM argument that trauma does not cause dissociation. Space constraints require limiting the answer to three areas, but readers are encouraged to read the full published debate in *Psychological Bulletin*. First, there are simple explanations for the FM theorists finding an overlap, or correlation, between dissociation and fantasy-proneness. The measure of fantasy-proneness that they frequently use, the Creative Experiences Questionnaire (Merckelbach et al., 2001), which was created by an FM theorist, includes some items similar in content to those on the DES, the most widely used self-report measure of dissociation. It is not surprising that these two scales are correlated, given they contain some similar items. Yet this simple statistical explanation is generally overlooked by the FM theorists.

Second, another measure used by the FM theorists that they state assesses dissociation, the DES-C (Wright & Loftus, 2000), uses the DES items yet requires respondents to make judgements about how often they experience each dissociative symptom compared with others. The FM theorists have not validated this measure with individuals with DDs. It is questionable whether these individuals, who often have difficulties with self-awareness and social cognition (Harricharan et al., 2021; McKinnon et al., 2016), can accurately make these comparisons. Thus, the FM theorists' conclusions about their research using this measure are suspect (see Chapter 4).

Third, there is another methodological explanation for the studies the FM theorists claim indicate that dissociative individuals exaggerate their symptoms. The measure of so-called exaggeration that they use, the Structured Inventory of Malingered Symptomatology (SIMS; Smith & Burger, 1997), contains scales with items that are common among traumatized people, including scales assessing depression, amnesia, and neurological symptoms (e.g., Schiavone et al., 2018). The neurological symptoms include temporal-lobe epilepsy-like symptoms, which are common among dissociative individuals (Schiavone et al., 2018). Endorsing items increases one's scores on the SIMS; high scores are interpreted as evidence of malingering. As experimental researchers, rather than clinicians with trauma expertise, the FM theorists seem unaware that high levels of depression, amnesia, and neurological somatoform symptoms are common among trauma survivors. For example, some seemingly neurological symptoms often associated with temporal lobe epilepsy (e.g., visual anomalies, auditory hallucinations; see Tables 2.1 and 2.2) are common among traumatized individuals, even though they are thought by many to be rare (Schiavone et al., 2018). Furthermore, the SIMS has poor validity for highly dissociative individuals, with an unacceptably low specificity of 14% in a study that used the SIMS to distinguish DID individuals from DID simulators and healthy control participants (Brand, Barth, et al., 2021). Researchers have found the SIMS includes genuine symptoms of mental illnesses including psychosis, depression, PTSD, and head trauma, leading researchers to conclude, "The SIMS is a pseudopsychological test" (Cernovsky et al., 2019, p. 121). The authors of a review of the SIMS found that the SIMS total score correlated .60 with self-reported PTSD symptoms; they concluded, "The SIMS is a fatally flawed psychological test with alarmingly high iatrogenic rates. Its use constitutes malpractice" (Cernovsky & Diamond, 2020, p. 30). In summary, the FM authors rely on measures that do not adequately assess what they purport they assess, and they do not recognize these limitations in interpreting their studies.

Beyond methodological problems, the FM theorists often cite studies that support their theory while overlooking those that refute their theory. For

TABLE 2.1. Complex Dissociative Disorders Versus Trauma Spectrum Disorders

	Primary psychosis	Complex DDs	PTSD	Temporal lobe epilepsy
Auditory hallucinations	Often	Often	Often	Possible
Internally vs. externally perceived voices	Either	Either	More likely internal	
Onset of voices	After age 18	Before age 18		
Number of voices	Typically one	Typically multiple	Typically one	
Child voices	Possible	Often		
Nonauditory hallucinations	Possible	Often	Often	Often
Trauma-related content	Sometimes	Sometimes	Sometimes	
Schneiderian first-rank symptoms	Often	More often		
Trauma exposure	Often	Often	Necessary	
Dissociative symptoms	Possible	Necessary	Common	Common

Note. DD = dissociative disorders; PTSD = posttraumatic stress disorder. Adapted from "Psychotic-Like Symptoms and the Temporal Lobe in Trauma-Related Disorders: Diagnosis, Treatment, and Assessment of Potential Malingering," by F. L. Schiavone, M. C. McKinnon, and R. A. Lanius, 2018, *Chronic Stress, 2*, 2470547018797046 (https://doi.org/10.1177/2470547018797046). Copyright 2018 by F. L. Schiavone, M. C. McKinnon, and R. A. Lanius. Adapted with permission.

TABLE 2.2. Temporal Lobe Dysfunction in Trauma-Related Disorders

	Trauma-exposed	PTSD
Structural	Decreased volume (right) Reduced cortical thickness	Decreased volume (right)
Functional	Altered resting state activity	Decreased blood flow (reexperiencing symptoms) Increased blood flow (dissociative symptoms)

	BPD	Dissociative depression
Structural	Decreased volume (right)	Unclear
Functional	Right hypometabolism	Unclear

	Depersonalization disorder	DID/OSDD
Structural	Decreased volume (right)	Decreased volume
Functional	Right hypometabolism	Left increased perfusion (in dissociated self-state)

Note. BPD = borderline personality disorder; DID = dissociative identity disorder; OSDD = other specified dissociative disorder; PTSD = posttraumatic stress disorder. From "Psychotic-Like Symptoms and the Temporal Lobe in Trauma-Related Disorders: Diagnosis, Treatment, and Assessment of Potential Malingering," by F. L. Schiavone, M. C. McKinnon, and R. A. Lanius, 2018, *Chronic Stress, 2*, 2470547018797046 (https://doi.org/10.1177/2470547018797046). Copyright 2018 by F. L. Schiavone, M. C. McKinnon, and R. A. Lanius. Reprinted with permission.

example, Giesbrecht et al. (2008) cited only two studies that used objective criteria to support their claim that trauma and dissociation are not related. Both studies had small, nongeneralizable samples (e.g., 30 psychiatric forensic inpatients). To reach their conclusion—that trauma did not cause dissociation—they overlooked the 10 studies with larger and more generalizable samples that met Dalenberg et al.'s (2012) rigorous inclusion criteria, all of which *did* support the TM hypothesis.

The meta-analyses and other evidence reviewed in the four-part *Psychological Bulletin* debate so thoroughly supported the TM theory that FM theorists subsequently conceded that *some recovered memories are likely to be accurate* and that *trauma treatment does not generally cause a worsening of dissociation* (Lynn et al., 2014). These concessions represent a significant softening in the more extreme arguments put forward by the FM theory.

Despite the concessions, FM theorists (Merckelbach & Patihis, 2018) subsequently challenged much of what was already established in the prior debate. In a new debate that spanned five papers published in *Personal Injury and Law* about TRD, Brand, Dalenberg, and colleagues (Brand et al. 2018; Dalenberg et al., 2020) once again corrected oversights, errors, and misstatements made by the FM proponents. For example, Merckelbach and Patihis argued that there were no empirical data about the interrater reliability of DD diagnoses, and the TM authors responded with data from six studies that showed strong interrater reliability for DD diagnoses. Similarly, the TM authors documented the FM selective reporting of research. For example, Merckelbach and Patihis failed to mention studies that show that dissociative individuals are not prone to developing false memories (e.g., Brand, Vissia, et al., 2016; Dalenberg et al., 2012; Kluemper & Dalenberg, 2014; Vissia et al., 2016).

Dalenberg et al. (2020) concluded that such biased reporting of research, refusal to acknowledge studies that counter their beliefs, and ad hominem attacks on the TM authors fell below standards of scientific discussion. They interpreted this pattern to indicate that the FM authors show motivated skepticism rather than openness to scientific discovery.

Two other causal pathways to dissociation subsequently proposed by FM authors are sleep problems and affect dysregulation. To argue that sleep problems cause dissociation, they cite a study that found decreases in dissociation occurred as sleep improved among inpatients. The FM theorists failed to emphasize in their reviews (e.g., van der Kloet, Merckelbach, et al., 2012) that in the original study (van der Kloet, Giesbrecht, et al., 2012), *the severity of childhood trauma predicted dissociation before and after treatment*. Moreover, childhood maltreatment predicted sleep disturbances—specifically, what they referred to as narcoleptic symptoms, which, in turn, predicted dissociation. Furthermore, structural equation analysis found that childhood maltreatment remained a strong predictor of dissociation, beyond the influence of narcoleptic symptoms ($r = .44$). Additionally, nightmares are symptoms of PTSD, which commonly co-occurs with DDs. Patients with DD often have complex sleep disorders related to their trauma history, including phobic and traumatic responses to night, sleep, and beds related to traumas that occurred in similar settings (Spiegel et al., 2011). Although their data support the TM, these findings are rarely acknowledged in FM publications. The FM theorists overlook evidence that sleep abnormalities are caused by posttraumatic and dissociative factors, rather than the other way around.

The FM theorists also suggest that affect dysregulation might represent an alternative cause for dissociative symptoms largely based on Briere and Runtz (2015), who found reports of dissociation among individuals who did not report having experienced traumatic events. The severity of dissociation was correlated with affect dysregulation. Yet the FM theorists (e.g., Merckelbach & Patihis, 2018) fail to note that Briere and Runtz found rates of clinically significant dissociation in their nontraumatized sample to be extraordinarily low (1.3%). This low level of clinical dissociation should have weakened their claim that significant dissociative symptoms are likely to occur in the absence of any trauma exposure. Furthermore, emotion dysregulation is predicted by trauma exposure and is highly related to dissociation. In fact, improving emotion regulation is a major focus in the Treatment of Dissociative Disorders (TOP DD) studies and thought to have been a contributor to reductions in dissociation (see Chapter 7 and Brand, Schielke, et al., 2019, 2022; Schielke et al., 2022). Nonetheless, when directly compared with measures of distress, dissociation has been shown to have a more specific association with childhood trauma history (e.g., Frewen et al., 2017). The TM theorists posit that dissociative symptoms develop as attempts to regulate trauma-related emotion dysregulation and distress.

The TM theorists attempted to foster scientific discussion about dissociation by summarizing areas of agreement between the models, including

> that trauma exposure is associated with depersonalization and, occasionally, memory errors; reports of dissociative symptoms may be elevated due to non-trauma factors; error rates for diagnosing DID are low; and multiple sources of information are required for assessing any symptom, including dissociation, in forensic contexts. (Dalenberg et al., 2020, p. 3)

They further acknowledge that both models agree that trauma exposure can be associated with fantasy processes (Dalenberg et al., 2012; Merckelbach et al., 2001). Specifically, the TM theorists acknowledge that engagement in fantasy can be a method of coping with trauma. For example, a woman reported that when her father came into her bedroom and raped her, she regularly imagined she was outdoors, smelling a lilac bush. This form of fantasy could be characterized as dissociation because it disconnected her from a recurring traumatizing event from which she could not escape. Thus, it provided some small buffer from the horror and betrayal of her father attacking her when she was a preschooler. However, her use of a dissociative type of fantasy did not cause her to be confused about the reality that her father had repeatedly raped her.

The TM recognizes that the correlations between antecedent trauma and dissociation are often in the moderate to large range. This indicates that there are other factors contributing to the development of TRD, including biological, attachment, hypnotizability, and cultural factors, which are reviewed next.

BIOLOGICAL CONTRIBUTIONS TO DISSOCIATION

Posttraumatic effects on memory, cognition, and logical reasoning are well documented for different types of trauma. Emotional dysregulation manifested as rapid shifts in affect and mental state produce neurobiological disruptions in an individual's sense of self and integrative and regulative capacities (Putnam, 2016). Neuroimaging studies indicate there are patterns of brain activation that differentiate dissociative, "hypoaroused" posttraumatic presentations from highly emotional, "hyperaroused" presentations of "classic" PTSD (Lanius et al., 2010). The body of research showing distinctions between hypoaroused, dissociative PTSD and hyperaroused "classic" or "simple" PTSD contributed to the inclusion of the dissociative subtype of PTSD to the fifth edition of the *Diagnostic and Statistical Manual of Mental Disorders* (American Psychiatric Association, 2013). Experimental activation of dissociative responses to recall of trauma is associated with decreased autonomic arousal, especially decreased heart rate. This is consistent with the theory that dissociative reactions in humans are similar to the "freezing" behaviors seen in some animals in response to predators.

Researchers are searching for brain-based measures of dissociation that could augment self-reports of dissociative symptoms. A thorough review identified biomarkers that are consistently found in pathological dissociation (Roydeva & Reinders, 2021). Lebois and colleagues (2021) found that after controlling for childhood trauma and PTSD, the default mode network (DMN) and frontoparietal control network show the strongest ability to predict dissociation. The DMN is involved in self-referential processes and social cognition, allowing one to draw inferences about oneself and mentalize others and providing an embodied sense of self in space and over time (reviewed in Lanius et al., 2020). The DMN is involved in altered autobiographical memory-related reexperiencing, emotional states such as guilt and shame, and perceptual alterations such as depersonalization and derealization in individuals with PTSD. Dissociative individuals show widespread functional alterations in the DMN during rest and trauma-related conditions compared with healthy control individuals; these alterations are thought to contribute to the clinical disturbances underlying sense of self in PTSD (Lanius et al., 2020).

For example, the DMN shows decreased connectivity during rest, which may contribute to a lack of a sense of self, and increased connectivity during subliminal (e.g., the word "rape" flashed so rapidly on a screen that the individual is not aware a word was shown) trauma stimulus among individuals with PTSD, which may contribute to heightened threat perception and reactivity. These alterations explain why in PTSD, especially when it is related to childhood maltreatment, individuals experience impaired sense of self as indicated by statements such as "I do not know who I am." The DMN does not complete maturation until adulthood; therefore, childhood trauma may be particularly influential in creating hypersensitivity to threat in the DMN (Lanius et al., 2020). Lanius et al. (2020) offered a fascinating clinical implication based on this research: The decreased activation of DMN when at rest may contribute to feeling dissociated and deadened, and the heightened DMN activation during threat may be a driving force for individuals with PTSD engaging in high-risk behavior—to "wake up" their DMN so that they feel alive and energized rather than numb and empty.

Neurobiological research in DID is yielding intriguing results, although more studies are needed, particularly with diverse participants. Studies show brain activity differences between self-states across various paradigms, neural correlates of switching between states, and patterns that may characterize the process of self-state integration (e.g., Lebois et al., 2019). DID patients' pathological dissociation scores on the Multidimensional Inventory of Dissociation (Dell, 2006a) have been estimated with moderate success using only brain functional network connectivity (Lebois et al., 2021). Brain structures and activity in DID patients have been compared with healthy controls and to professional actors; actors cannot accurately simulate DID brain activation patterns (e.g., Reinders et al., 2012; Schlumpf et al., 2014). This research indicates that DID is a severe disorder on a continuum of trauma disorders. Furthermore, these studies refute the FM notions that DID is merely based in role-playing or fantasy.

A trauma victim's genes may be altered by trauma through epigenetic mechanisms such as stress-induced DNA methylation. These trauma-induced genetic changes may be transmitted to future generations, providing a genetic contribution to the intergenerational pattern of family violence. Twin studies suggest that between 50% and 60% of the variation in dissociation is due to genetics (Becker-Blease et al., 2004; Jang et al., 1998). Possible gene targets have been identified in trauma-exposed children and adults, providing further evidence of the myriad biological contributions to TRD (see King et al., 2020).

DISORGANIZED ATTACHMENT

Disorganized attachment appears to be an important factor in the development of TRD. The Minnesota Longitudinal Study of Parent and Children is one of the gold standard studies of the effects of childhood neglect and abuse (Ogawa et al., 1997). The study focused on children of low-income families, from infancy through emerging adulthood. Maternal psychological unavailability, disorganized attachment style, and infant attention span accounted for 30% of the variability in dissociation at age 19. Age of trauma onset, chronicity, and severity of trauma had more modest effects when attachment style was taken into consideration. Using structural equation modeling, Carlson (1998) analyzed the Minnesota study's data and found that aspects of the caregiving relationship, including child abuse in infancy, directly contributed to dissociation at age 19 as well as indirectly contributed to dissociation through disorganized attachment (Carlson, 1998).

In another longitudinal study, when children were 19 years old, maternal unresponsiveness, withdrawal, and attachment disorganization were more strongly predictive of dissociation than overtly hostile or threatening behaviors, or even the infants' own disorganized attachment (Lyons-Ruth et al., 2006). These parental behaviors may be "hidden traumas," which are experienced in infants' brains as a significant threat to survival due to the infant's total dependence on the caregiver. Neither of these studies included individuals with DDs, so it is unclear to what extent these results capture the impact of extreme, chronic childhood abuse as is found in complex DDs.

There is, however, good reason to believe that disorganized attachment may contribute to the development of complex DDs. The contradictory behaviors seen in infants with a disorganized attachment style (e.g., walking toward the mother with the infant's face turned away from her) resemble the disorganized, conflicting attachment seen among self-states in complex DDs (e.g., Liotti, 1992). Disorganized attachment may represent a vulnerability factor for the development of complex DDs, particularly among children who are exposed to severe trauma. Indeed, self-reported disorganized attachment partially mediated the relationship between child maltreatment and dissociation (Briere et al., 2019). Even after controlling for anxious and avoidant attachment, dissociation was significantly linked to disorganized attachment. The combination of parental maltreatment or fearfulness of the child interspersed with, at times, relative safety and connection are likely to be likely to lead to confusion. Briere et al. (2019) concluded: "These experiences may lead to contradictory, unintegrated working models of self and others, resulting in the fragmentation, confusion, and lapses in attention characteristic of both DA [disorganized attachment] and some dissociative presentations" (p. 492).

Research by D. P. Brown and Elliott (2016) supports the role of insecure attachment, particularly disorganized attachment, in the development of complex DDs. The authors studied 45 adult survivors of childhood sexual abuse who had been placed in an orphanage where two priests had been relocated by the Catholic Church after previous allegations of committing sexual abuse (D. P. Brown & Elliott, 2016). Dr. Brown was hired as a forensic expert in a lawsuit against the Catholic Church to evaluate the adult survivors who reported having been physically and/or sexually abused at the orphanage. Although some remembered the physical abuse, all had forgotten the sexual abuse, and most of the victims had not reported the sexual abuse in childhood. The lawsuit settled against the Church for most of the victims before trial. The 45 adults were given an exhaustive 16-hour battery of psychological measures including tests for malingering and the Adult Attachment Interview (AAI; George et al., 1996). Insecure attachment (mostly disorganized) was significantly associated with depersonalization and derealization. Those who had secure attachment rarely showed symptoms of dissociation, leading the authors to suggest that secure attachment may protect traumatized children from developing significant dissociative symptoms, even if they experience childhood trauma.

Furthermore, D. P. Brown and Elliott (2016) collected data on AAIs from 60 reliably diagnosed DID patients and found that more than 90% had "cannot classify" as their primary attachment and more than 90% had "unresolved status" with respect to trauma or loss. The few who did not have unresolved status had resolved loss or trauma in psychotherapy. The authors concluded, "These data strongly suggest that pervasive disorganization and specifically disorganization around the exploration of trauma or abuse essentially defines the mind of the DID patient" (p. 192). They theorized that the self-states express different unmet attachment needs in individuals with disorganized attachment. Brown and Elliott concluded that "the combination of disorganized attachment aggravated by later childhood abuse predicts the development of dissociative disorders in adulthood" (p. 193). Further, they suggested that "simple PTSD" results from single or even multiple traumas if insecure attachment is not present. However, if early childhood insecure attachment is aggravated by later abuse or trauma, complex TRDs (including somatoform symptoms, complex dissociative symptoms, and multiple addictive behaviors) are likely to develop, along with additional comorbid psychiatric disorders.

In summary, the attachment and trauma literatures suggest that attachment patterns in relationships, including that between the therapist and patient, are crucial to address in treatment.

CULTURE

Culture influences the development and expression of psychiatric disorders, including TRD and DDs, although this is an area that has not yet been extensively researched. There are cultural variations in environmental factors, such as the degree of oppression, gender roles, and spiritual customs and beliefs, that influence perpetrators of abuse as well as their victims. These variables can influence the type of trauma one is exposed to as well as symptomatic expression (Şar et al., 2017). Family structures vary culturally as well, including boundary structures, family roles, and sexual norms and expectations. These family variables impact whether trauma occurs in the family, and if so, how family members respond to it. Societal variables such as degree of oppression, community violence, and traditions may also influence symptom expression (Şar et al., 2017). For example, in some cultures, possession states are a variation of DID, whereas in other cultures this presentation is rarely if ever seen. Despite cross-cultural differences, some factors such as the role of attachment and neglect in the etiology of DDs play a consistent role around the world. For example, in a study of Turkish college students, emotional neglect predicted a DD diagnosis, including DID (Şar et al., 2006). In a South African study, emotional neglect by parents or siblings was the strongest predictor of an adult diagnosis of a DD, including DID (Krüger & Fletcher, 2017).

HYPNOTIZABILITY

High hypnotizability is a nonpathological, genetically derived capacity that renders an individual more susceptible to hypnosis. As such, it could also be considered a biological contributor to dissociation because when a highly hypnotizable person experiences trauma, they may be at particular risk for developing a complex DD (reviewed in Dell, 2017). DID patients and patients with chronic complex PTSD are high in hypnotizability (Dell, 2017; Şar et al., 2017; Wieder et al., 2022).

In summary, although dissociation is transdiagnostic, it is particularly likely to be chronic and severe enough to cause dysfunction in traumatized individuals, particularly when insecure attachment, and biological, cultural, and/or hypnotizability contributors are also present.

DID TREATMENT AND PATIENT WELL-BEING

Another often-repeated FM conjecture that requires careful examination is the notion that DID treatment harms patients, supposedly by iatrogenically creating self-states, or the belief therein, among suggestible individuals (Gee et al., 2003; Lilienfeld, 2007; Lynn et al., 2012; Powell & Gee, 1999). An examination of Lilienfeld's opinion piece "Psychological Treatments That Cause Harm" revealed he failed to cite any treatment studies that showed treatment of DID patients caused harm (Brand, Loewenstein, & Spiegel, 2014). Rather, he cited opinion pieces written by other FM advocates. He also challenged techniques used by clinicians to foster awareness of self-states among individuals with DID. It was not possible for Lilienfeld to cite research showing DID treatment is harmful because no study has found this to be true. Lilienfeld made inaccurate statements including that most cases of DIDs are found by a small number of therapists who are supposedly DID specialists; other FM theorists argue that the disorder is diagnosed primarily in North America, both of which are myths that have been repeatedly disproven (Brand, Sar, et al., 2016). For example, hundreds of international clinicians who were not DID specialists participated in prospective treatment studies with DID (and DD not otherwise specified) patients in the TOP DD studies (Brand, Classen, Lanius, et al., 2009; Brand, Schielke, et al., 2019). Brand and Loewenstein (2014) analyzed data from one of the TOP DD studies to determine whether patients showed signs of worsening as assessed by identity alteration, hearing voices, or amnesia over 30 months in outpatient treatment. All three dissociative symptoms declined with treatment, with identity alteration and hearing voices decreasing significantly, although, as seen in Figure 2.1, the decline in amnesia only trended toward being significant. If treatment increased fragmentation and amnesia, the opposite pattern would have emerged. In contrast to FM theorist claims that treatment itself causes harm, the authors concluded, "Indeed there are data

FIGURE 2.1. Mean Amnesia and Identity Alteration Over Four Assessments in Dissociative Disorder Patients in Treatment of Dissociative Disorders Study Participants With 95% Confidence Intervals

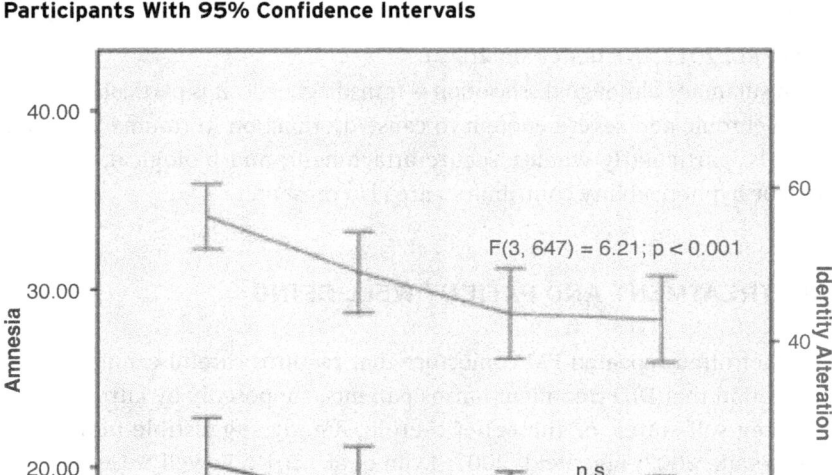

Adapted from "Does Phasic Trauma Treatment Make Patients With Dissociative Identity Disorder Treatment More Dissociative?" by B. L. Brand and R. J. Loewenstein, 2014, *Journal of Trauma & Dissociation, 15*(1), p. 59 (https://doi.org/10.1080/15299732. 2013.828150). Copyright 2014 by Taylor & Francis (www.tandfonline.com). Adapted with permission.

that iatrogenic harm may result from *depriving* DID patients of appropriate treatment" (p. 22, emphasis added).

Research investigating the impact of betrayal trauma—that is, trauma perpetrated by someone a child depends on—also supports the TM. For example, in international samples, betrayal trauma was more strongly linked with DID features than was nonbetrayal trauma (Fung et al., 2022). Childhood betrayal trauma predicted 7.8% of the variance in dissociative amnesia and 1.2% of identity dissociation, after controlling for nonbetrayal trauma, age, and depression.

Similarly, as noted earlier, a meta-analysis of DD treatment studies showed that dissociation decreased with treatment specifically tailored toward treating trauma-related difficulties such as dissociation (Dalenberg et al., 2012). Additionally, another meta-analysis of eight DD studies found moderate to large within-subject, pre–post standardized Hedge's *g* effect sizes in seven groups of symptoms (Brand, Classen, McNary, et al., 2009); see Table 2.3. To provide comparison data, Brand et al. (2009) conducted a meta-analysis of six treatment studies in which at least one fourth of the adult sample had experienced childhood sexual abuse. The effect sizes were comparable to those in the DD studies, suggesting that DD patients benefit from treatment roughly as much as other patients who experienced childhood sexual abuse.

In conclusion, there is no empirical support for the FM claim that treating DDs harms patients. As is discussed in Chapter 7, expert guidelines and expert recommendations about treatment interventions indicate that the standard of care for complex DDs is a carefully paced, staged approach that stabilizes patients' safety and symptoms in the first stage of treatment, followed by in-depth trauma processing after the stabilization stage. Patients provided treatment that is consistent with this standard of care have shown reductions in nonsuicidal self-injury, hospitalizations, treatment costs, and symptoms of PTSD and dissociation, as well as improved emotion regulation and improvements in other adaptive capacities (e.g., Brand, Schielke, et al., 2019). However, treatment that is not consistent with the expert guidelines and recommendations can overwhelm patients with emotions or traumatic

TABLE 2.3. Comparison of Effect Sizes for DD Studies and Individual Treatment Studies for Childhood Trauma

Outcome	Effect size for DD treatment studies comparing pre- and post-treatment data	Effect size for individual treatment studies of childhood trauma
Overall outcomes	.71	.82
Depression	1.12	.98
Dissociation	.70	.94
General distress	1.09	.49

Note. Data from a review of dissociative disorders treatment studies and six treatment outcome studies of individual therapy for adults in which at least 25% of the sample reported childhood abuse (data from Brand, Classen, McNary, et al., 2009). DD = dissociative disorders. From "Dispelling Myths About Dissociative Identity Disorder Treatment: An Empirically Based Approach," by B. L. Brand, R. J. Loewenstein, and D. Spiegel, 2014, *Psychiatry*, 77(2), p. 175 (https://doi.org/10.1521/psyc.2014.77.2.169). Copyright 2014 by The Washington School of Psychiatry. Reprinted by permission of Taylor & Francis Ltd., http://www.tandfonline.com on behalf of The Washington School of Psychiatry.

memories before they have the capacity to manage them. If the FM proponents had reviewed DD treatment research, they would have found evidence that treatment is beneficial, although more research is still needed in this area.

The Impact of the Fantasy Model

The FM myths about traumatic memories, dissociation, and the "harmful" impact of treating DID have received considerable coverage in the media and within the mental health field. The FM narrative has found its way into many undergraduate and graduate psychology textbooks, often without a balanced presentation of empirical evidence about TRD, child abuse, and traumatic memories (Brand, Kumar, et al., 2019; Gleaves, 2007; Kissee et al., 2014; Wilgus et al., 2015). These textbooks are read by hundreds of thousands of students each year. Misrepresentations and bias can negatively affect students' understanding and attitudes about trauma and trauma survivors, their career choices, and the way they respond to disclosures about trauma and dissociation by their peers and loved ones. These students are tomorrow's health care and mental health providers, attorneys, first responders, teachers, professors, politicians, police, and jurors. As a consultant, I have repeatedly heard about individuals in treatment for TRD who have become highly distressed after hearing professors and clinical supervisors talk dismissively or derisively about dissociated trauma memories and TRD or after reading the unbalanced FM narrative featured in textbooks. Academic psychology textbooks have rightfully been challenged about their historical endorsement of myths and stereotypes about race and gender. It is time to challenge the myths perpetuated by the mental and medical health care fields, textbooks, and training programs about trauma and TRD.

Recent years have seen a greater willingness among survivors to speak publicly about child abuse and sexual assault, such as the #MeToo movement. Trauma survivors' disclosures of trauma have led to prosecution in highly publicized cases of sexual assault and harassment in businesses, athletic teams, scouting organizations, educational institutions, places of worship, government agencies, and other institutions. The growing awareness about trauma and dissociation needs to fuel widespread changes that provide greater prevention of trauma, as well as protection and support to trauma survivors. These changes urgently need to take place in the education and training of mental health professionals as well.

Most clinicians have received little if any systematic training in complex trauma and dissociation (see Chapter 1). As a result, few are well trained in research-supported methods for assessing and treating TRD. If clinicians read textbooks that contain inaccurate, biased information about trauma and TRD, they may develop negative and harmful beliefs about traumatized individuals. Clinicians who have been taught or supervised by mentors who believe the FM perspective may be less effective and empathetic and may act dismissive or shaming when working with traumatized individuals.

Sadly, research reveals that dissociative patients are an underserved group who are sometimes distressed and even mistreated rather than helped by clinicians. A survey of 276 dissociative individuals from 17 countries found that 97% had encountered barriers to obtaining mental health treatment (Nester, Hawkins, et al., 2022). Most (52%) reported a barrier to treatment was not being able to find a provider with availability and trauma training. Forty-two percent of the sample reported that they had encountered clinicians who expressed disbelief about their reports of dissociative symptoms, childhood abuse, or both. Some participants reported that clinicians had mocked them when they discussed dissociation. Others had clinicians tell them they were faking dissociative symptoms. Participants reported clinicians had been invalidating and shaming; one provider ended sessions abruptly if the patient dissociated.

It is highly improbable that a clinician would respond this way to non-dissociative disorders; for example, abruptly ending a session if a patient hallucinated or experienced a panic attack or worsening depression during session. It is unlikely that patients would be told that they were exaggerating their reports of hallucinations, panic attacks, or depression. It is discriminatory for clinicians to mistreat dissociative and traumatized individuals. Many of the invalidating responses reported in the Nester et al. study (Nester, Hawkins, et al., 2022) reflect notions put forth by the FM proponents. That is, these clinicians may believe the FM myths that dissociative patients are especially fantasy-prone and suggestible and that they exaggerate their symptoms or trauma history. Research-based training about complex trauma and TRD is urgently needed to counter these myths and foster respectful, research-informed methods of working with traumatized patients, including those with TRD.

In some situations, patients may in fact purposefully or inadvertently exaggerate their history or symptoms, including but not limited to trauma and dissociation. It is also possible that traumatized individuals may under-report their trauma history or symptoms, as has been found in research; for example, only 26% of children reported sexual abuse to adults in a population study (Bottoms et al., 2016; Lahtinen et al., 2018, 2022). However, in the study by Nester et al., there were no reports of clinicians invalidating or shaming clients for underreporting symptoms or trauma. In fact, it appears that some clinicians expect symptom and trauma exaggeration rather than underreporting among dissociative individuals; this is consistent with the unsupported FM notions. Therefore, the FM perspective may be contributing to dissociative patients being invalidated, mistreated, and turned away from treatment by clinicians who subscribe to its unfounded notions. This may lead to a "trauma denial-based care environment, re-traumatization, and delayed protection and clinical intervention" (Fung et al., 2022, p. 16).

Clinicians who question the validity of patients' reports of trauma or symptoms need to consider the basis for their questions carefully. If the questions stem from FM myths, clinicians should strive to learn more about complex trauma, and they should examine their beliefs for biases based in myths rather than science, as with any misunderstood, underserved, stereotyped, or discriminated group. Sensitive, respectful, trauma- and research-informed methods of interacting with all patients are essential, including when working with individuals who are suspected of exaggerating or minimizing their symptoms or life experiences.

The preponderance of scientific evidence, when fairly and accurately reviewed, supports the TM theory of dissociation, not the FM. The FM authors initially suggested that fantasy-proneness, suggestibility, and treatment that attended to dissociation caused individuals to report they experienced dissociation, rather than trauma-causing dissociation. When research did not provide much support for those causal relationships, the FM theorists shifted their focus and suggested that sleep problems and emotional dysregulation might cause dissociation. However, these new notions were put forth without recognizing that the underlying, primary driver of dissociation, sleep problems, and emotional dysregulation in their studies could have been trauma. Pathological dissociation is caused by trauma, often in combination with attachment problems, biological alterations, cultural influences, and hypnotic contributions. It is time that the mental health field provides research-informed assistance to individuals with TRD, rather than dismissive myth-based reactions that can cause harm and delay access to beneficial treatment.

In summary, individuals with TRD are often underserved and misunderstood. They are sometimes even mistreated by the mental health system, in part due to myths and misconceptualizations about dissociation. It is the ethical and professional responsibility of clinicians and researchers to help, rather than overlook, shame, or denigrate those who have already been harmed and who seek assistance from the mental health field. Contrary to the warnings of the FM authors, iatrogenic harm is more likely to result from treatment by clinicians who believe and practice according to debunked myths about TRD or those who do not act in accordance with trauma- and dissociation-informed assessment and treatment guidelines.

3

THERAPEUTIC APPROACH TO ASSESSING TRAUMA EXPOSURE AND TRAUMA-RELATED DISSOCIATION

Traumatized individuals often develop symptoms and adaptations that create challenges for assessors. They often experience overwhelming emotion and traumatic intrusions, which they attempt to prevent by consciously avoiding thinking and talking about trauma, dissociation, substance use and other means. The process of assessment can trigger trauma-related symptoms, resulting in states of overwhelm and feeling too much, or, alternatively, too little. Trauma survivors also often vacillate between remembering too much or too little of their trauma, so their ability to access and report experiences can vary. To gather assessment data that accurately represent the client's full capacities, struggles, symptoms, and the contextual aspects of their lives, assessors need to work within the client's "window of tolerance" of emotion while assessing trauma exposure and its sequelae (Ogden et al., 2006; Siegel, 1999). Clinicians who are tuned in to the profound level of shame, mistrust, terror, betrayal, hurt, sorrow, anger, and related emotions that clients may experience are better able to pace assessment appropriately.

This chapter discusses these issues and describes practices that foster a collaborative working relationship with clients so that they feel understood,

https://doi.org/10.1037/0000386-003
The Concise Guide to the Assessment and Treatment of Trauma-Related Dissociation, by B. L. Brand

supported, in control, and safe. Different assessment methods may be useful depending on whether the client has experienced one-time or time-limited versus complex trauma, the individual's level of resources, and the severity of trauma-related dissociation (TRD). In this chapter, I address the process of assessing for dissociation in relatively unstructured initial intake interviews and the process that can be useful in formal psychological assessment. In Chapter 4, I address in more detail the content of assessing for dissociation using validated self-report measures and semistructured interviews.

Most assessments in clinical practice occur during an intake interview in the first few meetings with a client. Intake interviews are relatively unstructured and can be highly informative if the client is carefully observed and thoughtfully interviewed. Nonetheless, such interviews are prone to subjective interpretations by a clinician, including errors and oversights. Some clinicians prefer to allow the client to talk freely, determining the focus. This approach is likely to miss crucial information about topics clients may forget to mention or prefer to avoid, including issues related to safety, unhealthy self-soothing (such as substance use), trauma (including possible ongoing interpersonal violence), and dissociation. Many graduate programs do not train students in conducting initial diagnostic interviewing. I strongly recommend following a routine intake interview format so that these easily avoided topics are not missed. The intake outline I give to students in my classes about diagnostic interviewing includes initial questions about trauma exposure and possible trauma-related reactions (see Appendix A; this outline is also available online at https://www.apa.org/pubs/books/assessment-treatment-trauma-related-dissociation). When trauma and/or dissociation are identified in the intake interview, further assessment is recommended. Whenever possible, clinicians need to follow up on signs and symptoms noted in initial interviews by using structured interviews or evidence-based assessment measures that deepen their understanding of clients and guide treatment planning to best address the client's needs.

CLINICAL ASSESSMENT AS A FORM OF LISTENING AND INTERVENTION

Traditional psychological assessment emphasizes information gathering using empirically validated psychological instruments administered for the purposes of diagnosis, treatment planning, evaluation, and increased understanding of the client. The process involves assessing for and synthesizing the client's strengths and weaknesses, past and current life experiences, skills, and sociocultural circumstances. Trauma assessments typically cover these areas as well as assessing, understanding, and describing the patient's functioning, adaptations, and symptoms as seen through the lens of their trauma exposure and within the particular context of their lives.

Historically, psychological assessment favored information gathering wherein the evaluator, usually a psychologist, was seen as the "expert" who compared the individual's test scores to nomothetic norms to derive conclusions. However, these assessments were often dehumanizing and potentially harmful to clients (Fischer, 1985). This is particularly true in cases of trauma. Today, emphasis has shifted to "collaborative" and "therapeutic assessment" (e.g., F. B. Evans & Finn, 2017; Finn & Tonsager, 1997). Collaborative assessment involves engaging the client in clarifying the reasons for the assessment and observing test behaviors and responses, and fostering and encouraging the client to voice their experience. When conducted in this manner, assessment empowers the client to choose how they are seen and understood, both by themselves and by the assessor.

Assessment using a sensitive and trauma-informed perspective, which considers the experience and impact of trauma on survivors, involves encouraging the client to share reactions to past experiences as well as to the assessment process itself. A sensitive, trauma-informed approach to assessment fosters better insights into the client's struggles as well as their strengths and should be consistent with the principles and processes of collaborative or therapeutic assessment. This type of assessment enables trauma survivors to gain a better understanding of themselves and develop an awareness that their reactions and symptoms make sense in light of their life experiences. This type of assessment can be a powerful intervention itself and facilitate change (Newman et al., 2012).

Assessments administered by clinicians who are knowledgeable about trauma can "enhance evidence-based listening" (Newman et al., 2012, p. 51). The questions posed, the tests and interviews used, the process of engaging with and responding to the client's reactions and revelations, and the interpretation of those reactions and testing data should be informed by knowledge of the research and clinical literature on trauma. While this chapter addresses therapeutic assessment, forensic assessment requires different methods including maintaining neutrality rather than taking a collaborative, therapeutic approach, so these are addressed in Chapter 6.

Laura Brown (2023) suggested that clinicians recognize symptoms as indication that the traumatized person cannot yet bear to know and feel fully what they have endured. For example, "sleep disturbance" is often due to the person not being able to tolerate the horrifying nightmares of trauma that they face when they sleep. TRD is a sign that there are potent aspects of trauma that the client cannot yet fully face. Assessors also need to be aware of the pronounced power differential we have in our assessment meetings as we ask a person to become vulnerable, share things that may be disorganizing, exceptionally painful, and that they barely can think about much less understand. Brown advised that assessments should be conducted in a less authoritative, "colonizing" manner than they usually occur. Typically, the clinician is clearly "in charge" with the focus on symptoms—that is, what is "wrong with you." Instead, when possible, she suggested allowing the person to start wherever they can and with what they feel is most important for us to know. This approach is empowering and respectful, when feasible. However, in situations where symptoms need to be ascertained and diagnoses determined, strive to reduce the power differential between clients and assessors.

"SEEING" AND ADDRESSING TRD

TRD can occur anywhere, including in the therapy office. Dissociation can obscure or sever the connections between overwhelming trauma and one's internal experiences, affecting one's awareness of their body, relationships, and environment. Clinicians and traumatized individuals may not be able to recognize dissociation, or its ties to the trauma(s) that led to its development, unless clinicians have been trained to watch carefully for and inquire about dissociation.

Observing Dissociation

Sometimes there are observable signs of possible dissociation. For example, a client who drops their head so that their face is not visible for an extended period may do so because they feel ashamed, which may become overwhelming and lead them to dissociate. Prolonged staring, or a faraway, glassy, unseeing look may also indicate the client is starting to dissociate. Catching these signs early helps keep the client from going into a deep state of dissociation from which it is more difficult to rouse. The clinician can point these signs out to the client and gently ask them to describe their internal experience ("Can you describe what you are feeling?" and then "What are you noticing in your body?"). If the client acknowledges dissociation (e.g., feeling far away, tingly, or spacey), the clinician can suggest they use grounding techniques (described in the next section). After the client is better grounded, the clinician should encourage them to explore what they were thinking and feeling just as they began to dissociate. Repeatedly tracking and exploring moments of dissociation in this manner helps the client develop skills in identifying dissociation and the underlying phobic avoidance of vulnerability, connection, emotions, and trauma-related experiences.

Grounding Techniques

If a client becomes highly dissociated either during assessment or treatment sessions, clinicians can guide them in using grounding techniques to help them return to a state of normal consciousness where they are aware of their surroundings. Repeatedly using their name is helpful, as is using a kind but loud voice. For example, a clinician might say,

> Sam, you are in my therapy office, it is (insert date) and you are safe here. It looks like you are dissociating, so it will help to get grounded. Sam, focus on your feet on the ground. Begin to press your toes down firmly. That's good. Now start to work on moving your legs. Good, now start moving your fingers (and so on).

Continue to guide the person to move and look around the room, using all their senses to get reoriented to the present and anchored in their body. Encourage them to feel the chair or their clothing or something comforting from current reality (e.g., a ring given to them by their partner). If they are still having difficulty after grounding, consider asking them to list attributes about themselves and their lives (especially positive developments and/or strengths that are conflict-free, such as a current pet). The emphasis should be on helping them differentiate "here and now" from the "there and then" of traumatic experiences. They can also drink something cold or hot, suck on ice or a flavorful mint, or smell something strong such as an orange. For more on grounding techniques and other essential techniques for working with highly dissociative clients, see Brand et al. (2022) and Schielke et al. (2022).

"Invisible" Dissociation

Many dissociative symptoms are internal experiences that are not easily observable. For example, a client may begin to perceive the office as shrouded in fog or see the therapist as sitting far, far away (both examples of derealization), feel dizzy (i.e., possible somatoform dissociation or anxiety), or become emotionally numb (i.e., depersonalization). A client with unimpaired hearing may suddenly be unable to hear what the therapist is saying due to the sound of "voices arguing" in their mind. Alternatively, a client may suddenly forget what they were just discussing with the clinician.

The clinician may wonder if the client is experiencing a small gap in their memory (i.e., micro amnesia), particularly if this occurs frequently or if the client cannot recall something they said or did during an earlier session that the clinician observed.

To differentiate whether dissociation is causing the memory gaps (rather than anxiety, neurological conditions, or another issue), watch carefully over time to determine whether there is a pattern to the amnestic gaps, such as gaps occurring only when the client talks about a relationship with an abusive person, or a particular emotion or experience. Many highly dissociative clients attempt to hide amnesia by remaining silent or guessing at what was being discussed and, in the process, subtly or not so subtly shifting topics. Notice these shifts in the conversation and inquire about them. Shifting topics may occur so often that the clinician suspects attention-deficit disorder or possibly even flight of ideas (although this usually occurs without the pressured speech seen in mania).

Periods of amnesia outside the office are easily missed unless the clinician asks and the client acknowledges that they cannot recall important auto-biographical information such as periods of time, even up to days or weeks that are seemingly "gone" from their memory. An example of such a gap would be a client being able to remember their teachers from Grades 1 to 3, no memory of teachers for the next two grades, followed by recall for teachers in subsequent grades. Gaps might yield important information about times of stress or trauma, so follow-up queries are indicated (e.g., "What was going on in your family during those years? In your neighborhood? Who were your closest friends then?").

Gaps in memory may be further detected by asking who their best friends and pets were throughout their life, how their childhood bedroom(s) and home(s) looked, and if they recall major life events such as graduation from high school or college, their own wedding, birth(s) of their children, and so on. It is important to determine if the client can report "memories" because they have seen photos or been told about these life events, as opposed to actually remembering being present at the event or in a given setting. Clinicians can ask, "Do you remember actually being there at that event, or is it something you know happened but don't actually recall being present?" Individuals with complex dissociative disorder (DD) may know about their important life events without having the lived experience that they themselves were involved and present. As with all psychiatric disorders, medical issues such as head trauma, neurological conditions, or substance use must be considered and ruled out as causing dissociative symptoms.

Individuals who have experienced complex chronic trauma may feel deadened, numb, and disconnected from other people. This can be misinterpreted as depression or negative symptoms of schizophrenia. However, if this deadened feeling alternates with trauma-related symptoms such as surges of intense emotion, terrifying intrusions of traumatic imagery, memory gaps, and dissociative symptoms, complex trauma and TRD should be considered and assessed.

In the preceding examples, follow-up assessment with a standardized, broad measure(s) of dissociation can clarify which disorder is causing the reported symptoms or observed signs. If clinicians do not sensitively ask about and further assess these unseen and often terrifying experiences, clients are left alone to deal with them, just as they may have been left alone after traumatic experiences in childhood.

Ignoring dissociation does not make it go away, contrary to what has been argued by some behaviorist authors and fantasy model theorists who do not recognize the traumatic origins of TRD (e.g., McHugh & Putnam, 1995). Research and clinical experience indicate that TRD does not disappear once it has become chronic, although there may be periods of time where it is less severe or less observable (Kluft, 1991; Loewenstein et al., 2017). Numerous clients have told me that they simply stopped talking about and hid dissociation from clinicians who did not understand or believe in TRD, yet they continued to suffer the symptoms. Although trauma treatment can result in improvement in posttraumatic stress disorder (PTSD) as well as depersonalization and derealization, treatment must specifically focus on underlying dissociative states in those with complex DD to resolve these symptoms (Jepsen et al., 2014).

BARRIERS TO SHARING LIVED TRAUMATIC EXPERIENCES

As these examples show, dissociation is sometimes not easily visible to the clinician, and it is often unrecognized by the client. Additional barriers can also preclude clients with TRD from sharing their experiences. Some individuals may have an awareness of these experiences, yet find them so frightening, perplexing, or shame-inducing that they may avoid thinking about them or revealing them to the clinician (Dorahy et al., 2017). They may sense that acknowledging dissociation means acknowledging things (i.e., abuse) they prefer to avoid thinking about.

It is crucial that assessors and clinicians understand how utterly terrifying it may be to experience emotions and bodily sensations connected to traumatic events, as well as to reveal these experiences to professionals. Additionally, even experiences that are positive can be threatening for those who have been purposefully violated by others. Experiences including being praised or noticed by others, seeking social support, and wanting connection may provoke fear and shame due to experiences of being taunted, bullied, or taken advantage of by past abusers. It is beneficial to grasp the enormity of the "ask" when we encourage traumatized clients to become aware of and share their emotions, fragmented memories, and disowned body sensations and needs with us. The fear of being real, feeling real, and feeling connected within themselves and to others is profound (Chefetz, 2015).

Clients may have been told that no one will believe them, people will think they are "crazy," or they will be harmed or abandoned if they reveal the trauma (e.g., Goodman-Brown et al., 2003). They may also fear the clinician's response, suspecting they will not be believed or will be judged or misdiagnosed. Sadly, these threats and fears are often well founded. Many who muster the courage to reveal that they were traumatized have not been believed, and some have been threatened with abandonment or violence for speaking out, particularly when the disclosed trauma was incest (Goodman-Brown et al., 2003).

For example, mothers of incestuously abused children sometimes respond to these revelations by claiming the child is making it up. Some are willing to admit their child is being abused but do not confront the abuser or protect the child due to financial dependence on the perpetrator, their own trauma-based pattern of submission to violence or unresolved dissociation, their attachment to the perpetrator, or other issues. Some sexual abuse victims are blamed for being "seductive," even though they were just children. These responses compound the damage wrought by the trauma. Unhelpful responses to adults disclosing childhood sexual abuse result in increased shame that then can exacerbate PTSD, depression, and distress (DeCou et al., 2017).

Unfortunately, some of these unhelpful and shaming responses can occur within a dissociative individual's relationship with a clinician. As noted in Chapter 2, many dissociative individuals have encountered clinicians who expressed disbelief in their history of trauma or dissociative symptoms (Nester, Hawkins, et al., 2022). Some individuals report that clinicians have made unhelpful statements about dissociation such as, "I can't help you until you can feel again." Research shows that individuals with DDs suffer from extremely high levels of shame and that when ashamed, they withdraw into and attack themselves (Dorahy et al., 2017). DD individuals attempt to avoid shame and difficult memories by engaging in behaviors including distraction and substance abuse. Negative responses from clinicians exacerbate dissociative individuals' tendency to experience shame, with some potentially responding with heightened hopelessness, increased urges to self-injure, or suicidal ideation.

CLINICIANS' CONCERNS ABOUT ASSESSING DISSOCIATION

Clinicians may feel wary of asking clients to share their disowned, trauma-related symptoms and experiences. This wariness is understandable given the enormity of pain and fear that chronically traumatized individuals experience. The majority of traumatized individuals, including those who experienced childhood abuse, do not find that trauma assessment questions cause undue distress if trauma is assessed sensitively (Carlson et al., 2003; Cromer et al., 2006; Newman et al., 1999; Walker et al., 1997; Yeater et al., 2012). In fact, many traumatized individuals find it reassuring to know that their trauma history might serve to help inform researchers or benefit other traumatized people.

Clinicians sometimes fear triggering a shift in dissociative self-states in individuals with dissociative identity disorder (DID). These individuals are, by definition, in a dissociative self-state every minute of every day, and they switch frequently, so we do not need to fear triggering a switch. Switching is a natural phenomenon of DID, although it is often unrecognized by clients and clinicians, and occurs much more often and subtly than both realize (Loewenstein et al., 1987). Therefore, switching is not something that clinicians need to fear, although given the stigmatizing and inaccurate portrayals of DID in the media, it is understandable that clinicians may be anxious about working with these individuals (Brand & Pasko, 2017). Additionally, assessment and treatment approaches based in research and informed by expert guidelines are widely available, so practitioners whose assessments and interventions fall below the standard of care, resulting in harm to dissociative patients, may face ethics charges, complaints to licensing boards, and legal challenges.

It is important to be aware of and challenge stigmas and inaccurate assumptions we may hold about dissociative individuals, particularly DID, because individuals with this disorder are so often misrepresented in media as violent, sociopathic, and dangerous. Only a fraction of individuals with DDs have had criminal justice involvement; furthermore, dissociation, PTSD, and emotion dysregulation do not predict involvement with the criminal justice system among individuals in treatment for DDs (Webermann & Brand, 2017), although men with DDs may be more at risk to be violent than women, as is the case in general for men (Loewenstein & Putnam, 1990). In more than 30 years of practice in settings such as inpatient units, jails, and prisons, including with death row inmates, I have not been attacked by a client. However, I strive to be attuned to my own and the client's emotional state and notice when a client becomes agitated. In those situations, after attempting to help the client become more regulated, including attempting to help them get oriented to who I am and what the current situation is, I end treatment and assessment sessions if I feel it is safer to do so. Individuals with DID are much more likely to be victims of violence caused by others or inflicted on themselves as nonsuicidal self-injury (NSSI) or suicide attempts than to be perpetrators of violence directed at others.

As clinicians, not asking about trauma and trauma-related symptoms may serve as a reenactment of the unwillingness to see, know, and protect the child that enabled an abuser(s) to harm child victims of abuse. We must be aware of our own fears about working with traumatized clients and manage them, with the support of consultation and our own psychotherapy, if needed, rather than allowing our fear and avoidance to act as barriers to providing sensitive assessment and treatment to traumatized clients (Chefetz, 1997b; Loewenstein, 1993).

Some clinicians may be concerned about "causing dissociation." Although asking about dissociation can provoke the defense (e.g., the person may feel spacey when they describe this symptom), that does not mean clinicians are causing the person to be dissociative. It's no different from asking about symptoms of depression: Inquiring about symptoms of depression may cause some clients to cry, but it does not cause depression. It is important that we manage our own anxiety, realizing that dissociative individuals dissociate whether we ask them about it or not. We do not "make" someone dissociative just by asking them about dissociation any more than we "make" depression, hallucinations, or suicidal ideation happen by asking about these symptoms.

Some may be concerned about creating "false memories" of abuse by asking about trauma. As noted in Chapter 2, however, a review of the scientific evidence determined that dissociated memories of abuse are as accurate as are continuously recalled memories, and although some details of abuse may be inaccurately recalled, the core of the memory is typically accurate (e.g., Becker-Blease & Freyd, 2017; Brewin & Andrews, 2017; Dalenberg, 1996; Dalenberg et al., 2012; Dalenberg & Palesh, 2010).

Studies conducted in laboratories indicate that a small group of people may begin to believe in trivial made-up stories that did not occur if told by researchers that it occurred. However, no research indicates that participants would begin to believe false abuse experiences; such experiments would not be ethical. Rather, researchers can trick a small number of individuals into reporting that they believe they experienced a common, briefly upsetting event that did not actually occur (i.e., getting lost in a mall or knocking over a punch bowl). These lab findings about minor distressing events are not equivalent to the charge from the fantasy model theorists that therapists can implant false memories of abuse. Importantly, patients who have recalled previously dissociated trauma memories of abuse are "remarkably less suggestible" (Leavitt, 1997, p. 265) than individuals in a control group of patients. The patients who did not have a history of sexual abuse were more at risk for altering their memories than those who had been abused. Similarly, individuals with DID are not more suggestible or prone to false memories than other individuals (Vissia et al., 2016). Taken together, these and other studies suggest that the risk of creating false memories of abuse have been exaggerated. Nonetheless, it is important that clinicians are not leading or suggestive in the questions about trauma and dissociation and that their procedures are consistent with expert recommendations and guided by research. I address this later in the chapter.

THE IMPORTANCE OF A THERAPEUTIC RELATIONSHIP IN ASSESSMENT

What we can offer as assessors is the courage to see, truly listen to, and develop a therapeutic relationship with the traumatized person, including those with TRD. We can offer them a way out of their isolation, numbness, shame, and confusion about their experiences by helping them make sense of the problematic symptoms and behaviors they have developed as adaptations to living in chaotic and hurtful environments. If, after conducting the assessment process, we are going to continue working with the individual by providing treatment, we can offer them a carefully paced path of healing that guides them in recognizing and learning to manage trauma-related difficulties including TRD (see Chapter 7). It is our caring presence combined with our knowledge about trauma's impact and methods for healing that can enable clients to make gradual sense of their past and learn to tolerate being present and real in the current moment, and, over time, to develop hope for their future. If we are in the role of assessor and therapist, we may help guide them to "finding solid ground," which is an adjunctive program developed specifically for stabilizing TRD, which is discussed in Chapter 7 (Brand et al., 2022; Schielke et al., 2022).

COMPARING A THERAPEUTIC APPROACH TO A STANDARD ASSESSMENT APPROACH: THE CASE OF "CINDY"

A collaborative, therapeutic approach that is guided by clinical and empirical evidence about TRD can provide a deep understanding of clients. Assessments that lack this approach or are conducted by assessors who are not familiar with TRD can inadvertently contribute to the client being misunderstood, misdiagnosed, and even more mistrustful of clinicians than they were before they were assessed.

A clinical vignette follows that I developed by merging aspects of assessment consultation cases. "Cindy," a survivor of pervasive childhood neglect, physical abuse, and repeated incest, had had psychological testing conducted during treatment for depression in her late 20s to determine why she was so "treatment resistant." Despite her fear that the female psychologist would think she was "crazy," Cindy had bravely admitted she had heard voices since late childhood. She struggled with somatic symptoms, including chronic headaches and excruciating, yet strangely variable, muscular and pelvic pain. Treatment for irritable bowel syndrome, fibromyalgia, and migraines had not resulted in significant relief, nor had adequate trials of antidepressants or cognitive behavioral treatment significantly had a significant impact on her depression. No measures of trauma-related difficulties were used in the assessment. Cindy was not asked about a history of trauma. She barely allowed herself to think about or remember odd experiences, such as finding she had cut herself with no memory for having done so; she did not reveal these unsettling events, nor did the psychologist inquire about them. The psychologist interpreted her Minnesota Multiphasic Personality Inventory–2 (MMPI-2) and other testing data as indicating that Cindy suffered from paranoid schizophrenia and needed to be hospitalized. Despite the psychologist's alarm at the severity of her symptoms, from Cindy's perspective, she was "how I always am but more depressed some days," meaning she was at her baseline level of high suicidal ideation and frequent NSSI.

The diagnosis of paranoid schizophrenia and the psychologist's concern were jarring and inconsistent with Cindy's sense of herself. The psychologist did not attempt to elicit Cindy's reactions to her feedback, much less to review and share examples of some of the items she endorsed. If she had asked Cindy about some of the endorsed items on the MMPIs, for example, those in Bizarre Experiences on the Schizophrenia scale, she might have learned that the elevations were caused by flashbacks and a fear that Cindy was losing her mind. Cindy's elevations on the Schizophrenia, Paranoia, and Depression MMPI-2 scales, and her endorsement of items such as being alienated from her family, hearing voices, and feeling depressed, are common among trauma survivors and consistent with research on the profiles of individuals with DDs (e.g., Brand & Chasson, 2015; Brand, Chasson, et al., 2016). Unfortunately, the psychologist was aware neither of this research nor the impact of trauma.

Working collaboratively, the psychologist could have started with the easier-to-agree-with findings (Level 1 findings in Therapeutic Assessment;

Finn, 2015). Cindy was so upset and ashamed about the results and the way in which they were delivered "at her" that she refused further testing for years, even after she had begun treatment at a trauma-informed program. She was furious with herself for having allowed herself to be vulnerable, and she felt objectified, much like she had felt as a child when she had been sexually abused by a male neighbor and ridiculed and beaten by her mother.

Years later, after extensive discussion, Cindy reluctantly agreed to participate in collaborative, trauma-informed psychological assessment. This psychologist, Dr. Evans, started by asking Cindy about her reactions to the prior assessment. He planned with her how to make this experience different, with an emphasis on providing her with as much safety and control as possible. For example, Dr. Evans encouraged Cindy to tell him any time she wanted to stop for a break or if she needed to end an assessment session early due to feeling overwhelmed or exhausted. Dr. Evans asked Cindy what she most wanted to learn about herself and what she was most afraid of learning. The process was carefully paced; when the psychologist noticed Cindy might be beginning to feel strong emotion or starting to dissociate, he gently invited Cindy to check in with herself to see how she was feeling. At first Cindy replied in a monotone voice, "fine." Dr. Evans asked if was OK to ask a bit more, to which Cindy agreed. Dr. Evans suggested the best way to deal with dissociation was to slow down and check in with her body because it held her feelings (Armstrong, 2002). This was a new experience and allowed Cindy the opportunity to observe how her body expressed what was going on within her. She learned she felt cold and "far away" when asked about her relationship with her mother. She was anxious about noticing this connection, but it also made sense to her, given her mother's abuse.

Dr. Evans processed how Cindy was doing after each measure, and when she was feeling too much or too little, he encouraged her to determine whether she needed to tune into her body, take a break, use relaxation techniques, or use grounding techniques (with or without his guidance). Following the procedure recommended by Armstrong (2002) for working with dissociative individuals, after each test was complete, Dr. Evans inquired what was going on internally when Cindy's answers seemed confused, potentially thought-disordered, or potentially indicative of dramatic, personality-disordered emotional responding. Cindy shared that most of these responses, particularly those on the Rorschach, involved trauma-based associations, triggers, or an influx of responses from "the voices."

The Rorschach can be particularly challenging to traumatized individuals because it "goes against the grain of dissociation," requiring individuals to "delve into their internal store of association, the very thing that dissociation has helped them avoid" (Armstrong, 2002, p. 13). For those with TRD, the Rorschach can be a triggering assessment measure, yet it offers incomparable clarification about diagnostic dilemmas, making it a rich informative measure for understanding trauma and dissociation. This was the case for Cindy, who saw several traumatic images, including a tall, towering male who was threateningly showing his "thingy," that is, an erect penis. Cindy became visibly frightened and pushed the card away. With encouragement, she was able to complete the test. The Rorschach was particularly informative as it clarified that what looked like a possible psychotic disorder on the MMPI-2 (Schizophrenia T = 87, Paranoia T = 85, Psychopathic Deviate T = 80, Depression T = 75) was more accurately understood as a "traumatic thought disorder" (Armstrong, 2002). That is, her thinking became disorganized (INCOMs and FABCOMs; note these are Rorschach scores, as are others that follow in parentheses) and perception became distorted (low X+%) when she experienced traumatic intrusions (perceptions scored as Blood, Aggression, Morbid, Sex, and Anatomy responses; Armstrong & Loewenstein, 1990), yet she was able to recover and reestablish logical thinking and perception.

Armstrong (2002) described this poetically:

> When one considers that the essence of trauma and resulting dissociative avoidance is the need to protect oneself from a reality that has behaved in a chaotic and non-logical fashion, one can understand why these scores may reflect a 'traumatic thought disorder' rather than a psychotic thought disorder. (p. 17)

Cindy did not recall two responses she had reported when she was asked about them in the inquiry stage, which suggests dissociative amnesia and a possible complex DD (Brand, Armstrong, et al., 2006). This and other indications of amnesia and frequent shifts in her style of speaking, sophistication of thinking, and vocabulary (i.e., a man's "thingy" as well as "an Indian totem, like those found in the Pacific Northwest") and different styles of relating to the psychologist (e.g., sometimes serious and overly polite, other times more fearful and passive) suggested possible shifts in dissociative self-states.

These behavioral observations and the possibility of DID were supported by data from Cindy's Trauma Symptom Inventory–2, Structured Clinical Interview for *DSM-IV* Dissociative Disorders–Revised (Steinberg, 1994b), Posttraumatic Checklist for PTSD-5 (Blevins et al., 2015), Multiscale Dissociation Inventory (Briere, 2002), and Dissociative Experiences Scale (Bernstein & Putnam, 1986). Taken together, the results suggested Cindy suffered from DID, PTSD, major depression, generalized anxiety disorder, and probably "psychological factors affecting other medical conditions" (due to the impact of high stress and trauma reactivity impacting her gastrointestinal and pain conditions and dissociative factors contributing to her chronic migraines).

More important than the diagnoses themselves, the assessment indicated that Cindy's lack of progress in treatment was partially due to profound dissociation interfering with her ability to reliably stay grounded so she could learn and access information, skills, and insights gained in sessions. Traumatic intrusions severely impacted her ability to process information. Cindy's sense of herself was profoundly damaged, compounded by her sense that she could not protect herself from attacks that she expected would surely come from others. NSSI was one of the only ways she knew how to stop the flood of shame and other emotions and appeased some self-states that urged her to commit suicide.

Dr. Evans and Cindy's therapist discussed how best to convey the results to Cindy. They decided to share them together in a joint session with Cindy, followed by a few sessions with Dr. Evans to allow her to slowly take in the feedback. Providing feedback in a collaborative fashion gave Cindy a voice in sharing her sense of how the results fit with her sense of herself. In the first feedback session, she was relieved to learn that she did not have schizophrenia, although she was both frightened and yet not surprised to learn that the assessment suggested she had a DD, PTSD, and severe depression and anxiety. Only in later sessions was the diagnosis of DID mentioned, so that the feedback was not "dumped" on her too rapidly to assimilate.

Eventually, after hearing that the testing suggested she had compartmentalized self-states that had developed to protect her from the child abuse, Cindy discussed her ambivalent reactions with Dr. Evans and with her therapist. She made slow but steady progress over the next year, guided by the assessment recommendations that treatment needed to prioritize safety, stabilization of her self-destructive urges and behavior, and self-awareness and skill development (specifically, teaching her to identify, tolerate, and manage when she was dissociating and slipping into the traumatic past, and ways of "finding solid ground" in present reality; Brand et al., 2022; Schielke et al., 2022). Cindy and her therapist gradually worked on crucial concepts such as realizing that all parts of herself were important and needed to be respected. She slowly developed awareness of her parts and ways of communicating with them. In therapy, she and her parts learned how they could help in present reality to negotiate safe ways to deal with the trauma-based thoughts and feelings that led her to sometimes want to hurt herself or die (see Chapter 7 and International Society for the Study of Trauma and Dissociation, 2011).

ASSESSING DISSOCIATION IN INITIAL DIAGNOSTIC INTERVIEWS

Every client should be assessed for childhood and adulthood traumas. Almost all people can be asked about this in the initial intake interview. If clients are not directly asked, they often do not share this crucial information (Agar et al., 2002). In some highly unstable clients, assessing trauma may need to be deferred until they have stabilized enough to tolerate these questions. It is beyond the scope of this concise guide to provide detailed information about assessing trauma exposure (see Armstrong, 2017; Briere, 2004; Dalenberg & Briere, 2017).

Trauma exposure questions should come after a level of rapport has been developed. Interviews typically initially focus on the reasons the client is seeking assessment (or treatment), gathering information about vegetative symptoms (e.g., insomnia, poor appetite, and difficulty concentrating), then shifting to developmental history including questions about one's family. It is important to ask nonleading questions about trauma, starting with general, standard questions (e.g., "How was discipline handled in your family?") and then following up on responses that may indicate abuse using the client's own words ("You said you were 'whooped.' Who whooped you?" followed by, "What did they whoop you with?").

Armstrong suggests asking where the client felt safe growing up (Armstrong, 2017). If the client shows surprise and indicates they always felt safe, it is unlikely they experienced developmental trauma. If the client indicates feeling safe at school, the possibility of familial trauma and neglect can be explored, along with inquiring about how learning, teachers, and friends may have helped them develop resilience. If the client indicates they did not feel safe anywhere, the issue of having a troubled family, neighborhood, school(s), or a combination of these should be explored. Inquire about experiences of childhood physical, sexual, and emotional abuse; neglect; and bullying, as well as victimization in adulthood (e.g., interpersonal violence, sexual assault, stalking), noninterpersonal trauma (e.g., car accidents, natural disasters, fires), and historical trauma (discussed subsequently). It is essential to ask about any family or caregiver mental illness including substance abuse, as well as incarcerations or lengthy separations.

Clients may be understandably reluctant to discuss trauma for fear of becoming overwhelmed. Informing the client at the beginning of the assessment about the procedures as part of the informed consent process makes the process more predictable and less frightening. Let clients know that they will not be required to discuss trauma in detail. Share the reasons for asking about their history, including trauma history. Inform them that they can tell you if they are beginning to feel overwhelmed or need a break and that you will check in with them often to see how they are doing. Although most clients are relieved to hear this, some may interpret this to mean you are telling them to "keep silent about trauma." This type of trauma-related response makes it clear why it is important to inform clients at the beginning of the assessment about this approach and the reason for it.

It is important to avoid discussing in detail any trauma at this early stage because survivors may become highly activated and distressed. The therapeutic relationship is not sufficiently developed, nor does the assessor know the client's severity of trauma-related symptoms, capacity for managing emotions, engagement in risky or unsafe behaviors, and degree of interpersonal support or possible lack of safety in their relationships or community. Some clients may feel obligated to disclose more detail than they can tolerate sharing unless they are explicitly encouraged to pay attention to and observe their own limits. Clients can be advised, "It's important in this first session to share just a brief amount about any highly stressful or traumatic experiences you may have had so that you do not become overwhelmed with feelings or memories about the experience. Please share only the 'headlines' rather than all the details of the experience at this point. We can discuss more of what happened at a later time" (Loewenstein, 2006). Sharing the "headlines" with an empathic listener can be powerfully helpful, particularly when the assessor offers an understanding of trauma's impact and the ability to heal from trauma.

Determine the extent and pace with which each survivor can discuss trauma without becoming overly activated, shut down, dissociated, or triggered. Otherwise, they may become flooded during or after the meeting, and some may engage in distress-relieving unhealthy behaviors, such as self-injury or substance abuse. Signs of hyperarousal include shaking, hyperventilating, and flushed face. Signs of dissociation or hypoarousal include barely breathing, fixed staring, pallor, and collapsed posture. If any of these occur, the assessor should stop and help the client ground themselves, as reviewed earlier.

Clients are often unaware of the early warning signs that they are becoming hyperaroused or hypoaroused. Thus, clinicians should frequently ask the client how they are feeling emotionally and whether they notice any physical sensations that may be signs of distress or dissociation. Inquire whether the interview is going too fast or into too much depth, and if indicated, ask the client how the pace can be made more comfortable. Some trauma survivors have a remarkable ability not to notice or attend to their bodily needs. I have conducted day-long interviews with clients who did not eat, drink, or use the restroom throughout the entire day, despite frequent encouragement. Such denial of physical states is useful information for planning treatment.

All trauma survivors should be assessed for symptoms of dissociation, generally starting with the most common symptoms (i.e., depersonalization, derealization, amnesia). Clarify duration, frequency, and precipitants for dissociative symptoms. Give the client choice and control when possible. Add questions about less common dissociative symptoms (e.g., identity alteration, fugue) if one or more common symptoms are endorsed. Confirm with the client that the symptoms do not occur solely in the context of substance use or withdrawal, head injury, seizure, or other medical comorbidities.

When clients endorse symptoms in the interview or on self-report measures, ask for concrete recent examples to ensure the client is considering pathological dissociation and correctly understanding terms. For example, clarify that when they report "blanking out" they are not just daydreaming, and when they endorse hearing voices, they are not confusing their own thoughts with auditory hallucinations.

The opposite can also occur, most commonly when clients who have dissociative self-states describe these states' input as "just my own thoughts" rather than as voices. To clarify whether the thoughts are related to self-states, inquire as to whether the thoughts are different from their typical thinking (e.g., having highly depressive, morbid thoughts when they do not feel depressed), values (e.g., thoughts and impulses about stealing, having an affair, cursing at someone, and so on, when it goes against their typical values), and behavioral patterns (e.g., a passive, conflict-avoidant person having almost overwhelming urges to scream at their boss, an adult who typically acts reserved having a strong desire to hide under a table). Differentiating thoughts resulting from self-states versus obsessive or scrupulous thinking can be challenging. If these phenomena are dissociative in nature, they should occur in the context of other dissociative and trauma-based phenomena and complex trauma history, often with comorbid disorders, and frequent NSSI or suicidal ideation.

If the client experiences frequent depersonalization or derealization, it is advisable to do more in-depth assessment. One option is using Loewenstein's (1991b) office mental status exam for a less formal assessment of dissociation (see Exhibit 3.1 for an abbreviated, adapted version). The questions in this interview are helpful in assessing dissociation; however, this interview has not been assessed empirically and does not yield interpretative scores. Clinicians should solicit examples of symptoms endorsed to clarify if they are dissociative experiences, as well as to ascertain whether they occur exclusively in the presence of a medical condition or under the influences of substances.

EXHIBIT 3.1. Office Mental Status Interview for Assessing Dissociation

Trauma

- As a child, where did you feel safe? Who was kind or supportive of you?
- Who made the rules in your family, and how were they enforced?
- Did you witness violence between family members?
- Have you ever had unwanted sexual contact with anyone? As a child? Teenager? Adult?
- Flashbacks; intrusive symptoms; sight, sound, taste, smell, touch: Do you ever experience events that happened to you before as if they are happening now?
- Nightmares: How often, since when? Do you awaken disoriented? Find yourself somewhere else?
- Are there specific people, situations, or objects that trigger you? Are these associated with time loss?
- Are you a jumpy person? Easily startled?
- Do you avoid people, situations, or things that remind you of traumatic or overwhelming events? Can you block out feelings?

Depersonalization and Derealization

Depersonalization

- Do you ever feel disconnected from your emotions?
- Do you ever feel like your thoughts are not your own?
- Do you have the experience of feeling as if you are outside yourself or watching yourself as if you were another person?
- Do you ever feel disconnected from yourself or as if you were unreal?
- Do you ever feel detached from your body, as if it (or part of it) does not belong to you?
- Do you ever look in the mirror and not recognize yourself?

Derealization

- Do you experience the world as unreal? As if you are in a fog or daze?
- Do you ever feel like you are in a dream?

Amnesia

- Do you have gaps in your memory of your life? Missing parts of your memory of your life history?
- Do you remember your childhood? When do those memories start? First memory? Next? (May inquire whether client can remember the names and faces of teachers, favorite friends, pets, their bedroom and home throughout developmental years)
- Do you ever find yourself in a place and not know how you got there (fugue)?
- Do you find objects in your possession (e.g., clothes, groceries, books) that you do not remember acquiring? Out of character items? Items a child might have?
- Do you find writings, drawings, or artistic productions in your possession that you must have created but do not recall creating?

(continues)

EXHIBIT 3.1. Office Mental Status Interview for Assessing Dissociation
(*Continued*)

Intrusion/Overlap/Interference From Dissociative Self-States (due to passive influence)

- Do you have thoughts or feelings that come from inside or outside you that don't feel like yours? Are outside your control?
- Do you have impulses or engage in behaviors that don't seem to be coming from you?
- Do you ever feel like thoughts are being blocked or taken out of your head?
- Do you hear voices, sounds, or conversations in your mind?

Analgesia

- Are you able to block out physical pain? Wholly? Partly? Always? Sometimes?

Somatoform symptoms

- Do you ever get physical symptoms/pain that your doctors can't medically explain?

Identity Alterations Questions

- Do you find that sometimes you can do things with amazing ease that seem much more difficult or impossible at other times?
- Does your taste in food, music, or personal habits seem to fluctuate?
- Does your handwriting change frequently? A little? A lot? Childlike?
- Are you right-handed or left-handed? Does it fluctuate?
- Do people tell you that you act so differently that you seem like a different person sometimes?

Note. Adapted from "An Office Mental Status Examination for Complex Chronic Dissociative Symptoms and Multiple Personality Disorder," by R. J. Loewenstein, 1991, *The Psychiatric Clinics of North America, 14*(3), p. 569 (https://doi.org/10.1016/S0193-953X(18)30290-9). Copyright 1991 by Elsevier. Adapted with permission.

I strongly recommend following informal clinical interviews with structured, validated self-report questionnaire(s) about dissociation. Informal interviews are screening measures, not diagnostic measures. High scores warrant additional assessment, preferably using a standardized, validated interview for DDs or other validated measure(s) that assesses the multidimensional symptoms of dissociation (see Chapter 4).

THE IMPACT OF SINGLE VERSUS COMPLEX TRAUMA

A distinction is often made between a trauma that occurs once or is time-limited, or noninterpersonal (e.g., accidents), versus chronic, complex trauma. *Complex trauma* refers to severe, repeated trauma; most often, it refers to developmental trauma that begins in childhood and may continue into adulthood (e.g., Ford, 2021). Chronic developmental trauma is associated with complex neurobiological, relational, and psychological dysregulations (e.g., Ortiz et al., 2022). Following this differentiation, many experts distinguish "simple" or "classic" PTSD from "complex" PTSD (Bisson et al., 2020; Courtois & Ford, 2013; Herman, 1992b). Not only are child maltreatment and adversity implicated in a range of psychological and negative health outcomes, but they are also linked with poorer response to psychotherapy and psychiatric medication (e.g., Nemeroff et al., 2003; Thomas et al., 2019).

These distinctions are important because individuals who experience a single, time-limited trauma are relatively less likely to develop PTSD, compared with those with a history of complex traumas, although many single traumas, particularly interpersonal trauma such as sexual assaults, can cause PTSD (Briere, Agee, et al., 2016). Single traumas may result in initial symptoms that resolve without intervention. Most people recover from noninterpersonal single traumas without developing PTSD, and their initial symptoms resolve relatively rapidly. However, a significant subgroup suffers long-term effects with some developing chronic problems that can endure for decades (e.g., Holgersen et al., 2011). Those whose initial symptoms do not rapidly decline may need intervention so that they do not struggle with PTSD for years.

Childhood maltreatment is a risk factor for revictimization later in life. Therefore, many survivors of child maltreatment have experienced or will experience adult victimization. Furthermore, dissociation predicts adult interpersonal victimization (Webermann et al., 2021). Repeated traumas are likely to exacerbate the impact of earlier traumas and contribute to particularly complex outcomes (Briere & Scott, 2012; Ford & Courtois, 2020b).

The development of PTSD or other symptoms such as depression or anxiety after single or complex trauma depends on a variety of factors. These factors include characteristics of the event and intraindividual variables including the person's coping style, others' reactions and level of support, previous trauma, and preexisting psychological disorders. Those who experience dissociation during or shortly after the trauma are more likely to develop PTSD. A meta-analysis found evidence that seven variables predicted the development of PTSD: prior trauma, prior psychological adjustment, family history of psychopathology, perceived life threat, social support following trauma, peritraumatic emotional reactions, and peritraumatic dissociation (Ozer et al., 2003), although peritraumatic dissociation was the strongest (weighted $r = .35$). This implies that these variables should be reviewed when assessing survivors, with particular attention paid to assessing peritraumatic dissociation.

Cumulative interpersonal traumas have been shown to be the strongest predictors of PTSD, whereas cumulative noninterpersonal traumas are generally less potent (Briere, Agee, et al., 2016). As reviewed in Chapter 1, numerous studies show a cumulative, additive impact of various adverse childhood experiences increasing one's risk for childhood and adult mental and medical conditions (e.g., Felitti et al., 1998). Studies support and extend these initial "additive" risk findings to show patterns of synergism (i.e., rather than the "dose" from multiple traumas being additive, their combined impact becomes multiplicative). Analyses using data from the National Comorbidity Survey—Replication showed that seven of eight childhood adversities predicted more complex adult psychopathology (Putnam et al., 2013).

Adults who had experienced four or more childhood adversities had much greater risk of complex psychological symptoms. Sexual abuse was the most potent of all the adversities, particularly for women. Furthermore, synergistic patterns occurred in women when they had experienced sexual abuse, whereas synergistic patterns occurred in men when they had experienced childhood economic hardship. Parental depression or anxiety was synergistic with sexual abuse for both genders and with physical abuse for women. The authors concluded that overarching diagnostic categories such as complex PTSD appear warranted for individuals with complex psychopathology related to extensive childhood adversities. Recent research has replicated these results with a sample of more than 10,000 youth, supporting the particularly damaging impact of sexual abuse combined with a range of other adversities (Putnam et al., 2020).

Aspects of individuals' sociocultural context are important to consider because many individuals experience frequent events that can accumulate, resulting in vulnerability to trauma reactions. Social maltreatment and oppression such as racism, sexism, homophobia, and transphobia likely influence marginalized individuals' responses to trauma. This may contribute to the development of more complex reactions to what seems like a single, "simple" trauma. Many authors believe that identity-based microaggressions should be considered a traumatic stressor because research, including meta-analyses, indicate these experiences can have serious deleterious impacts (e.g., Allwood et al., 2021; Lui & Quezada, 2019). Individuals with minoritized identities often face greater exposure to traumatic events and have higher rates of PTSD (e.g., Roberts et al., 2011; Shipherd et al., 2011).

Historical traumas, defined as collective maltreatment by a dominant culture that extends over generations, have damaging effects including PTSD, substance abuse, anxiety, depression, violence, suicide, and vulnerability to illnesses (reviewed in Briere & Scott, 2012). In North America, historical traumas have affected many racial, ethnic, and religious minorities including Black, Indigenous, Asian, Latinx, Muslim, and Jewish people, as well as many immigrants. Eadie and Briere (2023) argue that although females are not typically thought of as a group separately affected by historical trauma, they have been exposed to gender-based violence and discrimination for centuries, with higher rates of PTSD, depression, anxiety, eating disorders, and suicide attempts than males. The differential risk of women developing these disorders has been linked to women's higher exposure to sexual victimization, interpersonal violence, and discrimination, including in the workplace and educational institutions. It is crucial that assessors consider and inquire about social maltreatment including the impact of historical traumas to gain a comprehensive understanding of an individual's trauma history.

ASSESSING SINGLE VERSUS COMPLEX TRAUMA

Individuals exposed to single traumas typically resolve their acute symptoms, although some develop acute stress disorder, symptoms of depression, anxiety, insomnia, or increased substance use. They should be interviewed using a semistructured diagnostic interview to assess for symptoms of acute stress disorder (if the trauma occurred in the past month) and PTSD (if the trauma occurred more than 1 month ago), along with the other disorders generally assessed in a careful initial diagnostic interview occurring at the start of psychotherapy.

In complex trauma cases, the initial diagnostic interview should include those standard areas, but as noted in Chapter 1, assessment should also extend to the following broader impacts:

- affective dysregulation (e.g., dissociative numbing alternating with hyperarousal and emotional flooding; problems with anger, anxiety, shame)

- behavioral dysregulation (e.g., impulsive, self-destructive, and aggressive behavior; substance abuse; high-risk behaviors)

- identity disturbance (e.g., compartmentalization of self or self-fragmentation, difficulties with body image and eating disorders)

- disruption in meaning (e.g., seeing others and the world as traumatizing and untrustworthy and the self as damaged and blameworthy for trauma)

- interpersonal problems (e.g., avoidance of relationships; chaotic, violent, abusive relationships; enmeshed relationships)

- somatization and medical problems (e.g., gastroesophageal reflux disease, irritable bowel syndrome, chronic fatigue, headaches, heart disease, auto-immune disorders)

In summary, dysregulation and disruption—of arousal, emotion, behavior, identity, meaning, relationships, and body—are the central issues to assess and treat among clients who have experienced complex trauma (Brand & Lanius, 2014; Briere & Scott, 2015; Courtois & Ford, 2013; Frewen & Lanius, 2015; van der Kolk et al., 1996).

ASSESSING FOR POSSIBLE COMPLEX DISSOCIATIVE DISORDERS

Judith Armstrong developed a method for assessing possible complex DDs that involves a collaborative testing procedure, careful observation and documentation of clients' behavior, a battery of psychological tests, and attention to the assessor's countertransference (Armstrong, 1991, 2002). Assessors should carefully watch for behaviors identified by Armstrong in Table 3.1, noting precisely when they occur. This helps decipher the topics or situations that overwhelm the client's ability to regulate emotion, perceive accurately and think clearly, or that trigger dissociation. A single behavioral sign or data point is insufficient to determine whether the individual has a complex DD (or any other disorder). Rather, a pattern of dissociative and trauma-based responding is more indicative of a complex DD. Testing and behavioral data should be reviewed, nondissociative hypotheses should be considered and ruled out, and the *Diagnostic and Statistical Manual of Mental Disorders* stipulated list of symptoms must be present to meet diagnostic criteria for a DD.

Armstrong (1994) identified DID as an alternative developmental pathway, rather than a developmental arrest, the latter being more characteristic of borderline personality disorder. Armstrong hypothesized that DID is a sophisticated posttraumatic adaptation that may develop when a child grows up in an environment where adults act erratically—sometimes violent, sometimes neglectful, and sometimes nurturing. The child learns to treat themselves and their parents (or whoever was abusive and neglectful) as if they were different people, according to the highly variable behavior the adult is demonstrating at a given moment. Predicting others' behavior is nearly impossible when adults are highly inconsistent, so the child develops different patterns of behavior, feeling, and thinking that emerge depending on the adult's state. This adaptation allows the child to shift as needed to fit the ever-changing moods and behaviors of their caregivers. Context-bound

TABLE 3.1. Dissociative Behaviors Checklist

Fluctuations	Behaviors suggestive of dissociative interference
Activity level–abrupt increase/decrease in activity	*Clearing gestures*–gestural attempts to clear thoughts (e.g., shaking head, sweeping hand)
Affect–abrupt major alterations in mood or affective expression	*Distracted*–delimited, momentary inattention
Developmental fluctuation–age regression/ progression (e.g., childlike behavior in an adolescent or adult, adultified behavior in a child)	*Hiding gestures*–hides part of face from view (e.g., covers mouth with hand; buries face in clothing, arms, or behind hair)
Fluctuation in relatedness–sudden, marked alteration in attitude or level of interaction toward tester	*Eye movement*–eyes rolling upward so much that pupils are almost not visible, closed eyes, rapid blinking. Interpret this category conservatively. Focus on duration, extensiveness, and frequency to distinguish from eye irritation or efforts at concentration.
Somatic fluctuation–report sudden complaints of physical symptoms during testing (e.g., headaches, heart palpitations, exhaustion); include sudden difficulty hearing examiner or seeing test material	*Interference*–reports or shows evidence of blocking (e.g., "going blank")

Trauma-based reactions	Emotion
Sexualized behavior–sexually suggestive activity (e.g., masturbatory or sexualized pelvic or chest movements)	*Fearful*–statements of fear and/or anxiety related to testing; also include behaviors associated with fear or panic (e.g., silent huddling, rapid and shallow breathing, sudden paleness)
Startle response–startling to either test or nontest stimuli (e.g., to examiner's voice, a door shutting, phone ringing)	*Overstimulation*–statements of feeling flooded/overwhelmed, maybe associated with temporary inability to continue to respond to test
Trauma associations–spontaneous associations to past trauma; identification of test item with past abuse	*Rocking*–sideways or front-back rocking
	Distance–moves unusually close to or draws away (often fearfully) from testing materials; emotional distance such as complaints of deadness or disconnection

Dissociation	Amnesia
Staring–intensely focused, fixed staring and/or blank, vacant gaze, generally accompanied by immobility	*Disowning*–actively denies giving or seeing a response previously reported
Unresponsive–appears unable to respond to examiner or test stimuli (i.e., person has "far away" look); Do not include volitional noncooperation	*Amnesia*–sudden inability to recall major aspect of experience (e.g., forgets a Rorschach response they gave just a few minutes earlier)

Note. Adapted from "Deciphering the Broken Narrative of Trauma: Signs of Traumatic Dissociation on the Rorschach," by J. G. Armstrong, 2002, *Rorschachiana*, 25(1), p. 19 (https://doi.org/10.1027/1192-5604.25.1.11). Copyright 2002 by Hogrefe. Adapted with permission.

disconnectedness develop over time. The child does not learn to smooth transitions between these disconnected states, so state changes remain abrupt and disconnected throughout life (Putnam, 1997).

Assessment does not result in an "X-ray of the truth" (Armstrong, 1996). Instead, the results are influenced by the interpersonal experience between assessors and patients, the rapport between them, how open and self-reflective the patient feels they can be, and other variables. Armstrong (1996) noted that just as an X-ray can provide meaningless information if the patient moves or if it is poorly focused, a frightened or resistant patient will give confusing responses that yield misleading or "fragmentary" interpretations.

Because standardized assessment mandates facilitating the most accurate possible evaluation of the client's capabilities, failing to invite all self-states of a person with dissociative states to participate in assessment violates standardization (Armstrong, 1993). Dissociative phenomena are not "noise" to be eliminated, but rather, in Armstrong's words, the "music" of the patient that needs to be understood through amplification. Despite individuals with complex DDs often believing they will be "abused, invaded, shamed, controlled, and betrayed by people" (Armstrong, 1996, p. 11), if all self-states are invited to participate in a collaborative type of assessment, it is possible to encourage openness to learning about oneself. Armstrong (1996) advised using an invitation before starting the assessment: "Sometimes people feel they have different sides, aspects, or moods. Is that true for you?" If the client acknowledges this is true, ask them to describe how they experience it. Then, using their words so that suggestion is minimized, ask whether they would be willing to express all aspects of themselves in the assessment. In addition to what has been just described, Armstrong suggested periodically inviting the person to "listen inside" to see if any part of them has any concerns or questions.

Armstrong's (1996) method includes discussing with the client how they arrived at their answers and any reactions they had after completing each test. Projective tests are particularly informative with dissociative individuals because themes of abuse, betrayal, and dissociative coping (e.g., characters who sleep, go away mentally, dream, fantasize, pretend, or hide who they really are) often emerge. Characters may be described who divide into more than one person or have two heads. Protective characters who defend someone or something that is vulnerable may be described.

PTSD-like responding, where traumatic intrusions alternate with distancing, dissociation, and avoidance may be illustrated on the Thematic Apperception Test or Rorschach. The Rorschach is a particularly rich method of assessment for TRD, although it can trigger traumatic associations. However, with support from the clinician, even most highly dissociative individuals can complete the

Rorschach. The information it yields is often unparalleled because it shows the individual's ability to think, feel, and defensively protect themselves in real time, without requiring clients to be aware of and able to report these shifting capacities. Chapter 4 includes more information about the Rorschach patterns found in individuals with DDs.

CONCLUSION

I have emphasized the complexity of TRD and the corresponding assessment process. It is crucial that assessors strive to make assessment safe and collaborative so that traumatized individuals are willing to allow themselves to be truly observed and understood. This demands courage and curiosity from individuals who have survived traumatic experiences by not knowing, feeling, and remembering all of what they experienced. Our willingness to listen and see goes against the imperative of disowning and fragmenting oneself. When done well, it is hoped that the results of our collaborative assessment will support our clients in becoming more self-aware and self-compassionate, eventually easing some of the shame and self-attack that may have reverberated in their lives through chronically repetitive, trauma-based patterns of poor self-care, high-risk behaviors, and limited self-awareness.

4 SELF-REPORT MEASURES AND INTERVIEWS FOR ASSESSING DISSOCIATION

This chapter provides an overview of measures used to assess trauma-related dissociation (TRD), including self-report screening measures, clinician-report measures, and clinician-administered interviews. Formal psychological testing is discussed, and suggestions are given for a battery of tests that can aid in clarifying what types of dissociation a person experiences, if any, and their severity. The chapter discusses evidence-supported methods for differentiating factitious, exaggerated, or malingered dissociation and presents two cases of clients who report TRD.

As discussed in Chapter 1, the core problems that should be assessed in individuals who have experienced complex trauma include affect, behavioral, and somatic dysregulation; dissociation; impaired self-concept; disruption in meaning; and insecure patterns of attachment (Cloitre et al., 2011). Assessing for these deficits as well as for patterns of comorbidity, attachment history, trauma-related adaptations, and strengths provides an understanding of traumatized individuals that informs treatment planning. Individuals' history of trauma exposure and immediate as well as later reactions to trauma should also be assessed including pretraumatic, peritraumatic, and

https://doi.org/10.1037/0000386-004

The Concise Guide to the Assessment and Treatment of Trauma-Related Dissociation,
by B. L. Brand

posttraumatic factors (e.g., peritraumatic dissociation, family environment, others' reactions to trauma; see Chapters 1 and 3). For information about assessing problems related to trauma other than dissociation, see, for example, Briere (2004), Briere and Scott (2012), and Dalenberg and Briere (2017).

Assessors also need to inquire carefully about distress-reduction behaviors, including nonsuicidal self-injury (NSSI), suicidal behavior, risky sexual behavior, compulsive eating issues and purging, aggression, stealing, and other potentially unhealthy or risky behaviors common in complex trauma (Briere, 2019). Sometimes these behaviors are attempts to block or distract from traumatic intrusions, change emotional and physical states (e.g., to switch from feeling ashamed to feeling numb), provide a sense of control, convey distress to others, and distract from and manage painful memories, emotions, and symptoms (Nester, Boi, et al., 2022).

Some dissociative clients use NSSI to punish themselves due to trauma-related beliefs that they are "bad" and "deserve punishment" or as a safer alternative to suicide (Brand, 2001; Brand et al., 2022; Nester, Hawkins, et al., 2022). They are often reenactments of trauma, sometimes symbolically (e.g., vomiting after binging as a method of expelling what could not be dispelled after oral sexual abuse), sometimes concretely (e.g., a client who had inadequate food or water due to neglectful parents may not allow themselves to eat or hydrate properly).

These behaviors are often anxiety-provoking for therapists. They likely developed in the context of overwhelming emotion due to poor attachment to caregivers or childhood maltreatment, when other methods of self-regulation were not yet developed and adults were not sufficiently protective and soothing. Furthermore, clients may have observed adults becoming highly dysregulated, violent, self-destructive, terrified, or abusive when distressed. Clients may have had few, if any, opportunities to learn safe self-soothing. Seen through this lens, distress reduction behaviors, along with avoidance and dissociation, are understandable. They were, and continue to be, survival mechanisms. Their resolution typically requires considerable discussion, understanding, and extensive focus in treatment (see Chapter 7).

Highly dissociative individuals frequently use dissociation when recalling distressing information; this in turn can lead to an underreporting of experiences. Furthermore, because memories from the earliest years of life are not verbally accessible, even a careful assessment of trauma exposure may not reveal an early trauma history. Trauma experts suggest that early trauma, including attachment trauma, may be an explanation for a lack of reported trauma history in individuals who have pathological dissociation (Briere & Scott, 2012).

During the assessment process with severe trauma survivors, clinicians are countering what may be a lifelong habit of not knowing, not feeling, and not connecting. Patients may show mixed nonverbal reactions of being both willing and yet uncomfortable with reflecting and sharing about themselves. This ambivalence and inconsistent reporting may lead uninformed assessors to suspect survivors are fabricating or malingering their symptoms or history. Although this is a possibility, the possibility of TRD interfering with consistent self-awareness and ability to recall and report experiences should also be considered.

Early in their working relationship, clinicians need to evaluate thoughtfully how deeply they want to delve into a client's trauma history. They cannot conclude that a highly traumatized individual does not have dissociative symptoms based on a single assessment session. It can sometimes take years for clients to be willing to discuss their internal experiences or become sufficiently aware of them; in such cases, it may be difficult to assess and diagnose a DD accurately. There are "windows of diagnosability" for complex DDs, with periods of symptoms being less pronounced or more hidden (Kluft, 1991). Behavioral signs may provide early indication of dissociative symptoms (see Table 3.1 in Chapter 3 of this volume and Loewenstein, 1991b). Dissociative individuals may not realize others do not experience these phenomena or that they are important to report to clinicians.

THE MOST IMPORTANT ASSESSMENT TOOLS

The process of assessing TRD is profoundly interpersonal. For an assessment to be of real use in understanding the individual, a tremendously important tool we assessors must use is a willingness and ability to *listen deeply and watch carefully*, guided by a sense of humility and awareness of the depth of the "ask" we are making when we invite a traumatized person to share themselves with us.

I have been invited to assess individuals who are incarcerated and facing possible death sentences for allegedly murdering someone, as well as inmates on death row. Before these meetings, I am often momentarily unsettled by the responsibility and the pressure to "get them to open up" so I can understand them accurately and fulfill my ethical obligation as a forensic expert and my moral responsibility as a person. The tests I take in with me are important, but among the most important tools I have are *calming myself* and *truly listening* carefully and with humility to their experience of growing up, living in the world, and, if it is deemed appropriate by the attorneys who have hired me, what they were experiencing leading up to and during the crimes.

As I enter death row, I am aware that I am a middle-aged White woman will all kinds of privilege that make my life much easier than the lives of most of the people I assess. On death row, I typically meet with someone who is a person of color, oftentimes whose life has been filled with struggle, chaos, stress, poverty, trauma, and limited options. It can feel insensitive to ask a total stranger who is incarcerated and surrounded by potential violence to tell me about their most vulnerable and awful moments, the behaviors they have engaged in, and choices they have made, which they rarely understand and, in some cases, do not remember. Often they are ashamed and deeply regret many aspects of their lives. How would any person feel, telling a stranger about our most painful and shame-filled life experiences?

Whether I am conducting the assessment for a forensic or a clinical purpose, I strive to start with the same orientation: humbly acknowledging to the individual the challenges of the task ahead of us, describing the procedures, asking their input about how to make it most manageable for them, giving them as much control as possible, and *listening and watching* with full presence and with genuine empathy.

CULTURAL ISSUES IN ASSESSMENT

Cross-cultural and diversity issues need to be considered in assessment and treatment of TRD (Lewis-Fernández et al., 2007). Bodily and psychological complaints are linked to physiological and psychological factors that are influenced by trauma and shaped by one's culture. These two domains are related, and deciphering "which one" is causing a given symptom can be misleading because they are intrinsically entwined (Briere & Scott, 2012). In many cultures, distress often shows up in bodily symptoms more than psychological symptoms, so people seek medical or more traditional or spiritual helpers rather than mental health clinicians. They may not recognize or want to discuss the link between psychological stress and physical symptoms. Although it can be difficult for individuals from individualistic cultures to talk about trauma, it is often even more difficult and may go against collectivistic cultures to do so (Schnyder et al., 2016). Discussing individual experiences that are shameful, particularly when they occurred within the family or wider community, may be experienced as bringing profound shame to one's family or group. For some particularly mistrustful or fragile individuals, a safe, collaborative relationship must be developed before asking about these secretive and painful experiences.

Assessments should be conducted by someone who speaks the individual's original language whenever possible; otherwise, much nuance and understanding may be lost. Filling out questionnaires about personal topics such as trauma exposure and symptoms may seem odd or completely wrong to do for some individuals—so much so that it may engender passive compliance (or refusal to complete the measures) and lead to little disclosure about one's experience. In some cultures, it is extremely difficult to address topics such as torture of refugees, interpersonal violence within the family, female genital mutilation, and physical punishment of children (Schnyder et al., 2016). Preliminary research indicates that many measures of dissociation show cross-cultural applicability with evidence of adequate psychometric properties, so if the individual is willing to complete measures, they may yield meaningful information (Lewis-Fernández et al., 2007). However, to fully understand and characterize cross-cultural experiences of dissociation, new measures need to be developed that reflect specific cultures, and much more attention to cross-cultural manifestations of TRD is needed.

TRAUMA-RELATED TRANSFERENCE AND COUNTERTRANSFERENCE

Individuals who have experienced trauma, particularly interpersonal violence perpetrated by loved ones and authority figures, are prone to "traumatic transference" reactions in which they perceive the clinician as uncaring, abusive, demeaning, or enacting some other trauma-based interpersonal dynamic (Dalenberg, 2000; Loewenstein, 1993). Assessors need to be empathetic and nondefensive during discussions about these potentially difficult exchanges, keeping in mind that discussing and working through these trauma-based interpersonal beliefs is a crucially important aspect of healing from trauma. Recognizing and managing traumatic transference, and the powerful feelings it can create in clinicians ("traumatic countertransference"), is critical for the successful assessment and treatment of individuals with TRD. If a client communicates that they feel minimized or judged, the clinician also needs to consider whether they may be subtly conveying doubt or judgment about a client's trauma history or symptoms.

At times, some individuals report events that strain credibility and seem fantastical. Even when the client seems to be exaggerating symptoms or to have embellished or fully fabricated some experiences, clinicians must proceed with respect, tactfulness, and thoughtful management. Consultation with clinicians experienced in assessing and treating TRD clients is beneficial, as is reviewing the clinical literature about traumatic transference and countertransference (Chefetz, 1997a; Kluft, 1994b; Loewenstein, 1993; Wilson & Lindy, 1994).

ADEQUATELY ASSESSING AND DOCUMENTING TRD

Multiple sources of information are particularly helpful when assessing TRD. These include information gained from interviews, behavioral observations, self-report measures, structured interviews, performance-based measures, and collateral sources (e.g., family, friends, partners, if the individuals provide written consent). It is common for individuals who are eventually diagnosed with a DD not to have been given this diagnosis by previous clinicians because so few clinicians have training in assessing dissociation (see Chapter 1). For this reason, it is essential to do an independent assessment rather than relying on past diagnoses.

Most clinicians gather diagnostic and psychosocial history information during relatively unstructured intake interviews. As discussed in Chapter 3, I recommend using a semistructured intake interview so that clinically relevant topics including trauma and dissociation are not inadvertently overlooked (see Chapter 3, Appendix A, and https://www.apa.org/pubs/books/assessment-treatment-trauma-related-dissociation for an example of such an interview). When trauma or dissociation (or both) are identified in the intake interview, further assessment using empirically validated measures or structured interviews is strongly indicated, when possible. Using evidence-based assessment measures increases the clinician and client's understanding of clients' symptoms and strengths (and personality if such tests are used) as well as their treatment needs. Furthermore, accurately documenting the nature and severity of clients' difficulties and an initial overview of their trauma exposure at the beginning of treatment is an important element of ethical practice and risk management.

For example, imagine a case in which the clinician failed to assess for trauma and dissociation, and the patient rapidly becomes suicidal and highly dissociative in the first month of treatment. If the clinician had instead conducted an initial diagnostic interview and documented a history of complex trauma and severe dissociative symptoms at the start of treatment, they could target these symptoms earlier in treatment. The thorough assessment would provide crucial information about treatment, making it less likely that the client would decompensate; but if they did, the provider's notes and procedures would assist in supporting the adequacy of care provided.

There is another important reason to conduct thorough initial intake interviews and validated measures of trauma and dissociation. Judith Herman

(1992b) cogently identified that each time society begins to be willing to tolerate acknowledging the painful truth about the prevalence and enduring impact of trauma, particularly the maltreatment of children, there is a backlash. Society becomes unwilling to see, believe, and acknowledge that trauma is common and damaging.

I was trained as a psychologist during the late 1980s and early 1990s, just as many individuals became courageous enough to acknowledge that they had experienced childhood sexual abuse. These disclosures, particularly when they involved incest, were initially shocking to many people, including many mental health professionals, because sexual abuse was hidden and considered a taboo topic. For a while, the media was awash with stories about child sexual abuse. It is incredibly uncomfortable to tolerate knowing that children are abused, especially because most perpetrators are parents (Sedlak et al., 2010). There was a subsequent backlash against such family secrets being revealed. People's reputations, relationships, and, in some cases, finances, were at stake and became more important to protect than the survivors of child sexual abuse. Initial media coverage that revealed many accounts of child sexual abuse shifted to a focus on families that had been reportedly harmed by false allegations of abuse. Denial and repudiation took over. McFarlane (2010) captured this defense against acknowledging child abuse: "The demand for idealization and social harmony erodes a willingness within the community at large to acknowledge and understand the brutality and exploitation that can sit behind the tidy gardens of suburbia" (p. 46).

Similarly, it becomes too awful for society to acknowledge that individuals who fight in wars, who are beaten by their partners, or who are tortured by political groups may be emotionally and physically scarred for the rest of their lives. This defensive tendency to deny is inherent in being human. If trauma survivors talk too much about their symptoms and suffering, they are often told that they are exaggerating, malingering, or being weak. Society goes through a process of denial similar to that of trauma survivors. That is, trauma "intrudes" in its consciousness, much like trauma survivors experience periods of intrusion, yet awareness of this trauma is terribly painful, and eventually it becomes intolerable (Herman, 1992b). Like survivors who try to "unsee" what they have witnessed and experienced by dissociating and avoiding contemplating it, society too enters a backlash period of avoidance, denial, and dissociation—and sometimes, the effects of the backlash are felt in the legal system.

In the early 1990s, lawsuits proliferated against clinicians who worked to help survivors heal from child sexual abuse. At that time, the trauma field was still learning how to assess for trauma and dissociation without being leading, and validated trauma measures were not yet widely developed and available. In cases where the clinician conducted an adequate assessment of trauma and dissociation, the medical records could document that the patient reported a history of child abuse, PTSD, dissociation, and comorbid symptoms as presenting problems. This clinical record would be important evidence that, if it becomes an issue, the clinician did not "implant" memories of trauma or "suggest" symptoms of dissociation to the client, as has been argued by supporters of the fantasy model of dissociation (see Chapter 2).

Thankfully, the most extreme claims made by the fantasy model theorists and a minority of clinicians have been replaced by more reasonable and defensible practices based in growing awareness about trauma and dissociation. As the field has developed research that challenges many of the myths about dissociated memories of trauma and the fantasy model of dissociation, and as clinicians have learned evidence-supported practices for assessing trauma and dissociation, lawsuits against therapists for such claims have dwindled. The False Memory Syndrome Foundation, an organization created by parents accused of sexually abusing their child, promulgated doubt about the reliability of memories of child abuse and challenged trauma therapy and the clinicians who conducted it. The term *false memory syndrome* was never scientifically supported nor included in the *Diagnostic and Statistical Manual of Mental Disorders* (*DSM*), although some high-profile fantasy model proponents such as Elizabeth Loftus testified about "false memories" for the defense of individuals, including Harvey Weinstein and Ghislaine Maxwell (found guilty of sex trafficking girls along with Jeffrey Epstein). After 27 years of garnering considerable attention in the media and from individuals accused of child abuse, the False Memory Syndrome Foundation shut down in 2019.

Following evidence-supported methods of assessing trauma and dissociation, including using standardized measures and documenting the assessment process and its results, protects clients as well as practitioners. Empirically validated measures of posttraumatic stress disorder (PTSD), trauma exposure, and dissociation are now readily available. I strongly suggest using assessment practices that are consistent with expert consensus guidelines and empirical evidence (e.g., Armstrong, 2017; Briere & Armstrong, 2007; Briere & Spinazzola, 2009; Dalenberg & Briere, 2017; International Society for the Study of Trauma and Dissociation, 2011). Assessment guidelines for individuals with complex trauma histories have been developed by a group of trauma experts in the Trauma Division of the American Psychological Association, including this author, and are in the process of being reviewed and revised (Christine Courtois, personal communication, April 28, 2022).

TRAUMA-RELATED DISSOCIATION SHOULD BE ASSESSED AS A COMPLEX PHENOMENON

Dissociation is a complicated construct with a range of phenomena that require assessment. Many measures aiming to assess dissociation in complex PTSD, and dissociative PTSD (DPTSD) evaluate only one or two types of dissociation. Briere, Dietrich, and Semple (2016) found that "dissociative complexity" (i.e., experiencing multiple types of dissociation) was higher among females, those with high cumulative trauma, and those with comorbidities including suicidality and substance use. This indicates that dissociative complexity is a clinically meaningful construct that needs to be assessed broadly. Thus, thorough assessment of dissociation requires assessors to select a single measure or a group of measures that adequately assess a wide range of dissociative phenomena.

The differential diagnosis of TRD, particularly differentiating DDs from other disorders is challenging, especially for dissociative identity disorder (DID). Table 1.2 in Chapter 1 presents clinical and research-supported differences between DID and bipolar, psychotic, and borderline personality disorders, which are often mistaken as or can be comorbid with TRD.

UNDERSTANDING UTILITY STATISTICS TERMINOLOGY

Research provides guidance on the accuracy of cutoff scores on self-report measures compared with the diagnoses made by clinicians, typically using validated interviews. Test outcomes are considered "positive" if the individual has the illness (i.e., DD) and "negative" if the individual does not have a DD. Test results may or may not match the reality of the person's actual DD status. *True positive* cases are those DD individuals who are correctly diagnosed in an interview as having a DD when, in actuality, they do have a DD. A *false positive* case occurs when a non-DD person is incorrectly identified as having a DD; this is also referred to as Type I error. A *true negative* case is a non-DD person identified as non-DD. A false negative is a DD person incorrectly identified as non-DD and is also called a Type II error. (Note that in discussions of malingering, utility statistics are often interpreted differently. See Chapter 5 and the discussion later in this chapter.)

Cutoff scores for assessment measures are the scores above which respondents would be classified as being likely to have a DD (or on a malingering test, classified as malingering). Anyone scoring at or above the cutoff should be referred for further assessment due to a high suspicion that they may have a DD. The *sensitivity* of a given measure is the proportion of individuals who actually have the condition of interest (i.e., a DD, or malingering), or said differently, the measure's ability to correctly identify DDs (or, in the case of malingering tests, the ability of the test to correctly identify malingerers). *Specificity* is the proportion of individuals who do not have a DD who are correctly identified by the measure as not having a DD (or, in the case of malingering, the test's ability to identify people with a genuine disorder as not malingering). There is always a trade-off between sensitivity and specificity, in that an increase in one score leads to a decrease in the other. A perfectly accurate measure would identify 100% of DD patients (100% sensitivity) and would never inaccurately classify people who do not have a DD as having a DD (100% specificity).

Positive predictive value (PPV) is the proportion of clients who scored at or above the cutoff and who, when assessed by a clinician, were found to have the disorder being examined (in this case, DPTSD or a DD). The dissociation screeners tend to have low PPVs, with only approximately 40% to 50% of those who score above the cutoff meeting diagnostic criteria for a DD when diagnosed via clinical interview. Because it is important that disorders are not missed by screeners, cutoff scores are selected to minimize false negatives (i.e., someone with a DD is classified as not having a DD). The result is that screeners purposefully have high false positive rates (i.e., someone without a DD is determined to have a DD) and therefore cannot be relied on for diagnoses. In contrast, the *negative predictive values* (NPV) for dissociation screeners are typically excellent. The NPV is the proportion of the clients who fall below the cutoff on the screener, and who, if assessed with a standardized interview, do not meet criteria for a DD. The screeners' NPV statistics are generally approximately 95%, meaning that only about 5% of those who are classified by a screener as not having a DD do indeed have a DD when assessed by interview.

The most accurate way to diagnose DDs is to have an assessor who is well trained in recognizing and diagnosing DDs conduct a structured or semistructured interview for dissociation; this is far more accurate (higher sensitivity and specificity) than self-report measures (Mueller-Pfeiffer et al., 2013; Mychailyszyn et al., 2021). With unlimited time and funding, all research participants and individuals undergoing assessment for TRD would be assessed by well-trained clinicians with a structured or semistructured interview for DDs. Unfortunately, pragmatics mandate that self-report screeners are often used rather than validated structured interviews.

Researchers and clinicians need to consider the risks and benefits carefully within the context of their assessment as they decide on cutoff scores. It is typically considered more important in clinical and research settings not to overlook a case of possible DD, so assessors typically elect to use lower cutoffs on self-report measures, then conduct follow-up interviews with anyone scoring at or higher than the cutoff.

SELF-REPORT SCREENING MEASURES OF DISSOCIATION

Clients who have experienced trauma should be assessed for dissociation beginning in the initial diagnostic interview(s) (see Chapter 3). When dissociative symptoms are identified, further assessment using an empirically validated measure(s) and/or structured interviews is strongly suggested. If the dissociation score is close to or higher than the cutoff on a screening or global trauma measure, further assessment for a DD is indicated, preferably with more detailed self-report measures as well as an interview for DDs. The self-report measures and interviews that focus exclusively on dissociation or include a subscale specifically addressing dissociation are reviewed here. Due to space constraints, only the most frequently used, empirically supported, and rigorously developed are described. Strengths and limitations are also listed. (See Table 4.1 for a summary. See Chapter 6 for TRD measures used with youth.)

How does one decide which measure(s) to use? Considerations may include the following: the individual to be assessed (their age; whether comparisons are needed that come from community vs. clinical vs. severely dissociative samples), whether a specified time period is desired (e.g., no time specified vs. 1 week vs. 1 month vs. current state at the time of the assessment or their state at the time of the trauma), whether validity scales and/or *T* scores are desired, whether a specific type of dissociation is of interest (e.g., depersonalization, somatosensory, vs. multiple types of dissociation), whether validity scales are needed to assess for response style, and to what extent very strong psychometric properties are needed (i.e., measures whose development was guided by test theory and assessed in a wide range of samples are most valid and reliable). Ethical practice requires using measures that have been validated on samples with characteristics similar to the person being tested, including whether research has been done validating the measure with highly dissociative individuals.

To guide informal interviews after completion of self-report measures, ask for examples of endorsed items, particularly those highly endorsed or that are suggestive of severe dissociation. Pose the questions with curiosity (e.g., "What is that like for you when this happens?") to stimulate openness, not shame (Briere & Armstrong, 2007). Follow-up questions clarify if the endorsed items and frequencies are being interpreted accurately. For

TABLE 4.1. Selected Self-Report and Interviews for Trauma-Related Dissociation

Validated measure	DOI or ISBN	Author/source	Normed on GP	No. of items/ validity scales	Reporting period	Types of dissociation assessed
			Interviews			
Peritraumatic Dissociative Experiences Questionnaire (PDEQ) (clinician-rated version)	Chapter 6 in 1-59385-035-2	Marmar et al., 1997; free in research article	No	19/no	At the time of the traumatic event	Peritraumatic depersonalization & derealization
Clinician Administered Dissociative States Scale (CADSS)	10.1023/ A:1024465317902	Bremner et al., 1998; free in research article	No	27/no	At the time of the interview	Depersonalization, derealization, amnesia, identity alteration
Dissociative Subtype of PTSD Interview (DSP-I)	10.1080/15299732. 2019.1597806	Eidhof et al., 2019; free as a supplement to the research article	No	Eight with additional follow-up questions/no	Past month	Depersonalization, derealization, blanking out, emotional numbing, amnesia, alterations in sensory perception, identity confusion
Structured Clinical Interview for Dissociative Disorders-Revised (SCID-D)	ISBN 978-1-61537-342-0	Steinberg, 2023; for purchase at https://www. appi.org/	No	272/no	Follow-up queries about onset and most recent symptoms	Amnesia, depersonalization, derealization, identity confusion, identity alteration

Measure	DOI	Availability	Validity scale	No. items/cost	Time frame	Constructs assessed
Dissociative Disorders Interview Schedule (DDIS)	None	Free at https://www.rossinst.com/ddis		132/no; yes/ no format may limit utility when feigning or factitiousness is a concern		Schneiderian symptoms, possession, depression, childhood abuse, borderline traits, amnesia, fugue, depersonalization, derealization, identity alteration
Selected self-report measures of dissociation						
Dissociative Experiences Scale (DES) (Note: There are also revised and brief versions, as well as a validity scale addition.)	10.1037/t07472-000	Bernstein & Putnam, 1986; free at https://www.isst-d.org/resources/	No	28/not in the DES-II, but a validity scale has been created	None specified	Absorption, amnesia, depersonalization, derealization, but yields only summary score
Multiscale Dissociation Inventory (MDI)	10.1037/t05179-000	Briere, 2002; available from author at jbriere@usc.edu	Yes	30/no	Past month	Disengagement, depersonalization, derealization, emotional constriction (numbing), memory disturbance, identity disturbance
Dissociative Symptoms Scale (DSS) (Note: There is also an eight-item version.)	10.1177/1073191116645904	Carlson et al., 2018; Free at https://journals.sagepub.com/doi/suppl/10.1177/1073191116645904/suppl_file/sj-pdf-1-asm-10.1177_1073191116645904.pdf	No	20/no	Past week	Depersonalization, derealization, gaps in memory or awareness, reexperiencing of sensations, cognitions, or behavior

(continues)

TABLE 4.1. Selected Self-Report and Interviews for Trauma-Related Dissociation (Continued)

Validated measure	DOI or ISBN	Author/source	Normed on GP	No. of items/ validity scales	Reporting period	Types of dissociation assessed
Multidimensional Inventory of Dissociation (MID) (Note: There is also a 60-item version.)	10.1037/t71132-000	Dell, 2006a; free at https://www. mid-assessment. com/	No	218/five validity scales (possible indications of psychotic, factitious, or malingered presentations, and borderline personality disorder traits)	None specified	Severe pathological dissociation; 23 types of dissociative symptoms and 12 dissociative factors
Somatoform Dissociation Questionnaire (SDQ-20) (Note: There is also a five-item version.)	10.1097/00005053-199611000-00006	Nijenhuis et al., 1996; free at https://www. enijenhuis.nl/eng	No	Five- and 20-item versions/no	Past year	Somatoform dissociation
Peritraumatic Dissociative Experiences Questionnaire (PDEQ) (self-report version)	Chapter 6 in 1-59385-035-2	Marmar et al., 1997; free in research article	No	10/no	At the time of the traumatic event	Peritraumatic depersonalization and derealization
Trauma Symptom Inventory-2 (TSI-2)	None	Briere, 2011; for purchase at https://www. parinc.com/	Yes	10 dissociative items/yes	Past 6 months	Depersonalization, trance, amnesia (as well as a range of trauma and attachment related difficulties)
State Scale of Dissociation (SSD)	10.1348/ 147608302169535	Krüger and Mace, 2002; free in research article	No	56/yes, five factors	State dissociation	Derealization, depersonalization, identity confusion, identity alteration, conversion, amnesia and hyperamnesia

Note. GP = general population.

example, if an item is endorsed at 80%, the client should be able to give several recent examples. If there is concern about the accuracy of the self-report, ask for additional examples. Individuals with severe amnesia can have amnesia for amnesia as well as amnesia for other symptoms, so consider this possibility if the individual cannot identify as many examples as might be expected (Loewenstein et al., 2017). In such cases, careful behavioral observation and an extended period of assessment may be needed. Particularly when there is concern about the accuracy of self-report, include objective measures with validity scales or standalone measures designed to assess exaggeration and malingering. In some cases, it may be helpful to seek input from individuals who know the client well (with written permission from the client).

Dissociative Experiences Scale

The Dissociative Experiences Scale (DES; Bernstein & Putnam, 1986) is a 28-item self-report measure that is the most widely used screen for dissociation. The DES items assess depersonalization, derealization, identity alteration, amnesia, trance, and ability to ignore pain. It does not specify a time frame. Sample items include "Having the experience of finding themselves in a place and having no idea how they got there" and "Finding new things among their belongings that they do not remember buying." It is scored by summing the items and dividing by 28 to create an average score. The first version of the DES required individuals to mark on a 100-mm visual analog line how often they experienced a given symptom. Scoring this version was imprecise, so the format on the DES-II was changed to the percentage of time a symptom is experienced (Carlson & Putnam, 1993). Many authors do not denote that they are referring to the DES-II, but that is the version that has been used in the past 2 decades; for simplicity's sake, I refer to the DES-II as the DES throughout this book. The DES demonstrates good to excellent reliability. Test–retest reliability in three samples ranged from .79 to .93 over 4 weeks to 1 year (Carlson & Putnam, 1993; van IJzendoorn & Schuengel, 1996). The DES's internal reliability is also excellent as measured by split-half reliability and Cronbach's alpha (average alpha = .93 in 16 studies; van IJzendoorn & Schuengel, 1996). The DES has excellent convergent validity with other dissociation measures and structured interviews (combined $d = 1.82$, $N = 5,916$; van IJzendoorn & Schuengel, 1996). It correlated strongly with the Semi-Structured Clinical Interview for Dissociative Symptoms and Disorders (SCID-D; $r = .76$ and $d = 2.33$, $N = 117$; van IJzendoorn & Schuengel, 1996). A confirmatory factor analysis found that all three DES factors (amnesia, derealization/depersonalization and absorption) were statistically and positively correlated with the four *DSM-5* PTSD factors ($r = .27–.46$; Armour et al., 2014). These moderate correlations show that PTSD and the DPTSD are related but not equivalent. The DES also shows convergent-related validity in that dissociation and related phenomena such as absorption and perceptual alteration are strongly related (van IJzendoorn & Schuengel, 1996).

The DES has excellent construct validity. For example, two meta-analyses indicate the DES has criterion-related validity with average scores falling on a continuum from low to high with the highest scores occurring in DID and other DDs (Lyssenko et al., 2018; van IJzendoorn & Schuengel, 1996). Distinguishing among PTSD, DD not otherwise specified/other specified dissociative disorder (DDNOS-1/OSDD-1), and DID is likely to be the most challenging discrimination to make using the DES. However, DES scores are higher in patients with DID compared with DDNOS. Studies have investigated the ability of the DES to discriminate between the presence of a DD using receiver operating characteristic (ROC) curves and the corresponding area under the curve (AUC). The AUC was .99 when distinguishing DDs from healthy control participants and ranged from .79 to .96 in distinguishing mixed psychiatric patients from those with DDs (Draijer & Boon, 1993; Mueller-Pfeiffer et al., 2013; Steinberg et al., 1991).

Culture plays a role in the expression of many psychological symptoms, including dissociation. However, the core symptoms of pathological dissociation are generally similar across cultures (Putnam, 1997). DES scores do not generally correlate with socioeconomic status, gender, or education (reviewed in Carlson & Putnam, 1993; van IJzendoorn & Schuengel, 1996). However, dissociation usually declines from early childhood to adulthood with the exception of individuals with DDs (Putnam, 1997). Some studies have found gender, racial, and ethnic differences on the DES, although these studies have typically been conducted with college students, did not control for trauma exposure, or used small samples (Barker-Collo, 2001; Douglas, 2009; Dunn et al., 1998). Larger samples have not typically found ethnic differences (Monnier et al., 2002) or they have disappeared after controlling for level of trauma (Zatzick et al., 1994). Thus, ethnic and racial differences appear to reflect life experiences, although research in racial and ethnic groups using large samples and trauma exposure measures are needed (Putnam, 1997).

Despite the evidence for the DES's ability to discriminate between different disorders and healthy controls and other indicators of construct validity, the DES is meant to be a *screening* instrument, not a diagnostic instrument. High DES scores signal the possibility of TRD and the need for further evaluation but do not serve as a diagnosis of a DD. A cutoff of 30 for an average DES score has a 74% sensitivity rate for DID and an 80% specificity rate (Carlson et al., 1993). Due to the low base rate of DID (assumed to be 5% for the Carlson et al., 1993, study), only 17% of patients scoring 30 or higher actually have DID, and 83% of those scoring higher than the cutoff would not have DID (Carlson et al., 1993). A DES cutoff of 15 or 20 is sometimes recommended for screening purposes (Foote et al., 2006; Mueller-Pfeiffer et al., 2013; Mueller et al., 2007; Rodewald et al., 2006; Steinberg et al., 1991). For example, a cutoff of 30 would have resulted in very low sensitivity of 42.9% resulting in 57% of the SCID-D diagnosed DID individuals being misclassified as not having DID (Mueller et al., 2007). However, the mean DES scores observed in persons with DDs are often much higher; see Figure 1.1 in Chapter 1 (Lyssenko et al., 2018).

The DES has been used to measure dissociation categorically with a taxon—that is, whether the person is or is not in the "pathological" dissociation cluster of eight items (Waller et al., 1996)—as well as dimensionally— that is, the average DES score (Waller et al., 1996). The DES taxon consists of the average of Items 3, 5 7, 8, 12, 13, 22, and 27. The taxon was derived empirically as the low base rate items that distinguished DD individuals from those without DDs. The DES taxon has lower base rates and lower reliability in nonclinical samples than does the DES (Dalenberg et al., 2012).

Although the DES assesses the severe experiences of amnesia found in DID, it does not assess well for the most common DD: dissociative amnesia. The DES does not assess memory gaps for part or all of a traumatic event(s). It only includes one item assessing for intrusive experiences such the internal dialogues in OSDD-1. These intrusions are better assessed by the Multidimensional Inventory of Dissociation (MID; discussed subsequently). It also does not assess dissociative conversion symptoms.

Some authors challenge the inclusion of absorption items on the grounds that absorption is more common in the general population and, they argue, it is nonpathological (Giesbrecht et al., 2008). Research does not generally support this view. Approximately 75% of DD patients were high on absorption in one study (Leavitt, 2001). DID patients were higher on absorption than patients with schizophrenia and other DD patients (Leavitt, 1999). Absorption is more strongly correlated with psychotic symptoms and general distress than is amnesia (Allen et al., 1996, 1997; Allen & Coyne, 1995). Dalenberg et al. (2012) argued persuasively that dissociation should be defined as including absorption because absorption may facilitate or be a low level of dissociation.

DISSOCIATIVE EXPERIENCES SCALE-REVISED

The DES–Revised (DES-R) was created to correct for skewness and lepto-kurtosis in the DES (Dalenberg et al., 1994). Items are retained from the DES, but the response scale changed to frequencies endorsed from "this never happens" to "this happens at least once a week." This change normal-ized the distribution without changing the relationship of the scores on the DES-R to other variables. The correlation between the DES and DES-R was .90 (Coe et al., 1995).

Dissociative Experiences Scale-Validity

The DES-Validity (DES-V; Abu-Rus et al., 2020) was created because the DES does not have a validity scale. The DES-V items are given along with the DES. The DES-V was developed using several types of checks for validity including structure, atypicality of endorsements, inconsistency, manipu-lation checks, and understanding of vocabulary. The DES-V's atypicality scale showed a strong ability to differentiate honest responders from those coached to feign dissociation; the feigners scored more than 5 times higher than did honest respondents and a group with PTSD. One point is given for each of the validity items that fall in the feigning range on atypicality, structure, and inconsistency. Using a cut-score of 1, the atypicality scale had a sensitivity of .90 and specificity of .71. However, before the DES-V should be used in clinical or forensic settings, replication with clinically diagnosed DD and PTSD samples is needed.

Brief Dissociative Experiences Scale

The Brief DES (DES-B; Dalenberg & Carlson, 2010) is an eight-item self-report measure based on the DES to measure the severity of dissociation in the last week. It was included in the *DSM-5* online assessment measures (https//www.psychiatry.org/dsm5) that were recommended to clinicians and researchers. The DES-B items assess derealization, identity alteration, amnesia, trance, and ability to ignore pain. An average score is created and ranges from 0 to 32, with higher scores indicating more frequent dis-sociation. Respondents endorse items on a 5-point Likert scale from 0 = *not at all* to 4 = *more than once per day*. Sample items include "I feel as though I were looking at the world through a fog so that people and things seem far away or unclear," "I find that I did things that I do not remember doing," and "I act so differently from one situation to another that it is almost as if

I were two different people." The DES-B is beginning to be used in research and shows promise in that high-scoring participants also elevate on associated characteristics such as PTSD, depression, insomnia, and emotion dysregulation (Geng et al., 2022)

Dissociative Symptoms Scale

The Dissociative Symptoms Scale (DSS; Carlson et al., 2018) is a 20-item measure that was developed to assess moderately severe dissociation in a wide range of clinical populations. It was not intended to assess the very severe dissociative symptoms found in DID and OSDD-1. Its development was unusually rigorous and guided by item response theory (IRT) analyses and structural analyses using four clinical and five nonclinical samples ($N = 1,600$). The DSS's four factors accounted for 60.1% of the variance, indicating dissociation is multidimensional (Briere, Weathers, et al., 2005). It showed very good internal consistency, 1 week test–retest reliability (because dissociation may vary over time in some samples, particularly acute trauma samples), and strong convergent, divergent, and construct validity. IRT analyses indicate that the items depict moderately severe dissociative symptoms, as opposed to the DES's combination of mild and severe dissociative items. This suggests that the DSS will perform well with nontraumatized as well as traumatized individuals. However, at the time of writing, the DSS has not yet been used with DD samples. Such research is needed.

The DSS assesses depersonalization, derealization, gaps in awareness or memory, and trauma-related reexperiencing of sensations, thoughts, or behavior. Respondents are asked how often they have experienced symptoms in the past week. There are four depersonalization items (e.g., "I felt like I wasn't myself"), four derealization items (e.g., "Things around me seemed strange or unreal"), three gaps in memory items (e.g., "I couldn't remember things that had happened during the day even when I tried to"), and four gaps in awareness items (e.g., "I found myself staring into space and thinking of nothing"). There are nine reexperiencing items including items assessing cognitive or behavioral reexperiencing (e.g., "I had moments when I lost control and acted like I was back in an upsetting time in my past") and assessing sensory perceptions (e.g., "I smelled something that I know wasn't really there"). The DSS scores are summed for a total score; subscale scores are the mean for the items in each factor to take into consideration differing numbers of items in the factors.

Consistent with DES studies, adolescents' scores tend to be higher, then decline until age 21, after which age was not significantly associated with

DSS scores. There were no differences in total DSS scored across gender in clinical or nonclinical samples. However, there were some small significant subscale differences according to gender. For example, in the clinical samples, women were higher than men on depersonalization/derealization (Carlson et al., 2018). DSS scores are highly correlated with DES scores, moderately correlated with trauma exposure, moderately to highly related with PTSD symptoms, and not significantly correlated with life stress, alcohol use, or socioeconomic status. Research is needed to determine if DSS scores vary by race, ethnicity, and other culturally relevant variables.

Dissociative Symptoms Scale–Brief

The brief version of the DSS (DSS-B; Macia et al., 2022) is an eight-item version of the DSS. DSS-B items were selected by identifying the two items from each DSS subscale that were most precise in measuring moderately severe levels of dissociation in clinical and nonclinical samples. The DSS's four-factor structure and subscales were adequately replicated. Its scores showed comparably strong reliability and validity to the DSS. DSS-B scores appear to have high levels of measurement invariance across ethnic and racial groups so that any differences found between groups are not due to differences in interpretation by the participants.

Somatoform Dissociation Questionnaire

The Somatoform Dissociation Questionnaire (SDQ-20; Nijenhuis et al., 1996) is a 20-item measure that assesses the somatoform experiences associated with dissociation during the past year. Responses are rated on a 5-point Likert scale from 1 (*applies to me not at all*) to 5 (*applies to me extremely*). Sample items include "My body, or a part of it, feels numb" and "I am paralyzed for a while." The SDQ-20 shows excellent internal consistency ($\alpha = .95$; Nijenhuis et al., 1996). Factor analyses indicate it has one factor (Nijenhuis et al., 1998). The SDQ-20 can discriminate DD from non-DD psychiatric patients. DID patients score higher than do those with DDNOS.

In a multisite study of 160 consecutive mixed psychiatric patients, interviewers blind to the results of the DES, SDQ-20, and MID conducted structured interviews for Axis I disorders, including DDs and personality disorders (Mueller-Pfeiffer et al., 2013). To assess the diagnostic ability of the screeners, ROC curves and AUC were assessed. The internal consistency of all three measures was excellent (DES = .94, SDQ-20 = .89, MID = .99). There were moderate intercorrelations between the measures' summary scores ($r = .74–.90$). The screeners showed similarly good discrimination between participants with versus without DDs (AUCs = .83–.84). The scales performed well in distinguishing DDNOS-1/DID versus no DD (AUCs = .86–.89) and had similar sensitivity and specificity at various cutoffs. Comorbid disorders did not confound the ROC curves with regard to presence of a DD. The authors concluded that there were not significant differences between the DES, SDQ-20, and MID in diagnostic accuracy although all three yielded high false positive rates.

Somatoform Dissociation Questionnaire-5

A five-item screen for DD, the SDQ-5, has also been developed. The SDQ-5 has a sensitivity of 94% and a specificity of 98% when distinguishing DD patients from mixed psychiatric patients (Nijenhuis et al., 1997, 1998).

Cambridge Depersonalization Scale

The Cambridge Depersonalization Scale (CDS; Sierra & Berrios, 2000) is a 29-item measure of the frequency of depersonalization during the past 6 months. Respondents report the frequency of depersonalization on a scale from 0 (*never*) to 4 (*all the time*). CDS has good internal consistency and split-half reliability, as well as criterion validity in that it can differentiate individuals with *DSM-IV* depersonalization disorder from those with anxiety and temporal lobe epilepsy (Sierra & Berrios, 2000). Factor analyses have found the CDS is multidimensional with two (Blevins et al., 2013), four (Aponte-Soto et al., 2014; Sierra et al., 2005), and five factors (Simeon et al., 2008). Sample items include "My surroundings feel detached or unreal, as if there was a veil between me and the outside world" and "Parts of my body feel as if they didn't belong to me."

Trauma Symptom Inventory-2

The Trauma Symptom Inventory–2 (TSI-2; Briere, 2011) is a global measure of the impact of trauma that includes a 10-item subscale measuring dissociation as well as two validity scales. The TSI-2 assesses symptoms during the past 6 months. The TSI-2 Dissociation subscale screens for depersonalization (e.g., "feeling outside of your body"), derealization ("feeling like things are not real"), trance, and amnesia. It does not assess for symptoms of dissociation specific to DID/OSDD-1.

Multiscale Dissociation Inventory

The Multiscale Dissociation Inventory (MDI; Briere, 2002) is a 30-item measure of dissociative experiences in the past month, with six subscales measuring disengagement ("spacing out"), depersonalization, derealization, emotional constriction ("not being able to feel emotions"), memory disturbance ("having blank spells"), and identity dissociation ("switching back and forth between different personalities"). The MDI assesses dissociative complexity with greater breadth than most self-report measures. The MDI uses a 5-point response scale (anchors *never* to *very often*). It does not have validity scales. Note that the identity dissociation items only assess frank switching and fragmentation of identity, not the more common and subtle intrusions that are more common features of DID. If DID is a consideration, a broader measure such as the MID should also be used in addition to or instead of the MDI.

The MDI is one of the only dissociation measures that has been normed on the general population. Standardization involved 444 individuals who reported having experienced trauma drawn from a population-based sample ($N = 620$), yielding T scores; this allows an individual's scores to be compared with the general population. Scores are interpreted as being clinically significant if they are three standard deviations above the population mean. Due to it being normed on a general population sample, only a small sample of individuals were included who were diagnosed with DID ($n = 13$). Replication with larger samples of individuals with DID is needed. T score cutoffs for the MDI are much higher than is typically seen in psychological tests due to clinical samples endorsing dissociative symptoms at approximately twice the severity of the general population; this is consistent with the results of meta-analysis (van IJzendoorn & Schuengel, 1996). The disparity between the frequency of dissociative symptoms in the two groups results in dissociative individuals having very high T scores. Because identity dissociation was rare in the standardization sample, the T score for that subscale must be very high (at a minimum of 95) before being considered clinically significant. Briere (2002) advised, "the assessing clinician should be prepared for T scores well over 100 for some individuals with major dissociation pathology" (p. 11). Assessors must understand this, or they may misinterpret very high T scores among individuals with DDs as indicative of exaggeration.

The MDI has very good internal consistency and validity (Briere, Weathers, et al., 2005). In a sample of 1,326 people gathered from the general population, clinical groups, and student populations, principal component analysis identified five moderately related factors on the MDI that shared an average of only 15% of common variance (Briere, Weathers, et al., 2005). MDI scores do not significantly differ by age, gender, race, or ethnicity (Briere, 2002).

Multidimensional Inventory of Dissociation

The MID is a comprehensive self-report measure of pathological dissociation (Dell, 2006a). Its 218 items measure a broad range of dissociation by assessing 23 types of dissociative symptoms. It uses an 11-point (0–10) Likert scale (anchors *never* and *always*) and takes 30 to 60 minutes to complete. Sample items include "Feeling like you are inside yourself watching what you are doing," "Your body feeling suddenly as if it really isn't yours," "Having blank spells or blackouts in your memory," and "Switching back and forth between feeling like an adult and feeling like a child." It includes subscales that might signal psychotic, borderline or other characterological issues, and PTSD symptoms. The 23 symptoms are broken into three theoretically derived groups: general symptoms of pathological dissociation (i.e., general memory problems, depersonalization, derealization, flashbacks, somatoform symptoms, trance); consciously experienced intrusions of another self-state (e.g., child voices, speech insertion, made or intrusive actions, temporary loss of well-rehearsed knowledge or skills); and amnesia, which involves fully dissociative intrusions into executive functioning (e.g., time loss, being told of disremembered actions, finding evidence of one's recent disremembered actions). The MID has 12 empirically derived dissociative factors (Dell, 2006a). The MID factors and symptom subscales are useful in identifying individuals whose profiles are similar to those of individuals with PTSD, DPTSD, OSDD, and DID, as well as individuals without pathological dissociation (Coy et al., 2020).

A unique feature of the MID is its inclusion of several validity scales that can assist in differentiating response styles, symptom overreporting, and signs of possible personality disorder (i.e., Defensiveness, Rare Symptoms, Attention-Seeking Behavior, Factitious Behavior, and Emotional Suffering). Although very useful in clinical assessments, the validity scales have not yet been used in research assessing malingering. The MID is lengthy due to the breadth of pathological dissociative symptoms it assesses. The MID has good to excellent internal consistency and test-retest reliability (Dell, 2006b; Gast et al., 2003; Somer & Dell, 2005). It provides a Diagnostic Impression, which has a predictive power of .89 in distinguishing DID and DDNOS-1b (OSDD in *DSM-5*) from other presentations (Dell, 2011). The MID accurately diagnosed 87% to 93% of DID cases (Dell, 2006a).

The MID does not specify a set time frame for symptoms. If concerning items are endorsed, it is important to determine whether they are current versus past experiences. For example, if someone acknowledges that they have exaggerated symptoms for attention, it is crucial to determine when they exaggerated symptoms. Sensitively discussing the situations in which they have exaggerated their symptoms or trauma history can reveal invaluable information about this means of soliciting care, which, if overlooked, can lead to complications in treatment if it is a current problem. Sometimes people state that the MID can diagnose DDs. Self-report measures for all disorders are only screens for disorders; as noted earlier, only clinicians can make diagnoses.

Another unique and important subscale is the MID-6's "I Have DID" subscale that can clarify to what extent an individual denies or identifies with having DID-like dissociated self-states. When very highly elevated, this scale indicates that caution may be warranted because the individual may be overly invested in having DID or that the disorder is a crucial aspect of their identity. This subscale can be particularly useful when individuals feel *strongly* that they have DID, yet they lack many of the typical co-occurring symptoms and history of profound trauma that are characteristic of DID. This is becoming an important differential issue, as some individuals who have seen social media portrayals of DID appear to identify strongly with having DID yet do not meet the criteria for it. Unusually high elevations in the "I Have DID" subscale combined with scores on the Amnesia subscales that are even higher than those expected among DID may signal a possibly factitious presentation (Paul Dell & Michael Coy, personal communication, May 8, 2022). See the case of "Tom" below and Chapter 6.

The MID-6 has good to excellent internal consistency ($\alpha = .84-.96$) and test–retest reliability over 4 to 8 weeks ($r = .82-.97$; Dell, 2006a). Its construct validity is indicated by its high correlations with PTSD symptoms ($r = .57-.72$). Mean MID scores correlate higher with the avoidance symptoms of PTSD than with the intrusion or hyperarousal symptoms. That suggests chronic use of dissociation may sometimes involve volitional, defensive avoidance of reminders of trauma, as well as automatic, nonconscious use of dissociation (Dell, 2006a). The MID shows excellent convergent validity with the DES ($r = .90$) and other measures of dissociation (Dell, 2006a). The MID distinguishes individuals with DID, DDNOS/OSDD, mixed psychiatric patients, and nonclinical adults, indicating excellent construct validity (which many authors call "discriminant validity").

Multidimensional Inventory of Dissociation–60

The 60-item MID (MID-60; Kate et al., 2021) is a 60-item self-report version of the MID. It was developed to shorten the MID administration time (from 30–60 minutes to 15–20 minutes). It uses an 11-point (0–10) Likert scale (anchors *never* and *always*). The MID-60 was derived from the five questions with the highest matrix loading for each of the MID's 12 factors (Dell & Lawson, 2009). Its factor structure is nearly identical to the MID. It has excellent internal reliability and good content and convergent validity. It yields 12 subscales, including amnesia (of the type found in DID, for example, "Coming to and finding you have done something you don't remember doing, e.g., smashed something, cut yourself, cleaned the whole house, etc."), subjective awareness of self-states ("Hearing a voice of a child in your head"), angry intrusions (e.g., "When you are angry, doing or saying things that you don't remember [after you calm down]"), persecutory intrusions (e.g., "Hearing a voice in your head that wants you to hurt yourself"), derealization/depersonalization, distress about severe memory problems ("Being bothered or upset by how much you forget"), loss of autobiographical memory (e.g., "Not remembering large parts of your childhood after age 5"), flashbacks, body symptoms (e.g., "Not being able to see for a while [as if you are blind] for no known medical reason), psychogenic nonepileptic seizures (e.g., "Having seizures for which your doctor can find no reason"), trance (e.g., "Going into trance for hours"), and self-confusion (e.g., "Feeling very confused about who you really are"). Its items assess phenomena specific to each DD and related experiences, including some PTSD and somatoform symptoms.

Dissociation Questionnaire

The Dissociation Questionnaire (DIS-Q; Vanderlinden et al., 1994) assesses a spectrum of dissociative experiences on a 5-point Likert scale from 1 (*not at all*) to 5 (*extremely*). It is a 63-item measure that was normed on 374 individuals from the general population. The DIS-Q was developed to evaluate the frequency of a wide range of dissociative phenomena from normal (e.g., daydreaming) to pathological (e.g., derealization; identity confusion) forms. It has four factors: identity confusion, loss of control, amnesia, and absorption. Items include "I have the feeling that my body is not (really) mine" and "At moments I cannot remember where I was the day (or days) before." Test–retest reliability over 3 to 4 weeks was good to excellent, as was the internal consistency. The DIS-Q discriminated DD patients from non-DD patients, although it was less able to differentiate DDs from PTSD.

Peritraumatic Dissociative Experiences Questionnaire

The 10-item Peritraumatic Dissociative Experiences Questionnaire (PDEQ; Marmar et al., 1997) measures dissociation at the time of a traumatic event.

It has well-established psychometric properties. There is also a clinician-administered version that has established internal consistency and validity (Marmar et al., 1997). Both versions of the PDEQ use a response scale of 1 (*not at all true*) to 5 (*extremely true*). The total score is the sum of the items, with scores above 15 indicating significant peritraumatic dissociation. Sample items include "I had moments of losing track of what was going on" and "My sense of time changed. Things seemed to be happening in slow motion."

State Scale of Dissociation

The State Scale of Dissociation (SSD; Krüger & Mace, 2002) is a 56-item measure of state dissociation at the time of completing the scale. It assesses responses on a 10-point scale between *not at all* to *very much so*. Items assess derealization, depersonalization, identity confusion, identity alteration, conversion, amnesia, and hyperamnesia (e.g., "This situation feels as if it has happened before in exactly the same way" and "It feels as if some past event is occurring again right now"). A five-factor model predicted 52.9% of the variance. It has good internal consistency and high split-half reliability. The SSD has shown high convergent validity with the DES, despite the latter being a measure of trait dissociation. SSD total and subscale scores vary according to diagnosis (e.g., DD vs. depression). The SSD is sensitive to rapid decreases in state dissociation (e.g., following a grounding exercise) across different patient groups, making it a good choice for repeated measurements and experimentally induced changes in dissociative state.

Scale for Tonic Immobility Occurring Post-Trauma

The Scale for Tonic Immobility Occurring Post-Trauma (STOP; Lloyd et al., 2019) assesses the presence and severity of tonic immobility that persists after trauma exposure. Tonic immobility is an evolutionarily derived, defensive reflex that is automatically activated in response to overwhelming threat (see Chapter 1). It results in the individual being physically immobile with increased muscle tone, loss of ability to move, analgesia, depersonalization, and derealization. Tonic immobility can reoccur after trauma exposure as a trauma-related altered state; it is generally terrifying to experience and associated with distress, including shame (Lloyd et al., 2019). Because it predicts the development of PTSD and poor prognosis to pharmacological treatment for PTSD, it can be important to assess and consider in treatment. The STOP assesses four latent constructs of the defense cascade and includes sensorimotor and perceptual alterations and dissociative experiences. The 30-item STOP has excellent reliability as well as good construct and convergent validity.

The 16-Item Maladaptive Daydreaming Scale

Maladaptive daydreaming is a recently recognized phenomenon that is somewhat correlated with dissociation and is therefore important to understand and differentiate from TRD. Maladaptive daydreaming is the pathological end of an absorptive trait spectrum spanning from immersive daydreaming to maladaptive daydreaming (see Chapters 1 and 2). It is linked to childhood trauma, may be a method of coping with childhood trauma or other states (i.e., boredom), and may possibly signal unresolved childhood trauma (Abu-Rayya et al., 2020; Somer, Abu-Rayya, et al., 2021; Somer, Somer, et al., 2016). However, most individuals who engage in maladaptive daydreaming report no trauma history. Clinicians need to be aware of maladaptive daydreaming and consider it in cases in which the client appears to be caught up in their inner world to a pathological extent. Clinicians must differentiate it from TRD.

The 16-item Maladaptive Daydreaming Scale (MDS-16; Somer, Lehrfeld, et al., 2016) assesses the percentage of time (between 0% and 100%) a symptom is experienced. Sample items include "Some people experience difficulties in controlling or limiting their daydreaming. How difficult has it been for you to keep your daydreaming under control?" and "Some people would rather daydream than do most other things. To what extent would you rather daydream than engage with other people or participate in social activities or hobbies?" Maladaptive daydreaming is strongly related to the DES ($r = .55$). However, this correlation is driven by the similarity between maladaptive daydreaming and absorption as assessed by the DES absorption scale ($r = .63$). Maladaptive daydreaming is not highly related to the DES's depersonalization/derealization ($r = .39$) or amnesia subscales ($r = .24$).

Dissociative Experiences Scale-C

The DES-C (Wright & Loftus, 2000) was meant to be an alternative version of the DES and is widely used by fantasy model theorists (see Chapter 2). The DES-C uses the DES items but asks individuals to rate whether they experience each dissociative symptom less or more than other people. The authors have not demonstrated that dissociative individuals can accurately compare their level of dissociation with that of others. The DES-C has poor concurrent validity; for example, it correlates only .25 with the DES (Wright &

Loftus, 2000). Furthermore, the measure has not been validated with DD samples. For these reasons, dissociation scholars challenge the ability of the DES-C to measure dissociation (Dalenberg et al., 2012). The fantasy model theorists found that the DES had a much stronger correlation with the State Scale of Dissociation than did the DES-C (.68 vs. .37, respectively) and with absorption (.69 vs. .41) among adults, although not among college students (Patihis & Lynn, 2017). Despite having found that the DES-C was not nearly as strongly related to other measures of dissociation as was the DES, Patihis and Lynn (2017) concluded, "In short, we detected no evidence that the DES II is a more valid scale the [sic] DES-C, with the exception of somewhat lower, yet still significant correlations, between the DES II and conceptually related variables in Study 2" (p. 401). Study 2 involved the adult sample (Patihis & Lynn, 2017). The DES-C's poor construct validity, together with the fantasy model theorists' minimization of findings that contradict their interpretations about the DES-C, raise serious doubts about the validity of conclusions reached by researchers who rely on the DES-C as a purported measure of dissociation.

Dissociative Subtype of PTSD Scale

The Dissociative Subtype of PTSD Scale (DSPS; Wolf et al., 2017) is a 15-item questionnaire assessing lifetime and past month depersonalization, derealization, loss of awareness, and dissociative amnesia. Participants rate the frequency of experiencing each symptom in the past month on a 4-point scale (*once or twice* to *daily or almost daily* as well as the intensity on a 5-point scale (*not very strong* to *extremely strong*).

Dissociation Tension Scale

The Dissociation Tension Scale (DTS; Stiglmayr et al., 2010) is a 21-item measure assessing somatoform and psychoform symptoms in the past 7 days. It contains an additional item about aversive inner tension. Items are the percent of time the symptom is experienced from *never* (0%) to *constantly* (100%). The DTS shows good convergent, discriminant, and differential validity. It has primarily been used with individuals with borderline personality disorder and has been shown to be sensitive to change in short time frames.

Additional Dissociation-Related Measures

There are many additional self-report measures of dissociation that are used less frequently, so they will not be discussed in detail here. The Questionnaire of Experiences of Dissociation (K. C. Riley, 1988) contains 26 items that are endorsed as "yes" or "no." The Tellegen Absorption Scale (Tellegen & Atkinson, 1974) measures the tendency to experience absorption, which has been operationalized as episodes of "total" attention that fully engage one's representational (i.e., perceptual, enactive, imaginative, and ideational) resources.

CLINICIAN-ADMINISTERED MEASURES ASSESSING LIMITED TYPES OF DISSOCIATION

Clinician-administered measures can augment the information gathered from self-report questionnaires. Several measures focus on a limited type of dissociation. These are described next, followed by the clinician administered structured interviews.

Peritraumatic Dissociative Experiences Questionnaire

The 10-item clinician administered Peritraumatic Dissociative Experiences Questionnaire (PDEQ; Marmar et al., 1997) measures dissociation at the time of a traumatic event. It has well-established psychometric properties. Various factor solutions have been found, including a two-factor solution (Lack of Awareness and Depersonalization/Derealization; Brooks et al., 2009). The PDEQ is a valid, reliable measure and works well with individuals with different degrees of peritraumatic dissociation.

Shutdown Dissociation Scale

The Shutdown Dissociation Scale (SHUT-D; Schalinski et al., 2015) is a structured interview to assess a person's vulnerability to dissociate. It consists of 13 items scored from 0 (*not at all*) to 3 (*five or more times per week*). The SHUT-D assesses aspects of the defense cascade (Schauer & Elbert, 2010), including items related to feeling insensitive to pain, feeling as if one cannot move, feeling dizzy or being unable to see, and fainting. It has shown adequate internal reliability, excellent test–retest reliability, and good predictive, convergent, and criterion-referenced concurrent validity.

The Clinician-Administrated Dissociative State Scale

The Clinician-Administrated Dissociative State Scale (CADSS; Bremner et al., 1998) is a 27-item scale measuring present-state dissociative symptoms. It consists of a self-report section and ratings scored by an observer.

The participant is asked 19 questions, each beginning with "at this time," and subjects respond with frequencies ranging from 0 (*not at all*) to 4 (*extremely*). A trained observer rates eight behavioral items (e.g., "Did the subject blank out or space out, or in some other way appear to have lost track of what was going on?") on a scale from 0 to 4. The items assess amnesia, depersonalization, and derealization. Self-report items include "Do things seem to be moving in slow motion?" "Do you space out, or in some other way lose track of what is going on?" and "Do you feel disconnected from your own body?" The CADSS shows good interrater reliability, construct validity, and predictive ability.

STRUCTURED INTERVIEWS FOR DIAGNOSING DPTSD AND DD

Two empirically validated interviews based on the *DSM* criteria are used to diagnose DDs, the Semi-Structured Clinical Interview for Dissociative Symptoms and Disorders (SCID-D; Steinberg, 2023) and the Dissociative Disorders Interview Schedule (DDIS; Ross et al., 1989). Due to space constraints, others that are less commonly used or not updated for the *DSM-5* are not discussed here (Simeon, Guralnik, & Schmeidler, 2001).

Semi-Structured Clinical Interview for Dissociative Symptoms and Disorders

The SCID-D (Steinberg, 2023) and its predecessors, the SCID-D (Steinberg et al., 1990) and the SCID-D-R (Steinberg, 1994a, 1994b), are interviews for diagnosing dissociative disorders. (Note that before the 2023 version, the interviews were known at the Structured Clinical Interview for Dissociative Disorders.) Throughout this book, these interviews are referred to as SCID-D. The SCID-D interviews yield scores for five subscales of dissociation, including amnesia, depersonalization, derealization, identity confusion, and identity alteration, as well as a total score. Two additional clinical areas are selected by the assessor for further inquiry (i.e., rapid mood changes, depersonalization, identity confusion, different names/person/childlike parts, internal dialogues, age regression and flashbacks, feeling of possession). Each subscale is rated on duration, frequency, and severity (absent, mild, moderate, or severe; range from 1 to 4) with a possible total score of 20. Most items require the interviewee to describe endorsed symptoms; this allows the interviewer to determine if the described experience is due to dissociation or to other nondissociative phenomena such as psychosis or developmental struggles. Administration, scoring, and interpretation of the SCID-D are described in the Interviewer's Guide (Steinberg, 1994a).

The authors of a meta-analysis summarized the SCID-D literature, noting that it has excellent interrater reliability (α = .76–.96), test–retest reliability (α = .72-.96), and good discriminant validity in distinguishing DID from feigned dissociation and schizophrenia, conversion disorders, and in distinguishing DD patients from non-DD psychiatric patients (Mychailyszyn et al., 2021). The meta-analysis included 15 studies with 1,194 individuals, 463 of whom had DDs. The effect sizes were large (Hedge's $g \geq 0.8$) in all comparisons. Specifically, the overall SCID-D score ($g = 3.12$) as well as each of the five subscales were able to differentiate DDs from non-DDs. Amnesia and identity alteration scores were particularly effective in differentiating DDs from non-DDs ($g = 2.16$ and 2.87, respectively). Depersonalization and derealization are common in a range of non-DD disorders, so it was not surprising that their effect sizes were somewhat smaller (i.e., $g = 1.63$ and 1.29, respectively). The SCID-D was also able to differentiate between clinical DID and factious DID ($g = -1.34$) and simulated DID ($g = 1.73$). The only exception to the pattern of large effects occurred when comparing depersonalization and derealization among individuals with DID to those with borderline or histrionic personality disorder who were referred for diagnostic clarification specifically due to the severity of dissociative symptoms (Boon & Draijer, 1993a).

SCID-D for the *DSM-5*

A French translation of the new edition of the SCID-D for the *DSM-5* and the *International Classification of Diseases–11th Revision* criteria was administered to 20 participants with a DD, 19 with a non-DD psychiatric disorder, and 10 healthy controls (Piedfort-Marin et al., 2022). There was 96% interrater agreement on DD versus non-DD diagnosis. Convergent validity was supported by high correlations between SCID-D total scores and scores on the SDQ-20 and DIS-Q. This translation showed good to excellent reliability, as well as discriminant and convergent validity.

DISSOCIATIVE DISORDERS INTERVIEW SCHEDULE

The Dissociative Disorders Interview Schedule (DDIS; Ross et al., 1989) is a structured interview developed to diagnose DDs. The version of the DDIS that has been used most often in research was linked to the *DSM-IV*. A new version linked to the *DSM-5* had not been validated at the time of writing. The DDIS includes some questions about BPD, major depression, somatization, and Schneiderian symptoms of schizophrenia, as well as explicit questions about childhood abuse (note that these are not behaviorally descriptive questions as is currently recommended, i.e., "Were you physically abused?"). The DDIS uses a "yes" or "no" response format, which makes it quick to administer (30–45 minutes). However, the absence of follow-up queries may contribute to false positive and negative classifications (Friedl et al., 2000). In the pilot study, the overall interrater reliability of the DDIS was .68, specificity was 100%, and sensitivity was 90% for DID (Ross et al., 1989). However, another study of 201 patients found that both depersonalization disorder and dissociative amnesia yielded somewhat lower interrater reliabilities ($\kappa < .60$; Ross et al., 2002).

Self-Report Dissociative Disorders Interview Schedule

The Self-Report DDIS (SR-DDIS) is based on the DDIS; it has a fair to good agreement rate with the DDIS (Ross & Browning, 2017). It has shown theoretically consistent linkages in cross-cultural research (Fung et al., 2022). For example, childhood betrayal trauma predicted 7.8% of the variance in dissociative amnesia and 1.2% of identity dissociation, as measured by the SR-DDIS, after controlling for covariates (e.g., nonbetrayal trauma, age, depression) among international participants (Fung et al., 2022).

Dissociative Subtype of PTSD Interview–I

The Dissociative Subtype of PTSD Interview–I (DSP-I; Eidhof et al., 2019) assesses the presence and severity of DPTSD in the past month. It examines depersonalization (five items) and derealization (three items) on a scale from 0 (*absent*) to 4 (*extreme*), as well as blanking out, emotional numbing, amnesia, alterations in sensory perception, and identity confusion. The interviewer also notes whether they observed any potentially dissociative symptoms. It has high internal consistency and good convergent and divergent validity. The DSP-I score accounted for twice the variance in PTSD severity when controlling for the number of traumas compared to the Clinician Administered PTSD Scale–5 (CAPS-5; Weathers et al., 2018). The broader range of dissociative symptoms assessed by the DSP-I appears to make the DSP-I more sensitive to DPTSD than the CAPS, which assesses only depersonalization and derealization.

PERFORMANCE-BASED MEASURES

Performance-based measures such as the Rorschach (Exner & Erdberg, 2005) and the Thematic Apperception Test (TAT; H. A. Murray, 1943) can help identify posttraumatic and dissociative reactions (e.g., F. B. Evans et al., 2023;

Kaser-Boyd & Evans, 2008; Morales & Viglione, 2022; van der Kolk & Ducey, 1989). Individuals with DDs often show trauma-based patterns on these measures that aid in differentiating them from other disorders, including borderline personality disorder and schizophrenia (Brand, Armstrong, et al., 2009). Performance-based measures provide an opportunity to observe the client *demonstrating* (rather than reporting on) reactions such as traumatic intrusions alternating with avoidance or dissociation, and psychological processes such as the ability to regulate thinking and emotions (Brand, Armstrong, et al., 2006; Brand, Armstrong, et al., 2009; Pica et al., 2001). PTSD and dissociative symptoms are often internal experiences that may be difficult to describe and rely on self-awareness, memory (which can vary depending on the state of the person), and willingness to report these phenomena. Thus, tools that allow assessors to observe trauma-based reactions firsthand are particularly valuable as a source of multimethod data. Dissociative clients may respond with themes of fragmentation, threat from others, and interpersonal isolation that portray their experience of self and others (Brand, Armstrong, et al., 2006; Brand, Armstrong, et al., 2009; Pica et al., 2001).

Individuals with complex DDs commonly show the following Rorschach patterns (Armstrong, 1991; Armstrong & Loewenstein, 1990; Brand, Armstrong, et al., 2006; Brand, Armstrong, et al., 2009):

- They generally will have high scores on the Traumatic Content Index (Sum of Sex, Blood, Anatomy, Aggression, and Morbid content divided by the number of responses). Scores are typically higher than 0.30 and often approximately 0.50 in DD clients.

- Complexity is maintained (high blends, low Lambda), along with an internalizing, obsessional style rather than an externalizing style of coping (the latter would be expected in borderline personality disorder).

- Although generally adequate, their thinking becomes less logical and their perception less conventional when traumatic percepts intrude; that is, they show a "traumatic thought disorder" rather than the thought disorder found in schizophrenia.

- Their form dimension (FD) responses are elevated, which indicates an ability to get distance from situations, including literally distancing from percepts on the cards. This is often associated with an ability to be self-reflective.

- Views of others are typically accurate and collaborative until trauma intrudes (M–, i.e., distorted human movement responses); sometimes they perceive people collaborating in hurting others (COP, i.e., cooperative action responses, are sometimes tainted by being paired with M–, AG [aggressive responses]).

- Individuals with DID may not recall the initial percepts they mentioned when they are asked to describe them further in the inquiry phase.

No studies have compared individuals who are feigning complex DDs with those with clinical DDs on the performance measures. Such research would be highly informative.

FORMAL PSYCHOLOGICAL ASSESSMENT WHEN DISSOCIATION MAY BE PRESENT

A comprehensive multimethod assessment provides an empirically grounded conceptualization of the client, which is informative for clinicians who seek to clarify diagnoses and personality features among traumatized clients (F. B. Evans et al., 2023). Ideally, a multimethod assessment should include a semistructured psychosocial interview, a validated structured interview targeting the specific referral or diagnostic questions (e.g., the SCID-D if DDs are considered), self-report symptom-specific tests (e.g., DSS, MDI, and/or the MID), possibly a multiscale personality inventory with clinical and validity scales (e.g., Minnesota Multiphasic Personality Inventory [MMPI], Butcher et al., 2001; Personality Assessment Inventory [PAI], Morey, 1991), and performance-based personality tests such as the Rorschach scored with the Comprehensive System (Exner, 2003) or the Rorschach Performance Assessment System (Meyer et al., 2017). Due to frequent concerns about the possibility of symptom exaggeration or malingering, it is wise to include measure(s) assessing possible malingering and effort, often referred to as symptom validity measures (described subsequently). It is critically important that assessors are informed about research with highly traumatized individuals, particularly on broadband personality tests and malingering tests. Traumatized individuals often score much higher than do nontraumatized individuals on tests such as the MMPI-2 and PAI, including on some validity subscales developed to assess symptom exaggeration (e.g., Klotz Flitter et al., 2003).

The referral questions, available research, and clinician's judgment about relevance for the case guide the selection of measures. I recommend including a trauma exposure measure to ensure a systematic, valid assessment of traumatic experiences, some of which may not have been reported to the treatment team. The Life Events Checklist for the *DSM-5* (LEC; Weathers et al., 2013) or the more extensive Trauma History Screen (Carlson et al., 2011) are examples. In some cases (e.g., client reports little recall for daily experiences), it may be useful to inquire about the individual's functioning and history from individuals who know them well, if the client gives written permission to do so. In forensic cases, such collateral interviews are essential (see Chapter 5). Assessors should keep in mind that some individuals within the client's support system may have been or may presently be manipulative or abusive to the client, and those individuals are obviously not being examined for their own possible response styles. Caregivers or partners who have been and/or continue to be abusive or neglectful are unlikely to admit to maltreatment and may give distorted representations of the client.

DIFFERENTIATING GENUINE CLINICAL PRESENTATIONS FROM FACTITIOUS, EXAGGERATED, OR MALINGERED DISSOCIATION

It is sometimes challenging to determine whether dissociative symptoms are genuine, factitious, exaggerated, malingered, or, even more difficult, some combination of these. Differences of opinion among clinicians about the veracity and etiology of a client's symptoms can lead to disagreements—and in some unfortunate cases, conflict—about diagnoses and treatment. Collegial communication and collaboration among the treatment team and a nuanced understanding of the client are essential. Objective, evidence-supported psychological assessment using multimethod data can provide clarity in these complex diagnostic dilemmas. The case examples that follow provide guidance about differentiating these presentations.

Validity Scale Research With TRD Samples

Validity scales are created with the goal of identifying individuals who may be exaggerating or malingering symptoms. These scales aim to detect whether an individual endorses too many symptoms or endorses atypical symptoms that are rare (in most populations), or if they endorse too many symptoms as being unbearable. (There are additional types of detection strategies used by validity scales that assess minimization of symptoms, inconsistency of reported symptoms, and other types of patterns and response sets, but these have not been found to be particularly problematic in TRD and so are not reviewed here.)

Individuals who experienced complex, chronic interpersonal trauma often suffer with a wide range of severe symptoms (see Chapter 1). Although the breadth and nature of their symptoms may be rare in some psychiatric groups, these symptoms have been documented for decades among individuals who have experienced complex trauma, particularly those who have the complex DDs (e.g., Boon & Draijer, 1993b; Brand & Chasson, 2015; Putnam et al., 1986; Schiavone et al., 2018; van der Kolk et al., 1996). For example, some somatoform dissociative symptoms may seem improbable to those who have not learned about the myriad somatic and neurological-seeming symptoms common in those with TRD (e.g., sudden numbness, blindness, deafness, or being paralyzed without medical cause; perceiving their body is changing in size, voice-hearing, visual anomalies; see Table 2.1, Chapter 2). Neurobiological research is beginning to clarify the physiological under-pinnings of some of these symptoms (Schiavone et al., 2018).

Individuals who survived complex interpersonal trauma and experience complicated, severe symptomatology are at risk for being misclassified as exaggerating or malingering due to their endorsement of items on validity scales that were thought to be rare or nonexistent in individuals with genuine clinical presentations (e.g., Brand & Chasson, 2015; Brand, Webermann, et al., 2016; L. S. Brown, 2009; Caldwell, 2001). These complexities make it challenging to determine whether reported TRD symptoms are genuine as opposed to factitious, exaggerated, malingered, or some combination of these. This differential diagnostic process should be informed by research about the testing profiles of individuals with TRD and those of individuals with factitious, malingered, or simulated TRD.

Measures That Have Shown Low or Mixed Utility With Highly Dissociative Samples

Unfortunately, some seemingly improbable and rare symptoms (e.g., dissociative experiences such as one's body seeming to change appearance or not recognizing oneself in the mirror) have been included on validity measures that were designed without an understanding of trauma's impact. As items are endorsed (or failed, depending on the measure) on these measures, the individual's score rises, thereby increasing the chance for being above the cutoff for malingering. This puts the individual at risk for being misclassified as malingering when they are accurately reporting symptoms.

An example of a malingering test that includes items commonly endorsed by complex trauma survivors is the Structured Interview of Malingered Symptomatology (SIMS; Widows & Smith, 2005). The SIMS is intended to be a malingering screen; its subscales assess amnesia, depression, and neurological-sounding experiences, psychosis, and low intelligence. All these symptoms except for low intelligence have been documented for decades among individuals with complex DDs (see Chapter 1). Despite temporal lobe epilepsy-like symptoms being common among dissociative individuals, some of these symptoms are included on the SIMS neurological subscale (Schiavone et al., 2018). Although the SIMS manual indicates that the items included are atypical among people with genuine depression, psychosis, and amnesia caused by brain dysfunction or injury, some of these are, in fact, common among nonmalingering trauma survivors (Cernovsky et al., 2019; Cernovsky & Diamond, 2020).

Interviews with nonmalingering trauma survivors who have completed the SIMS have revealed some trauma-related reasons for endorsing these items. For example, one item inquires whether one's mood worsens later in the day, because mood typically improves for depressed individuals as the day proceeds. Trauma survivors report having endorsed this item because abuse would occur after an abusive parent returned home from work; despite the passage of time, evenings may still be a conditioned trigger for low mood. An item on the SIMS Amnesia scale assesses whether memory for one's life and important events rapidly become a blur. This blurring of memory occurs for some individuals with DID when they switch self-states. Considering these trauma-related reasons for endorsing these and other SIMS items, it is not surprising that research shows that the majority (85.7%) of individuals with DID scored above the SIMS cutoff (Brand, Barth, et al., 2021). DID individuals scored higher than healthy control participants on every subscale except low intelligence, even after controlling for dissociation. The SIMS total score had excellent sensitivity for detecting feigned DID (96%), but, unfortunately, an unacceptably low specificity (14%), meaning it overclassifies nonexaggerating, genuine DID individuals as malingering. Thus, the SIMS does not appear to be a valid malingering test for use with highly dissociative individuals. (See Table 5.1 in Chapter 5 for the utility scores of other measures.)

Another important reason to know about dissociative individuals' performance on the SIMS is that the SIMS is often used in research by fantasy model theorists in support of their notion that dissociative individuals exaggerate symptoms. Fantasy model theorists claim that highly dissociative patients' high SIMS scores indicate that they are prone to symptom exaggeration and fantasy proneness (e.g., Merckelbach et al., 2015). In another study, they argued that because some asylum seekers score above cutoff on the SIMS, and endorse dissociative symptoms (e.g., sometimes not recognizing themselves in the mirror), clinicians should be cautious with asylum seekers because they may exaggerate symptoms (van der Heide & Merckelbach, 2016). Certainly, anyone in a high-stakes context may exaggerate symptoms. However, it is also exceedingly common for refugees to seek asylum due to being tortured or otherwise terribly traumatized in their home country (Chessell et al., 2019). Furthermore, as reviewed in Chapter 2, individuals with reliably diagnosed DID have been repeatedly shown not to be more suggestible, fantasy prone, or vulnerable to creating false memories compared with healthy control participants or individuals with PTSD. Even the fantasy model proponents have found this. Specifically, they concluded that "Dissociativity correlated with symptom over-reporting in the student samples, *but not in the clinical sample*" (emphasis added; Merckelbach et al., 2015, p. 165). Most (71%) of this clinical sample had DES scores above the cutoff of 30, signaling high dissociation. Merckelbach et al. (2017) subsequently admitted that the high correlation between SIMS scores and dissociation could be due to many SIMS items overlapping with trauma-related symptoms, although this conclusion is rarely mentioned in their other papers, and if it is, it is minimized (van der Heide & Merckelbach, 2016). The authors of a review of the SIMS found that the SIMS total score correlated .60 with self-reported PTSD symptoms as well as other genuine psychiatric symptoms (Cernovsky & Diamond, 2020). They concluded, "The SIMS is a fatally flawed psychological test with alarmingly high iatrogenic rates. Its use constitutes malpractice" (Cernovsky & Diamond, 2020, p. 30).

See additional discussion of biased reporting, motivated skepticism, and other lapses in logic and professionalism by the fantasy model theorists of research that challenges their model in (Dalenberg et al., 2020).

Similarly, the PAI Negative Impression (NIM) scale (Morey, 1991), which was developed to screen for possible symptom exaggeration and malingering, includes items that are related to trauma. For example, one item asks respondents if they sometimes feel like they have multiple personalities. It is not surprising that individuals with DID/DDNOS endorse this item because it is a symptom required under the *DSM*. It is also not surprising that they endorse another item about sometimes having only unhappy memories from childhood (Stadnik et al., 2013); see the PAI profiles in Figure 5.2 in Chapter 5. Stadnik et al. (2013) found dissociation significantly correlated with NIM among the DD/DDNOS sample, even after controlling for depression and borderline features. The DID/DDNOS patients were elevated on NIM, and to a lesser extent on another validity scale, MAL (i.e., Malingering Index), yet they were not elevated on the RDF (i.e., Rogers Discriminant Function) validity scale. This suggests that the RDF, and to a lesser extent the MAL, may be better PAI subscales for screening for possible exaggeration of symptoms in DD patients than the NIM.

Another example of a malingering measure that includes trauma-related items involves the Structured Interview of Reported Symptoms (SIRS/SIRS-2; Rogers et al., 1992). Examples of items that could be endorsed due to trauma exposure include three items on the Rare Symptoms subscale related to possible dissociative phenomena (i.e., feeling outside of one's body, one's face looking unfamiliar in the mirror, and major changes in the perception of one's body). Research has consistently shown that the SIRS misclassifies as possibly malingering approximately one-third of those who experienced complex trauma (Rogers et al., 2009) and approximately one third of individuals with DID (Brand, McNary, et al., 2006; Brand, Tursich, et al., 2014). Richard Rogers, an expert in malingering and the author of the SIRS, recognized that these and other SIRS items may be endorsed due to genuine trauma-related difficulties. As a result, he developed a Trauma Index, which consists of items that traumatized individuals do not typically endorse. The Trauma Index on the SIRS and the SIRS-2 (Rogers et al., 2010) does not overclassify traumatized individuals as feigning symptoms, even those who have DID (Brand, Tursich, et al., 2014; Rogers et al., 2009).

The TSI-2's Atypical Response does not perform well in differentiating simulated DDs from DDs. A study compared the TSI-2 profiles from 39 inpatients diagnosed with complex DDs (DID or OSDD-1) to those completed by 51 coached simulators (i.e., they were given fact sheets about DID; Palermo & Brand, 2019). Consistent with research on the TSI-2, the complex DD (CDD) patients elevated on most of the clinical scales and factors (Briere, 2011). There were significant differences between CDD patients' and simulators' TSI-2 profiles. Simulators failed to endorse some of the co-occurring symptoms common in CDD, including anxious arousal, depression, and suicidal ideation, while they overendorsed dissociation and dysfunctional sexual behavior. Despite these differences, the Atypical Response Scale correctly classified only 60% to 73% of participants, and its specificity scores were low. Nonetheless, the TSI-2 yields important clinical information such that it is often used in clinical and forensic evaluations, although for the latter, assessors will likely want to include additional assessment of malingering.

Many trauma experts urge caution when interpreting MMPI-2 validity scales among complex trauma survivors, including those with high dissociation, as well as scores on the MMPI-2 8 (Sc, Schizophrenia) subscale (Brand & Chasson, 2015; Brand, Chasson, et al., 2016; Elhai, Gold, Mateus, et al., 2001; Elhai et al., 2004; Wolf et al., 2009). Individuals with complex DDs usually also have PTSD, so research about feigned PTSD informs the detection of feigned DDs. Detecting feigned PTSD is challenging. For example, genuine PTSD patients were not distinguishable from those of feigners on the MMPI-2 validity scales (e.g., Bury & Bagby, 2002; Elhai, Gold, Sellers, et al., 2001). A meta-analysis of PTSD patients found extreme elevations on the MMPI-2 Fb (i.e., the Back Infrequency scale), F (i.e., the Infrequency scale), and Fp (i.e., the Infrequency-Psychopathology scale; Rogers et al., 2003). Among the MMPI-2 validity scales, Fp typically performs best in detecting feigned PTSD, particularly with survivors of child sexual abuse

(Elhai et al., 2004; Klotz Flitter et al., 2003; Rogers et al., 2003). Dissociation contributes to F scale elevations in dissociative samples (e.g., Brand & Chasson, 2015).

In addition to elevations on MMPI-2 validity scales, childhood trauma survivors are characterized by numerous elevated MMPI-2 clinical scales (see review in Brand & Chasson, 2015). For example, 11 of the Scale 8 items correctly differentiated 81% of adults abused in childhood from nonabused controls (Wolf et al., 2009). These endorsements reflected difficulty managing affect, impulses, and cognitive processes—including dissociation. In other words, these elevations were likely related to trauma rather than schizophrenia. "Trauma, forensic, and assessment experts agree that the extreme elevations on validity and clinical scales often reflect the array of symptoms, impairment, and distress common among those who experienced complex childhood trauma" (Brand & Chasson, 2015, p. 93).

Due to space constraints, three recent studies that have used the MMPI-2 with DID samples will be reviewed; interested readers can find published cases and older studies with the MMPI in Brand and Chasson (2015). (To date, no studies have been conducted with the MMPI-3 and highly dissociative samples.) Two of the studies by Brand and colleagues used the same participants, although different analyses examined different research questions. In the first study (Brand & Chasson, 2015), profile analyses compared a reliably diagnosed DID group ($n = 53$) with coached ($n = 77$) and uncoached ($n = 67$) DID simulators (see the MMPI-2 profiles in Figure 5.1 of Chapter 5). F, Fb, and Fp distinguished simulators from genuine DID patients, although, as is consistent with the PTSD literature, Fp performed best. The DID profiles found by Brand and Chasson were similar to the PTSD profiles from the Rogers et al. (2003) meta-analysis. Specifically, in the PTSD sample, F was 86.31 versus 90.99 for DID patients. The PTSD group's Fb was 92.31 versus 93.2 for the DID group, and the PTSD Fp was 69.02 versus 72.0 for the DID group. Similarly, DID participants' scores were lower than or similar to those obtained by PTSD patients who had experienced childhood sexual abuse (CSA; Ds2 was 75.62 in DID vs. 82.17 in CSA found by Elhai, Gold, Sellers, et al., 2001).

None of the validity scales studied by Brand and Chasson (2015) achieved a positive predictive power (PPP) higher than .66. A discriminant function analysis (DFA) combined validity and clinical subscale predictors and found a sensitivity of 83.0%, specificity of 86.0%, PPP of 68.8%, and overall diagnostic power of 85.3%. This DFA combination outperformed the single validity scales. The authors recommended using the formula identified by the DFA model instead of single MMPI indices. See the published study for cut scores and the classification equation with constants and coefficients. Despite exposure to accurate facts about DID, the DID simulators were not able to accurately feign DID. Furthermore, the DID profile was consistent with what would be expected with exposure to childhood trauma.

In the second study (Brand, Chasson, et al., 2016), the authors compared most and least common item endorsements on MMPI validity (i.e., F, Fb, and Fp) and clinical (i.e., 8 and 2 [D or Depression]) scales in the DID group to coached and uncoached DID simulators. The items most endorsed on the F subscale by the DID group included four items about negative feelings toward one's family of origin and single items about dissociation (Item 168), sexual difficulties, acknowledgment of mental health problems, self-destructive urges, and alcohol abuse. The most frequently endorsed Fb items by the DID group included four items about depression, three about self-destructive urges, three about fearfulness, and one each about dissociation, lack of family support, and believing one deserves punishment. The most frequently endorsed Fp items by the DID group included three items about negative feelings about one's family of origin, and one item each about fearing objects that could cause physical injury, sleep abnormalities, gender confusion, fear of the dark, lack of romantic love, and believing one's mind was being controlled. All these items are consistent with struggles or experiences of childhood trauma survivors. The MMPI items least likely to be endorsed by the DID group involved disregard for law enforcement, delusions, and sadistic traits. Strikingly, the items least commonly endorsed by the DID group tended to be among the most frequently endorsed by the DID simulators, particularly the uncoached simulators, who relied on their preexisting beliefs about DID, rather than the factual material about DID that was given to the coached group. The study's findings suggest that items least commonly endorsed by individuals with DID but frequently endorsed by simulators may be particularly useful to examine when attempting to differentiate clinical versus malingered DID on MMPI-2 validity scales.

On Scale 8, the DID group most frequently endorsed five items related to depression, four items consistent with trauma including possible trauma within the family, two dissociative items (i.e., Items 168 and 229), and items related to difficulty with sexual functioning and loneliness. The coached simulators matched these endorsements well. However, the uncoached group failed to endorse four items potentially suggestive of dissociation, three items about conflict or trauma within the family, and items measuring sexual dysfunction. The biggest difference in endorsements on MMPI-2 Scale 2 occurred with the simulators not endorsing somatic symptoms and memory difficulties.

The DID group's pattern of endorsement suggests that trauma and dissociation likely contributed to elevations on F, Fb and, to a lesser extent, Fp, which is consistent with links between these subscales and dissociation (e.g., Brand & Chasson, 2015; Klotz Flitter et al., 2003). Similarly, endorsements on Scale 8 in the DID group could relate to traumatization. The uncoached group incorrectly portrayed individuals with DID as delusional, sadistic, masochistic, lawless, and antisocial. These endorsements starkly contrasted with the items endorsed by the DID group and suggest that simulators may have been influenced by media portrayals of DID individuals as psychotic, dangerous, and often homicidal.

The third MMPI-2 study compared 30 women with DID with 43 DID feigners (Ambrose et al., 2023). Ambrose and colleagues found that dissociation was strongly correlated with clinical Scales 4 (Pd, Psychopathic Deviate), 6 (Pa, Paranoia), 7 (Pt, Psychasthenia), 8 (Sc, Schizophrenia), and 9 (Ma, Mania). Consistent with Brand and Chasson (2015), a profile analysis indicated the feigners scored higher than the DID group. Feigners scored the highest on Scales 4, 6, and 8. However, both groups scored above norms on all clinical scales except the DID group did not elevate on Scale 9. As in Brand and Chasson, DID patients elevated the highest on Scales 8 and 6 along with elevations on many of the validity scales analyzed in the study. As predicted, Scales 6, 8, and 9 had the largest effect sizes in differentiating the groups. Almost all (95.34%) of the feigners elevated more than 20 points on the average of the psychotic scales (6 and 8) compared with the average of the somatic (1 and 3) combined with the average of the mood (2 and 7) scales. Only one individual (3.3%) in the DID group showed the pattern of psychosis scales being much higher than somatic and mood scales; this pattern of feigners overplaying unusual symptoms may be useful to assess on the MMPI as well as other measures. The DID group did not differ from a PTSD sample on F, Fb, and Fp; thus, these "atypical" scales are less atypical in traumatized individuals. A discriminant function analysis of the validity scales accounted for 86% of the variance in DID status with Fp, S (Superlative), and F-K being robust predictors. This model classified 72 of 73 individuals correctly; one feigner was misclassified as being a DID patient. The authors conducted receiver operating characteristic curve analysis on seven validity scales; the area under the curve for Fp was .988, .929 for S, and .972 for F-K, which are excellent levels of discrimination. See the publication for cutoff scores. The authors concluded that the results indicate DID individuals show a profile of genuine symptoms that can be distinguished from simulated DID; furthermore, the study contradicts the notion that this DID was a hysterical or malingered condition.

Measures Showing Consistently Good Utility Scores With Highly Dissociative Individuals

At the time of writing, only one symptom validity test has been studied with highly dissociative individuals: the Test of Memory Malingering (TOMM;

Tombaugh, 1997). This test appears to be a test of memory, so if individuals were attempting to feign amnesia or memory problems, they would likely perform poorly on the TOMM. Low scores on the TOMM suggest possible malingering of memory problems or lack of effort on testing. Individuals with DID have dissociative amnesia for aspects of their autobiographical history, particularly traumatic events. Nonetheless, individuals with DID perform well on the TOMM. Brand, Webermann, et al. (2019) found that the DID group had higher TOMM scores on Trial 1 ($M = 47.55$, $SD = 4.62$) compared with the group simulating DID ($M = 34.19$, $SD = 10.68$), as well as on Trial 2 (DID I = 49.52, $SD = 14.20$ vs. simulators $M = 34.27$, $SD = 14.20$). The almost perfect scores achieved by the DID sample starkly contrast with the predictions of the fantasy model theorists, whose model implies that these individuals should have failed this test due to their supposedly exaggerated symptoms.

Two additional tests of malingering that have shown acceptable utility statistics in differentiating DID individuals to DID simulators: the Miller Forensic Assessment of Symptoms Test (M-FAST; Barth et al., 2023) and the SIRS/SIRS-2 Trauma Index. The M-FAST was able to distinguish 35 individuals with DID from 88 DID simulators when a slightly higher cut score was used. Specifically, when using the standard cutoff score of 6, the M-FAST misclassified 17.1% of individuals with DID as malingering. However, when using a cutoff score of 7, 93.6% of all participants were correctly classified and specificity improved (0.89) while maintaining adequate sensitivity (0.96). Notably, these results are likely due to the M-FAST not including many items that could be related to trauma.

As reviewed earlier, the SIRS/SIRS-2's Trauma Index (Brand, McNary, et al., 2006; Brand, Tursich, et al., 2014; Rogers et al., 2009, 2010) has been validated by two research teams using three complex trauma samples, two of which were individuals with DID. The Trauma Index consists of three subscales that are consistently unelevated among highly traumatized individuals: Symptom Combinations, Improbable or Absurd Symptoms, and Reported versus Observed Symptoms. The Trauma Index is calculated by summing the scores on these three subscales. If individuals score above the cutoff of 6, they are classified as possibly feigning. The Trauma Index can be calculated for either the SIRS or the SIRS-2 because the items and these subscales have remained consistent across the two versions of the SIRS.

In summary, trauma-informed research provides guidance about assessing exaggeration and malingering of TRD. Individuals who feign DID endorse media-based stereotypes of DID, which are relatively easily learned and feigned, and psychotic symptoms, yet they miss the subtle, lesser known symptoms and struggles such as depression and somatic symptoms (Ambrose et al.,

2023; Brand & Chasson, 2015; Brand, Chasson, et al., 2016; Coons & Milstein, 1994; Palermo & Brand, 2019). Social media may be contributing to more sophisticated malingered as well as factitious presentations of DDs because public access to information about DID has increased considerably with the dissemination of information and depictions on the over social media and the internet. I have seen a significant increase in requests for consultations regarding clients who present to clinicians with self-reported "diagnoses" of DID, yet their presentations are not consistent with the classic presentation of DID. Distinguishing whether these cases are factitious, malingered, or atypical DD, or a combination of these, is difficult. Their management may be even more difficult because if the clinician does not find evidence of DID, these clients may become angry and defensive. Even if they do not meet criteria for full DID, they may have experienced trauma and may have some genuine dissociative symptoms. This is addressed in more detail in the case of "Tom" later in the chapter and in Chapters 5 and 6.

Studies That Have Used Multimethod Assessment to Distinguish Malingering of DID

Two pilot studies compared genuine DID with simulated DID using multiple tests. Both found no veritable gain in using multiple tests. Welburn et al. (2003) compared DID patients' testing profiles on a battery of tests including the DES, SDQ-5, SCID-D, MMPI-2, and the Millon Clinical Multiaxial Inventory–III (MCMI-III; Millon, 1997) to the testing profiles of clinical staff who simulated DID, genuine patients with schizophrenia, and control participants. The DES and SDQ-5 differentiated DID and schizophrenia, but the screeners had high rates of inaccurately classifying feigners as DID patients. While DID simulators had more elevated DES and MMPI-2 scores than controls, the validity scales on the MMPI-2 (i.e., F, Fb, and F-K) and MCMI-III (i.e., X, Y, Z) did not distinguish the DID group from the simulated DID group. SCID-D profiles were the most effective in differentiating DID simulators from clinical DID (mean SCID-D total score 14.30 and $SD = 3.86$ vs. 19.08 and 1.24, respectively), as well as the individuals with schizophrenia ($M = 11.00$, $SD = 4.58$). The personality tests were not able to differentiate DID from the simulators. Importantly, the DID group scored higher than the group with schizophrenia on both tests' subscales intended to assess for schizophrenia, that is, Scale 8 on the MMPI and SS (Thought Disorder) on the MCMI. The Welburn et al. study is one of several that have supported the recognition of the SCID-D as the gold standard interview for assessing DDs.

Coons and Milstein (1994) used data from 112 consecutive admissions to a unit specializing in treating DID to determine how to distinguish the 101 genuine DID cases from the 11 factitious or malingered DID cases. The data included the MMPI, a mental status examination, intelligence testing, and collateral interviews. MMPI scores were available for only 50 DID patients. Consistent with Welburn et al.'s (2003) results, the MMPI did not differentiate the groups. (Note that to date, the only adequately powered studies of DID vs. simulated DID were able to detect differences between the groups on the MMPI-2; Ambrose et al., 2023; Brand & Chasson, 2015.) The groups were differentiated by the presence of well-known characteristics of malingering, including that DID malingerers often refused to allow collateral interviews and displayed extreme exaggeration during the examination. Furthermore, the malingerers reported significantly fewer subtle, comorbid psychiatric symptoms that are not well-known to occur in DID (i.e., decreased sexual desire, depression, auditory hallucinations, conversion symptoms) and even higher levels of well-known symptoms associated with DID than in the DID group (i.e., amnesia, fugue, substance abuse, self-mutilation, head-aches, visual hallucinations, delusions, somatic symptoms). Although not significantly different, the malingerers tended to display symptoms only while being observed, used DID as an excuse for behavior, and engaged in persistent lying (although individuals with DID are often accused of lying, so caution is warranted here). The malingerers also had numerous inconsistencies in their history; however, individuals with genuine DID may give somewhat differing accounts of their history when presenting in different states (e.g., in some states they acknowledge abuse by a parent, whereas in another state they may deny this). Additionally, the authors did not address how they distinguished somatic from conversion symptoms.

Despite relying on small samples, these studies yielded valuable insights into the differential diagnosis of genuine versus malingered DID. Studies using larger samples of SCID-D diagnosed DID patients versus DID simulators as well as known treatment-seeking DID malingerers, which use current versions of tests along with validated malingering scales, are urgently needed. Furthermore, research exploring the differentiation of exaggeration and malingering of other DDs besides DID is also urgently needed.

Synthesizing these studies with clinical experience, individuals with malingered and factitious DID presentations often lack the complex comorbidity expected in DID, as well as the typical avoidance of knowing about and discussing dissociation including self-states (e.g., Draijer & Boon, 1999; Kluft, 1987b; Loewenstein et al., 2002). Those with factitious DID often are intrigued and seem to enjoy thinking, writing, and talking about their "parts." They often report having DID with unusual and inconsistent features such as an unusual degree of awareness of their self-states with a lack of amnesia and absence of chronic, severe early childhood trauma. They may present in what they report are different states without any notable differences in behavior, manner of speaking, mood, memory, beliefs, or style of relating. They may show a lack of reactivity to potential triggers (e.g., not jumping in response to a loud, unexpected noise). They may change their behavior when they are not aware of being observed (e.g., outside the window of the assessor's office; in the waiting room or hallway) to suddenly acting strikingly different when they are aware of being observed (e.g., inside the assessor's office). They often show no convincing interest or investment in learning to manage their symptoms or changing their level of functioning. Although it is the weakest evidence among multiple sources of data, some malingerers' ways of interacting and sharing their story feel "false" and more like "drama" than "trauma" (Brand & Brown, 2023; L. S. Brown, 2009). Caution is needed when considering the assessor's reaction to the client because of our own potential biases, the many myths about TRD, and the impact of culture and context. Particularly in cases of suspected factitious or malingered TRD, assessors need to use a variety of sources of data with measures that have been validated with complex trauma survivors including those with severe dissociation. Consultation with colleagues who have expertise in TRD and differential diagnosis related to trauma in such cases is also highly recommended.

The Differential Diagnosis of Exaggerated or Malingered TRD

At the time of writing this book, some individuals who publicly identify as having DID have challenged the idea that patients presenting with highly atypical, dramatic, and publicized DID may not have DID. These individuals feel their experiences are minimized and discounted. Research aimed at learning about the various presentations of TRD is needed to understand the range of dissociation and how best to provide treatment to individuals with typical as well as atypical presentations of dissociation.

Coons and Milstein (1994) documented that approximately 10% of the consecutive admissions to their inpatient DID unit had factitious or malingered DID. A small subset of individuals feign TRD or exaggerate or even completely fabricate histories of trauma. Although the latter cases have been rare in more than 30 years of clinical practice, I have encountered some malingered cases of DID. It is important to have evidence-supported methods for identifying these individuals. This is a complex issue associated with a variety of motivations and styles of presenting.

Some traumatized individuals are so overwhelmed by their symptoms and feel so helpless in their ability to manage them that their testing profiles are unusually elevated (even beyond what the reviewed research indicates are typical scores among DD samples) and their presentations are dramatic in an effort to convey their desperation (Brand & Brown, 2023; L. S. Brown, 2009). These individuals can experience both genuine trauma-related symptoms along with a tendency to overstate the frequency or severity of their symptoms. Due to high levels of distress and poor emotion regulation, they may feel as if their symptoms are unendurable. Part of this type of dramatic presentation may be due to a lack of ability to notice and manage nuance and shifting degrees of emotion and symptomatology. These individuals may have features of histrionic or borderline personality disorder (Draijer & Boon, 1999).

Other trauma survivors are truly confused about their identities and may relate to feeling and acting so differently at different times that they believe they have dissociative self-states and DID. These individuals tend to describe more polarized, "good" versus "bad" self-states, and they tend not to be as conflicted about them as are individuals with traditional DID/OSDD-1 (Boon & Draijer, 1993a; Draijer & Boon, 1999). They show fewer or no signs of distress, avoidance, and dissociation while doing diagnostic interviewing for DDs, in contrast to many who have genuine DID (unless the latter have become educated about and accepting of their DD). These individuals may diagnose themselves with DID and refer to "parts" of themselves by name or in other ways present as having DID. (Note that some individuals who self-diagnose DID meet full *DSM* criteria for the disorder, whereas others do not; some may instead meet criteria for DPTSD or another DD.) These individuals often believe they have DID and they typically are not consciously attempting to feign the disorder. Boon and Draijer referred to this as "imitative DID" (Boon & Draijer, 1993a; Draijer & Boon, 1999). These individuals also often have personality features of borderline or histrionic personality disorder.

Additionally, some trauma survivors who experienced their distress or abuse being covertly or overtly minimized or denied may have adapted by escalating their pleas for help. This adaptation may result in elevations on validity scales that detect symptom amplification. Rather than "crying for help," as this style is often described, some may metaphorically be "screaming for help." Thus, they may recognize at times that they are overstating the frequency or severity of symptoms but believe that it is the only way people will listen to and help them.

Some people are consciously motivated to feign TRD, including DID, because they seek belonging, a way to understand their conflicting emotions, or a means of expressing their identity or gender issues. For others, DID is seen as a fascinating disorder, particularly now with skyrocketing visibility on social media platforms. The *DSM-5-TR* categorizes this presentation as factitious disorder (American Psychiatric Association, 2022). This is further described in the case of "Tom" that follows and in Chapters 2 and 6. As noted in the discussion of the MID, that test, as well as the SCID-D, may be particularly useful in discerning these cases from genuine clinical TRD and DID.

Finally, some individuals are motivated to feign TRD, perhaps especially dissociative amnesia or DID, for personal gain. The gain may be monetary, such as in a lawsuit or disability evaluation, or avoidance of legal sanctions or responsibility (e.g., time off work, being sentenced to life in prison without parole rather than given the death penalty). The *DSM-5-TR* refers to this as "malingering" (American Psychiatric Association, 2022). Malingering is differentiated from factitious disorder by the latter not being fully driven by the desire for external rewards. That is, there is some internal motivation for attention for factitious cases, such as desperation to receive help. The two are not mutually exclusive. To complicate differential diagnosis further, it is possible for an individual with some aspects of genuine TRD to also have some factitious or some malingered symptoms. The following cases illustrate how the assessor made differential diagnoses involving TRD. These cases are compilations of cases seen in my clinical practice.

The Case of "Jan"

"Jan" was a middle-aged woman experiencing significant mood lability. Her parents' marriage ended when she was 3, and her father, to whom she was close, died soon afterward. Jan reported frequent and severe child sexual abuse, including rape, by her stepfather beginning before she was in kindergarten. Her mother was physically and verbally abusive. In adolescence Jan had begun to cut herself and drink alcohol heavily to "to stop feeling." She became a successful professional, although her episodes of depression were sometimes so severe that she could barely get to work. Other times she worked obsessively and slept little. Sometimes Jan could not recall what she had done, including cutting herself, yet she insisted she had not relapsed into drinking. Sometimes she would present in her typical manner of being open and self-reflective, then become distant and "absent." Jan eventually revealed she heard a voice that sounded like her stepfather berating her and telling her she should cut herself. Although her psychiatrist and therapist agreed that Jan had PTSD, the psychiatrist believed she had bipolar disorder, whereas her therapist suspected DID. The treatment team sought psychological assessment to clarify Jan's diagnoses and treatment.

The psychologist conducted an assessment using the TOMM, M-FAST, PAI, TSI-2, LEC, DES, the SCID-D, a self-report measure of PTSD symptoms (i.e., Posttraumatic Checklist—5; Blevins et al., 2015), and the Rorschach. Jan was well under malingering cutoffs on the M-FAST and TOMM. On the PAI, Jan scored high on the NIM validity scale ($T = 77$), but she was not high on MAL or RDF, which is consistent with DDs (Stadnik et al., 2013). Jan jumped several times when she heard loud noises. She repeatedly rubbed her head, then looked "spaced out and far away." The psychologist had to call her name repeatedly to get Jan to respond. Jan could not recall what they had been discussing. Jan said, "I went . . . inside. It's quiet." This was a dissociative trance state.

On the PAI, Jan was very high on depression, anxiety, PTSD, and the social detachment and thought disorder subscales of schizophrenia. The TSI-2 and PCL-5 corroborated that Jan was struggling with overwhelming traumatic intrusions, avoidance, derealization, and depersonalization. Jan scored high on the DES (average = 45). On the SCID-D-R, Jan's responses indicated she struggled with severe amnesia, depersonalization, derealization, identity confusion, and identity alteration. Jan seemed uncomfortable as she revealed how she often felt that she could not control the behaviors and statements she made and that she was often amnestic for cutting. Twice on the SCID-D she did not recall symptoms she had initially reported to the psychologist.

Jan typically presented with sophisticated, articulate language and behavior during the assessment meetings. However, this style of presentation varied, particularly on the Rorschach. Some of her abridged Rorschach responses follow. (The comments in italics are added for clarification.)

Card I

1. A creature with a sinister look on its face. *(Although it is common to see faces, even frightening ones, the "sinister" creature is more threatening than that reported by most individuals.)*

2. A broken butterfly. [Inquiry: Looks like somebody punched holes in the wings and some of the wings are just bits and pieces. It's so broken you can't even find the rest of the pieces. (Holes?) If it were not a hole, these would be a different color. The background goes into infinity.] *(Her description of the butterfly being so badly broken that the pieces can't even be found hints at the possibility that she may have fragmented parts of herself due to being traumatized. Although it is important not to overinterpret a single reference to fragmentation or splitting, when such phenomena are*

repeated, it raises the possibility of dissociative compartmentalization. When this occurs, the individual may disconnect from traumatic experiences so they "can't even be found" or felt or known. The percept going off "into infinity" is an FD (Form Dimension) response, suggesting she may be distancing from the distressing percept of a terribly damaged butterfly.)

Card II

3. It's hard to say because I almost remember what I saw last time. I'm trying to block that out of my head. This is a lake. This is a bridge and a smaller lake. Here's a pathway going up to a castle in the sky. The red is like a gateway. This would be the banks of the lake. [Inquiry: This looks like water going into the lake? (eyes closed, dissociating). Because if it weren't, this would be blocked off, but it has to be water flowing into the lake this way. I just got distracted there. I'm sorry. I felt like this was blood. It didn't make sense to be in this picture. There can't be blood in this picture. (What makes it look like that?) It's far away. It could be a fallen tree making a nature's bridge but it's very narrow. The bridge is broken in the middle.] *(Her first two sentences show she is actively avoiding/dissociating a response given in a past Rorschach administration. She shifts from threatening percepts in Card I to a fanciful "castle in the sky," but that defensive maneuver is ruined by the intrusion of blood, which she is aware does not belong in this peaceful scene. Again, she uses a distancing FD response to attempt to get distance from the intrusive blood percept. The broken bridge may reflect how broken she perceives herself to be.)*

VI. (Other responses omitted due to space constraints)

7. (Closes eyes. Laughs. Head on table. Laughs.) I'm having trouble putting words . . . getting the words out. The first impression I had looking at this . . . the picture that you would find in a book about the anatomy of a female. These would be the legs spread apart. This would be the vaginal area and the anus and all that stuff. [Inquiry: Can't we not talk about this picture? (Try and say what makes it look like that if you can). (Eyes closed). It looks that way because it looks that way. (Where?) The whole thing. (Dissociating) *(She is so overwhelmed she can barely verbalize that she is seeing a woman's genitals and anus. She attempts to get distance by laughing, putting her head on the table, shutting her eyes, and intellectualizing the percept by making it an image in an anatomy book.)*

VII.

8. This could be something you would see on the wall in a cave. Maybe somebody carved out two faces. You might find this in the entrance of a cave where these two heads were the faces of the guardians guarding the cave. The cave was so massive that the path into the cave is very small. *(In this intellectualized response, she moves away from the previous traumatic images. She sees protective figures who are capable of guarding something hidden and small. This may reflect the phenomena of having protective self-states that "guard" something in need of protection.)*

Jan's perception of female sexual anatomy disrupted her thinking and ability to be articulate. Overwhelmed by the emotion that flooded her despite attempts at avoidance, Jan then began to dissociate. This percept was followed by imagery of a necklace, guardians guarding a cave, seahorses dancing, then another image of female genitalia followed by a "beautiful creature with many different colors, sparkles." Jan's Rorschach protocol shows trauma-based intrusions that she repeatedly defended against with intellectualized, fanciful images, and when that failed, she lapsed into dissociation. This pattern was reminiscent of how she had dissociated when her attempts to avoid her abusive mother and stepfather failed, and she "escaped" via dissociation. Jan's Trauma Content Index was 0.53, which is consistent with research on DID samples (Armstrong & Loewenstein, 1990; Brand, Armstrong, et al., 2006; Brand, Armstrong, et al., 2009).

In summary, the assessment clarified that Jan's shifting patterns of behavior, emotion, thinking, and amnestic gaps were due to DID rather than bipolar disorder. Space constraints limit further description of her testing, but the assessment consistently supported that she also suffered from complex PTSD and major depressive disorder. Her amnestic gaps appeared to be due to DID rather than relapsing with alcohol. The assessment indicated treatment needed to focus initially on supporting the containment of traumatic material, education about trauma's impact with particular focus on grounding, stabilizing NSSI, and healthier methods for regulating emotion.

The Case of "Tom"

The case of "Tom" illustrates using multimethod assessment to inform differential diagnosis in the context of suspected factitious or malingered DD. Tom's therapist, Ann, sought a consultation with a colleague with expertise in TRD because Ann did not see evidence of his having a complex DD, although Tom, a 17-year-old high school student, reported he had dissociative "personalities," which he referred by name (e.g., "Tommy," who was reportedly a little boy). Tom used the pronouns "we" and "us" when referring to himself instead of "I" and "me" and referred to himself at times in the third person as "Tommy." These behaviors may occur in DID. However, he did not show any changes in behavior, vocabulary, cognitive sophistication, mood, or manner of relating to the therapist when he reported he was "Tommy." He did not experience headaches or other somatic symptoms that are common in DID, including before or after he reported that he had "switched" states.

Tom's mother had brought him into therapy when he was a sophomore due to his crippling social anxiety, poor grades despite obvious intelligence, and minor cutting. He was awkward socially and presented with almost no eye contact, poor hygiene, and an inability to recognize when he had talked so long about topics that others had stopped listening. He lived with his mother but was not close to her. They barely saw each other because of her work schedule and because he spent so much time playing computer games and engaging with social media. He had no close friends other than online acquaintances. Tom had only met his father twice; his parents never married, and neither his father nor Tom was interested in having a relationship. Ann thought Tom had some features of being on the autism spectrum. His main interest was playing computer games for 5 or more hours per day as well as being involved in online groups.

Tom became involved with an online Reddit group where people talked about their "tulpas"—that is, fantasy "people" inside them, often based on comics, movies, or superheroes, or that relate to childhood imaginary companions that reportedly "grew up" (Somer, Cardeña, et al., 2021). Adults with DID sometimes experience their self-states as versions of the imaginary friends they had as children, which they did not outgrow as most nondissociative children do (Putnam, 1997; Silberg, 2013). Many of the people on the social platform reported that they had been diagnosed with DID. After 1 month of being highly engaged with the site, Tom began talking about his "personalities" in therapy and said he, too, had DID and that he was a "system" (of parts) rather than a person. He enjoyed talking about his "personalities" at length and introducing them to Ann.

Ann had not observed Tom being amnestic for anything he said or did in or out of session. Tom denied a history of trauma, including in his "personalities," other than having been bullied by boys at school in junior high. He remembered those events clearly. The bullying involved demeaning verbal abuse. Tom had not been physically or sexually threatened or harmed, although he had been terrified and terribly haunted by the boys' cruelty.

Ann noticed Tom often became anxious with notable sweating and hyper-ventilating when they talked about the bullying. He sometimes felt that his hands were growing larger (depersonalization) and his therapist was sitting a "mile away" (derealization) when they talked about the bullying. Tom worked hard to avoid thinking or talking about the boys' mistreatment. He felt like he was a "loser," just like the boys had shouted at him, and that he could not trust any peers to be nice to him.

Tom's mother did not have the resources for formal psychological testing, and Tom refused to meet with the consultant directly, so the consultant advised Ann to conduct an interview for DPTSD (i.e., DSP-I) and to have Tom complete the MID-60. Tom had an average MID score in the high range (i.e., 50), which might suggest DPTSD and possibly even DID or OSDD-1. However, some of Tom's validity scores were much higher than even typically found in DID and OSDD-1 (e.g., Rare Symptoms, Attention Seeking, Identity Confusion) as were other scales (i.e., I Have DID, I Have Parts, Child Parts, and Persecutory), which suggested a possible response style or personality traits that might impact his presentation. His I Have DID scale was higher than the I Have Parts scale, which is not typical in clinical DID and can suggest overidentification with having parts or factitious or malingered DID (Michael Coy, personal communication, May 9, 2022; Paul Dell, personal communication May 8, 2022). He also showed elevations on Depersonalization, Derealization, Trance, and Flashbacks, which were in the range expected with PTSD. He was lower on Memory Problems and Schneiderian first-rank symptoms than are DID and OSDD-1 individuals, although he reported forgetting what he did earlier in the day, not remembering what he ate at meals, and not remembering where he was the day before. He denied most of the frankly amnestic items on the Time Loss, Coming to, and Fugues scales.

Tom's memory problems seemed related to being distractible and caught up in his inner world and online life so much so that he missed conversations, had little awareness of his surroundings, and demonstrated poor recall for his daily activities. Follow-up questions indicated he lost track of time, sometimes for hours, when engaged online and while thinking about online conversations when he was offline. He scored in the range expected for DPTSD on the DSP-I with endorsements of depersonalization, derealization, absent-mindedness, numbing, and alterations in sensory perceptions. The consultant and Ann agreed that Tom had DPTSD and factitious DID. His sense of having DID seemed to stem from his being deeply confused about who he was, rather than consciously trying to deceive people, although he admitted he "went along" with others on Reddit because he wanted to fit in as they had treated him with kindness and, unlike his peers at school, they had included him. Further, he genuinely felt overwhelmed and terrified like a little child at times. He continued to insist he heard the voices of the bullies; this seemed to be a trauma-based internalization of their taunts and putdowns.

ASSESSING DISSOCIATION OVER TIME IN TREATMENT

Dissociation impacts treatment outcome for highly dissociative individuals. For example, Price et al. (2014) found that the degree of dissociation at the first session had considerable negative impact on treatment response in acutely traumatized individuals. These findings led the authors to recommend assessing dissociation initially as well as in future sessions. It is important to assess changes in the frequency, severity, and type of TRD experienced over time in treatment. This information clarifies to what extent dissociation may interfere with the ability to engage meaningfully, learn from, and recall what is discussed and learned in therapy, and thereby potentially impact the outcome. It is also important to assess a broad range of symptoms and level of functioning regularly over time in areas including emotion regulation, management of PTSD symptoms, self-compassion, and so on. Other resources discuss measures beyond those intended for TRD clients; the focus here is on measures specific to assessing progress in TRD clients (e.g., Briere & Scott, 2012; Courtois & Ford, 2013; Dalenberg & Briere, 2017).

A measure that can assess current state dissociation is the self-report SSD (Krüger & Mace, 2002), although its 56 items are likely unwieldy for use in every session. The DSS-B has only eight items, so it might be more realistic to use repeatedly, including at the start of each session.

Two measures assess the healthy capacities that are targeted in treating individuals with TRD. The Progress in Treatment Questionnaire–Therapist (PITQ-t) is a measure therapists complete about their patient, and the Progress in Treatment Questionnaire–Patient (PITQ-p) is a self-report measure completed by the patient (Schielke et al., 2017). The PITQ measures assess dissociative individuals' ability to manage their emotions, symptoms, and relationships safely and effectively as well as their ability to view themselves and others in a generally positive way. Both are in Appendix B. The measures have 32 similar items for each respondent, six of which are only completed by or for patients who report having dissociative self-states. Responses are rated on an 11-point scale from 0 (*never true*) to 100 (*always true*) with higher scores indicating better functioning. Both measures have demonstrated good internal consistency, adequate convergent validity, and good test–retest reliability. They were used in longitudinal treatment studies of DD individuals and found to be informative indicators of change over time (Brand, McNary, et al., 2013; Brand, Schielke, et al., 2019). The measures showed moderate convergent validity to measures of emotional dysregulation, dissociation, PTSD, and psychological quality of life. The PITQ-p demonstrated evidence of stronger relationships with established symptom measures than the PITQ-t.

CONCLUSION

Dissociative symptoms may potentially have significant impacts on functioning and treatment. It is imperative that dissociation is routinely assessed as a complex phenomenon among traumatized individuals by using measures that have been validated on TRD samples. In some cases, assessment for symptom exaggeration and malingering are indicated. As a working alliance is formed and treatment progresses with trauma survivors, it is important to continue assessing the extent and severity of dissociation, as well as other domains of functioning related to trauma's impact.

5 ASSESSING DISSOCIATION IN FORENSIC AND OTHER CONTEXTS IN WHICH MALINGERING IS CONSIDERED

Assessors with knowledge and experience in complex trauma and dissociation are urgently needed in forensic contexts due to the ubiquity of trauma. For example, posttraumatic stress disorder (PTSD) and trauma are highly prevalent in prison samples: 70% of female prisoners and 50% of male prisoners reported having experienced childhood sexual abuse (Briere, Agee, et al., 2016). In prison samples as well as the general population, the number of different types of trauma someone has been exposed to, particularly interpersonal trauma, predicts PTSD. Unfortunately, a lack of training about trauma and trauma-related dissociation (TRD) can lead assessors to misunderstand or overlook trauma-related reactions, sometimes leading to incorrect diagnostic conclusions and injustices. At the most extreme, some criminal defendants have been sentenced to death without the court being fully informed about severe and substantiated childhood abuse. This chapter presents assessment methods that are consistent with research and expert recommendations regarding assessing for TRD. Methods for distinguishing genuine versus imitative, factitious, and malingered TRD in forensic contexts are presented.

https://doi.org/10.1037/0000386-005
The Concise Guide to the Assessment and Treatment of Trauma-Related Dissociation, by B. L. Brand

TRAUMA AND TRAUMA-RELATED DISSOCIATION IN FORENSIC CONTEXTS

Trauma is frequently encountered in a variety of forensic contexts. Claims of injury causing pain and suffering occur in a variety of cases ranging from sexual assault, harassment, discrimination, personal injury, and disability. Forensic examiners may be asked to assess the impact and emotional damage resulting from specific trauma(s), including evaluating the relative impact of traumatic event(s) over the individual's lifetime (Dalenberg, Straus, & Ardill, 2017). Such assessment can help to determine the veracity of emotional harm claims in tort cases. Examiners may be asked to opine about the connection between alleged harm and reported trauma versus other possible causes such as prior traumas, malingering, or preexisting vulnerabilities including mental illness. Sometimes the argument is made in court that a sexual assault in adolescence or adulthood had few psychological effects or that symptoms of a sexual assault are due only to antecedent trauma. Research contradicts this, showing that child sexual abuse, as well as adolescent and adult sexual assaults, make independent, long-term contributions to later symptoms (Briere et al., 2020). Experts may be asked to opine about the presence, severity, and impact of trauma-related sequalae such as dissociation affecting the individual's ability to work (in disability assessments), to parent (in child custody and parent capacity in termination of parental rights determinations), and to benefit from treatment (in discussions about potential damages in tort cases and sentencing in criminal cases, among other roles; Rocchio, 2020).

In criminal cases, forensic examiners may be called on to assess whether an individual suffered from a severe mental illness at the time of an alleged criminal act, and if so, whether the disorder influenced their judgment or ability to control their behavior. Their testimony may influence whether the individual will be considered legally competent to stand trial, or whether they are legally insane versus partially or fully culpable of criminal acts.

As discussed in Chapter 1, dissociation can impact a wide range of higher level integrative and regulative capacities, thereby interfering with emotion regulation, thinking, memory, perception, emotional learning, control over behavior, and other psychological processes (Cavicchioli et al., 2021). When these processes are disrupted by dissociation, the individual is at risk for feeling detached from others, themselves, and possibly from the consequences of their behavior. In addition, the individual may misinterpret social situations, have limited emotional regulation, or show poor decision making, all of which can impact their functioning, choices, and behavior.

Dissociation is one of many possible responses to experiencing trauma. However, dissociative symptoms are transdiagnostic, and not all dissociation is trauma- or stress-related or pathological (see Chapter 1). The focus of this book is TRD. Information about TRD's prevalence, comorbid patterns, and differential diagnosis of various disorders from TRD and other trauma-related disorders is covered in other chapters.

Trauma and TRD can affect individuals in ways that are relevant in forensic contexts. For example, TRD predicts depression (Armour et al., 2014), non-suicidal self-injury (Ford & Gómez, 2015; Webermann et al., 2016), suicide attempts (Briere, Dietrich, & Semple, 2016; Foote & Park, 2008; Stein et al., 2013; Tamar-Gurol et al., 2008; Webermann et al., 2016), revictimization in adulthood (Webermann et al., 2021), posttraumatic stress disorder (PTSD) symptoms 3 years posttrauma (Mayou et al., 2002), and severe impairment (Stein et al., 2013). It can also be linked to poorer or slower response to treatment (Price et al., 2014), The scientific community, professional organizations, and the *Diagnostic and Statistical Manual for Mental Disorders* (5th ed., text rev. [*DSM-5-TR*]; American Psychiatric Association, 2022) recognize the existence of TRD and dissociative disorders (DDs) and recommend evaluating for these symptoms and diagnoses.

High levels of dissociation have been found in some violent individuals (Bradford & Smith, 1979; Moskowitz, 2004). Dissociative amnesia has been reported in approximately 25% to 45% of homicides (Bourget et al., 2017). Clinicians report that between 38% and 55% of patients with dissociative identity disorder (DID) have a history of any type of violence (see Webermann & Brand, 2017). Men with DDs are more likely to be violent than women with DDs, as is the case in general for men (Loewenstein & Putnam, 1990). Research is inconsistent about rates of violence in individuals with DDs. The inconsistent findings may be partially due to lack of clarity in older studies regarding whether patients who reported having "violent alters" were referring to self-directed (i.e., suicidal or self-harming) versus other-directed (e.g., homicidal or assaultive) violence. An older study of 21 men and 92 women diagnosed with DID found that the men had significantly higher rates of alcohol abuse. Forty-seven percent of the men and 35% of the women reportedly had engaged in criminal behavior, with 19% and 7%, respectively, reporting they had committed homicide (Loewenstein & Putnam, 1990). It is unclear whether the reported "homicide" was an internal (i.e., one self-state perceiving "murdering" another self-state) versus an external experience (i.e., directed at another person) or whether the individuals had *wished* they had killed someone but had not done so. Nonetheless, despite the subset of individuals reporting they had committed homicide, most of the participants reported they had not engaged in criminal behavior. Of those who reported criminal behavior, many said they had engaged in minor crimes, such as disorderly conduct or public drunkenness. The authors suggested that socioeconomic factors may have contributed to these unusually high rates of reported criminal behavior as their participants were largely economically disadvantaged.

In contrast, recent larger DD treatment studies have found significantly lower rates of criminal involvement. In a sample of 173 individuals in treatment for DDs, 0.6% of the patients reported having been incarcerated in the past 6 months (Webermann & Brand, 2017). Dissociation, PTSD, and emotion dysregulation did not predict involvement with the criminal justice system in this almost entirely (94%) female sample. Individuals with DDs are at greater risk for being victimized by others than being perpetrators. For example, whereas 29.6% of DD patients were victims of their partner's violence in the past 6 months, only 3.5% were physically victimizing their partner (and all participants who reported victimizing their partner were also being victimized; Webermann et al., 2014). A review of the research found that approximately 25% of individuals with DDs had been victims of any type of violent crime including physical or sexual interpersonal violence in the past 6 months to 1 year (Webermann & Brand, 2017). In studies on the prevalence of mental illness among violent offenders, violence is most common among individuals with substance use disorders, rather than DDs, schizophrenia, or other psychotic disorders (Webermann & Brand, 2017).

THE IMPORTANCE OF ASSESSING AND BEING KNOWLEDGEABLE ABOUT TRD IN FORENSIC CONTEXTS

In criminal cases, a lack of awareness about trauma and TRD has contributed to some individuals being tried and sentenced without the court learning about the role that trauma may have had on the defendant's development and behavior. For example, there are published cases in which defendants were sentenced to death without the court being made fully aware of substantiated, severe child abuse (e.g., Lewis et al., 1997). Some juveniles and adults have been sentenced to death without forensic examiners recognizing signs of TRD that were present across the lifespan; some of these defendants were diagnosed with DDs by researchers after they were already sentenced to be executed (Lewis et al., 1988, 1986, 1997). Sometimes the lack of consideration of trauma is so severe that questions are raised about the examiners' ethics. For example, in a study of 18 juveniles sentenced to death in Texas, the researchers wrote,

> Especially shocking were instances in which experts for the defense and family members who knew or should have known about the abuse and violence to which a subject had been exposed testified to the contrary. For example, in the case of Subject 12, whose father beat him so viciously that the police were called, a defense expert reported, "Family life was stable." (Lewis et al., 2004, p. 424)

Thankfully, awareness about the importance of trauma and TRD is growing. For example, the subtype of dissociative PTSD (DPTSD) was added to the *DSM-5* due to increasing awareness of the prevalence and impact of TRD. This awareness has led to a surge in research, including the development of validated methods for assessing TRD and DDs, and neurobiological studies that show that classic PTSD and TRD are associated with different patterns of brain activation and result in feeling flooded with emotion or detached and numb (e.g., Lanius et al., 2010; Roydeva & Reinders, 2021). Validated methods for assessing TRD and distinguishing it from malingering have been developed; these developments make evidence-based, accurate diagnosis of TRD in forensic contexts possible.

A history of trauma matters in forensic cases. A survey of capital cases demonstrated that a defendant's history of trauma and abuse was one of the factors considered seriously by juries (Shapiro et al., 2013). The courts have become increasingly aware of the potentially life-altering impacts of trauma. For example, the U.S. Supreme Court remanded to the Texas Court of Criminal Appeals the case involving Terence Tramaine Andrus because his attorneys had not adequately presented the devastating impact of child abuse and neglect on his development and behavior. The Court decided Andrus had demonstrated his "counsel's deficient performance" and that his counsel had failed to present a "tidal wave" of mitigating evidence about his childhood trauma and neglect (*Terence Tramaine Andrus v. Texas*, 2022, p. 18). Similarly, the Supreme Court found there was ineffective assistance from counsel in the failure to investigate and present the defendant's trauma history in *Williams v. Taylor* (2000) and *Wiggins v. Smith* (2003). Armstrong (2001) examined a defendant who had been convicted of the impulsive murder of two people. She found that he suffered from DID and a psychotic disorder, which significantly impaired his reality testing. Due to her finding of diminished responsibility, the man was sentenced to life in prison, rather than death. In an attempted murder case, the defendant was found not guilty by reason of insanity related to DID and other psychiatric disorders and sentenced to treatment at a forensic psychiatric hospital (*People v. Henderson*, 2015).

Forensic practitioners must practice within their areas of competency (American Psychological Association, 2013; Heilbrun et al., 2016). Those who are involved in trauma-related cases need to be aware of the current literature related to complex trauma, TRD, DPTSD, and DDs, including research-supported methods for assessing these disorders and differentiating them from exaggeration and malingering (e.g., Chapters 1 and 4, this volume; Bailey & Brown, 2020; Dalenberg, Straus, & Ardill, 2017; Ellickson-Larew, Escarfulleri, et al., 2020; Rocchio, 2020). They need to be able to inform triers of fact regarding a variety of topics including the nature and prevalence of trauma, complex trauma, PTSD, complex PTSD, DPTSD, TRD, and DDs (Brand et al., 2018; Brand, Schielke, & Brams, 2017; Rocchio, 2020). Furthermore, they need to be able to understand and explain these conditions and a range of trauma-based reactions, presentations, and comorbidities (see Chapter 1), as well as discuss myths and misunderstandings about TRD including the debate about its etiology (see Chapter 2). They need to be knowledgeable about trauma's impact on individuals' ability to relay their history, their responses to assessment and legal procedures, their presentation in forensic-related interviews and court appearances, and their ability to work with attorneys and others involved in forensic matters (Brand, Schielke, & Brams, 2017; Brand, Schielke, Brams, et al., 2017; Brand, Webermann, et al., 2016; Rocchio, 2020). They also need to be knowledgeable about forensic assessment and practice. Therefore, forensic examiners who intend to evaluate victims of complex trauma and mental health trauma experts in forensic assessments must have specialized training, professional consultation, and continuing education including current knowledge on emerging research to maintain the requisite competencies (Rocchio, 2020).

POTENTIAL CONFLICTS IN ROLES AND BIASES

Forensic experts need to be aware of the special roles and ethical requirements required in forensic practice (Rocchio, 2020). Their roles may include working as evaluators, consultants to attorneys, or scientific experts who provide scientific testimony (rather than assessing an individual). Forensic psychologists are required to follow the American Psychological Association's (APA's; 2017) *Ethical Principles of Psychologists and Code of Conduct* and the *Specialty Guidelines for Forensic Psychologists* (henceforth, "Specialty Guidelines"; APA, 2013). Other disciplines and specialties have ethical guidelines that must be followed; here, the emphasis is on forensic psychologists (Bush et al., 2020).

The Specialty Guidelines advise that experts serve as experts to the court, rather than being an advocate for the plaintiff, defense, or state. They suggest that psychologists must "maintain integrity by examining the issue or problem at hand from all reasonable perspectives and seek information that will differentially test plausible rival hypotheses" (APA, 2013, p. 15). The examiner must be neutral to the legal theories of the retaining attorney and provide an unbiased opinion about the forensic questions, regardless of whether the opinion supports, contradicts, or is neutral to the attorney's case (APA, 2013; Dalenberg, Straus, & Ardill, 2017). Attorneys sometimes ask clinicians providing treatment to traumatized clients to serve as a witness in a forensic matter due to their belief that the therapist can best explain the client's symptoms and disorders (Rocchio, 2020). However, treatment providers are only able to serve as fact witnesses for their clients, not expert witnesses, due to the conflicting roles, duties, and ethical responsibilities that differ between treatment providers and forensic experts (Greenberg & Shuman, 1997, 2007; Heilbrun et al., 2009).

Forensic experts are not immune from biases (Kassin et al., 2013). Regardless of who hired the expert, the expert must strive to be aware of and avoid potential conflicts and biases while maintaining an independent, scientifically grounded assessment (Bush et al., 2020; Heilbrun et al., 2009). Mental health professionals sometimes hold beliefs about TRD that are based in myth or outdated beliefs rather than up-to-date research (see Chapters 2 and 4). Such beliefs can have negative impacts, including leading to the misclassification of traumatized individuals as malingering when they are reporting genuine symptoms to the best of their ability, or to not recognizing when an individual is exaggerating or malingering their reported symptoms (Brand, Sar, et al., 2016; Brand, Webermann, et al., 2016).

Confirmation bias is the tendency to focus on and look for information that confirms one's initial hypothesis while ignoring contradictory information or alternative explanations (Kassin et al., 2013; Neal et al., 2022). Confirmation bias can impact forensic examinations if the expert consciously or unconsciously draws conclusions that support the view of the retaining party or that supports their own professional or personal view, regardless of evidence. Imagine a forensic case involving an individual who reports experiencing complex trauma and TRD and is examined by an expert who privately holds the belief that individuals who claim to suffer from dissociation are especially prone to fantasy and exaggeration. This examiner could be challenged that they showed confirmation bias if they did not use measures that have been validated with samples who have experienced complex trauma or dissociation, or if they distorted the scientific literature to support their preferred belief. Alternatively, an examiner might be influenced by confirmatory bias in the other direction if they did not rigorously assess for possible exaggeration and malingering or if they discounted evidence suggesting possible malingering. Forensic examiners need to consider evidence for a broad range of possible psychiatric disorders and hypotheses, including the possibility that the individual may have a trauma-related disorder or trauma-related damages, or that they may be exaggerating or fully malingering some aspects of their history or symptoms.

A good deal of literature on "debiasing techniques" can be used to counteract biases. Simple reflection on one's biases has not been shown to be an effective method for countering bias (Neal et al., 2022). According to a scoping review, one of the methods with strongest support for countering bias is a cognitive strategy called "consider-the-opposite" (Neal et al., 2022). Experts can ask themselves to form an initial judgment on a case, then consider possible alternatives that might be correct and reasons why they might be correct. This is discussed further later in the chapter. Examiners are advised to do this in all cases, including those wherein alleged trauma or TRD may be relevant. Examiners can present these considerations with transparency, showing that they developed their opinion by fairly considering a range of evidence and hypotheses.

Failing to assess adequately for or consider the impact of TRD in cases involving alleged trauma may lead to uncomfortable cross-examinations about the thoroughness of the assessment and possible bias. For example, a defense expert in a medical malpractice case opined that the plaintiff was exaggerating her symptoms. However, the plaintiff had been diagnosed with DID by her therapist before the suit. The defense expert did not acknowledge that the plaintiff's psychological test results were consistent with the literature on DID. The plaintiff's expert testified that the plaintiff's testing was consistent with the peer-reviewed literature on DID and that her scores were not unusual for someone with a DD. Consequently, the jury awarded a multimillion-dollar settlement to the plaintiff (*Rivera v. Bado*, 2014). Ignoring the trauma-dissociation link that has been repeatedly supported in rigorous research opens examiners to justified challenges of bias and "motivated skepticism" (Dalenberg et al., 2020).

CONDUCTING THOROUGH, FAIR FORENSIC ASSESSMENTS OF TRD

Given that TRD is widely accepted by the scientific community and is included as a symptom in borderline personality disorder, acute PTSD, PTSD, DPTSD, and the DDs in the *DSM* (American Psychiatric Association,

2022), examiners of individuals who may experience TRD (as well as other symptoms or possible disorders) must provide a broad, independent, evidence-based evaluation using scientifically validated measures and procedures (Bush et al., 2020; Heilbrun et al., 2009). Furthermore, ethical standards require the use of measures that have been shown to be reliable and valid with populations that are similar to the individual being examined (APA, 2013). For example, in the case of alleged damage due to sexual assault, a forensic examiner would ideally evaluate the individual's performance on measures that have been validated with individuals who have experienced sexual assault. If no research is available on samples similar to the individual being evaluated, this limitation needs to be made clear to the attorneys and the court. In such cases, the expert may need to be considerably more cautious about their interpretations of testing data and the certainty with which they draw professional opinions. Justice is best served when examiners on both sides of legal cases fully examine the issues at hand using appropriate, valid measures and procedures for the case (Brand, Schielke, & Brams, 2017; Dalenberg, Straus, & Ardill, 2017).

Claims of any psychiatric disorder or symptom, including TRD and DDs, can be evaluated only through a thorough forensic psychological evaluation that relies on multiple forms of data ("multimethod assessment") and examination of a variety of hypotheses about each case. The standard for forensic evaluations requires review of available data in developing a professional opinion. The examiner conducts a comprehensive forensic psychological evaluation including administration of validated tests (e.g., personality testing, malingering inventories, self-report measures, gold standard diagnostic interviews). As well, the examiner must review third-party information such as witness statements; police reports; collateral interviews of family members, friends of the defendant, teachers, coworkers, and others; legal records, including jail/prison records, prior court testimony and depositions; and available school, social service, medical, and psychiatric records (Bush et al., 2020; Heilbrun et al., 2009). It is particularly helpful to conduct collateral interviews with people who have known the assessee for years—preferably before, during, and after the incident in question, including family members, friends, coworkers, supervisors, therapists, and romantic partners. However, examiners need to be aware that some of these individuals may have harmed or failed to protect the evaluee in the past or present (Rocchio, 2020). Sometimes members of the family report highly discrepant accounts of events, including the behavior of parents or other caregivers.

UNDERSTANDING AND ASSESSING THE POTENTIAL IMPACT OF COMPLEX TRAUMA

Individuals who experienced childhood abuse or other types of complex and chronic interpersonal trauma are at risk for being misclassified as exaggerating or malingering symptoms due to the range of severe symptoms they experience. Although many such symptoms are thought to be rare, they are common in trauma survivors (e.g., Bailey & Brown, 2020; Briere & Scott, 2012; Wolf et al., 2009). As reviewed in Chapter 1, individuals with complex trauma, particularly those with complex DDs, typically experience a plethora of disturbances such as mood, anxiety, somatic, and seemingly neurological and psychotic symptoms, along with disturbances in identity, relationships, emotional and behavioral control, and memory. Although the breadth and nature of their symptoms may be rare in some psychiatric groups, these symptoms are well-documented and common among individuals who have experienced complex trauma, especially those who have complex DDs including DID (e.g., Boon & Draijer, 1993b; Brand & Chasson, 2015; Putnam et al., 1986; Schiavone et al., 2018).

Some traumatized individuals may be so overwhelmed by their symptoms, and their inability to manage them, that their psychological testing profiles may be unusually high and dramatic, reflecting an effort to convey their desperation (Brand & Brown, 2023; L. S. Brown, 2009). Those who are highly reactive to their current level of emotion or distress may not be able to reflect on and report their symptoms accurately over time because "now" is what preoccupies their experience. They do not have a reliable sense of how they were feeling a few days or weeks ago. This lack of accurate assessment can be exacerbated by dissociative amnesia because the individual may have gaps in their memory, perhaps particularly when they are overwhelmed. Additionally, some individuals have been in situations where their distress or abuse was covertly or overtly minimized or denied and may have adapted to the lack of concern by escalating their pleas for help; this may result in elevations on validity scales that detect symptom exaggeration. Individuals who report trauma or TRD may also purposefully exaggerate or malinger some or all their symptoms or history or present themselves as legally incompetent or insane when they are neither (Loewenstein, 2020).

Individuals with high levels of complex dissociative symptoms may be particularly at risk for being classified as exaggerating or malingering (e.g., Brand, Webermann, et al., 2016). Studies document a lack of training about dissociation and link this knowledge gap with misdiagnoses of DDs in the United States, Northern Ireland, and Australia, indicating a widespread lack of training about DDs (Dorahy et al., 2005; Leonard et al., 2005; Perniciaro, 2014). Skepticism and lack of training about dissociation often coexist. A survey of psychologists found that only 5% felt knowledgeable about DID, and 73% reported having received little or no training about DID (Mendez et al., 2000). Skepticism and lack of knowledge about the disorder were correlated, suggesting that more training about dissociation is critical in forensic assessment. Only 60.4% of U.S. clinicians could correctly diagnose DID when presented with a vignette clearly depicting the condition (Perniciaro, 2014). The most frequent misdiagnoses were PTSD (14.3%), schizophrenia (9.9%), and major depression (6.6%). Accurate diagnoses were most often made by clinicians who had treated a DID patient and who accepted the validity of DID. Of concern, clinicians were equally confident in their diagnoses, regardless of their accuracy. However, when clinicians have had training in TRD and give DD diagnoses, generally the diagnoses accurately match the client's symptoms (Nester et al., 2021).

These individuals' complex symptom presentations can obscure a DD. Along with a mixture of dissociative symptoms, individuals with complex DDs typically experience additional difficulties, including PTSD, treatment-resistant depression, substance abuse, eating disorders, somatoform symptoms, self-destructive and suicidal behavior, and personality disorder traits (e.g., Dell, 2002). They report higher levels of first-rank symptoms than do patients with schizophrenia, with the exception of audible thoughts and thought broadcasting (Kluft, 1987a; Ross et al., 1990). The individual may be partially conscious of some aspects of dissociation (e.g., hearing voices, thought insertion/withdrawal, "made" actions/impulses) as well as sometimes unaware of what they do in some states and completely unaware other times (e.g., time loss; Dell, 2006a).

In addition to general measures of personality, competent forensic evaluation of trauma including TRD requires the use of measures that evaluate the range of traumatic experiences and reactions (Brand, Schielke, Brams, et al., 2017; Dalenberg, Straus, & Ardill, 2017; Frankel, 2009; Frankel & Dalenberg, 2006; Rocchio, 2020). Measures should be included that address issues related to the case and have been validated with samples similar to the evaluee. Assessment measures should be selected based on evidence of adequate utility scores and error rates with traumatized samples. The possibility of exaggeration, malingering, and response sets must be considered and examined (Bush et al., 2020; Heilbrun et al., 2009).

Many tests designed to detect symptom exaggeration and feigning rely on detecting the endorsement of symptoms determined to be too numerous, unusual, or severe (Rogers & Bender, 2018). An example illuminates the risk of this approach. The Structured Interview of Reported Symptoms (SIRS; Rogers et al., 1992) is a widely used and validated measure for assessing malingering. However, several items on the SIRS are associated with trauma exposure; endorsement of these items increases one's scores and therefore the probability of being classified as possibly malingering. For example, three items on the Rare Symptoms subscale relate to possible dissociative phenomena (see Chapter 4). Research has shown that the SIRS misclassifies approximately one third of those who experienced complex trauma (Rogers et al., 2009) as well as one third of individuals with DID as potentially malingering (Brand, McNary, et al., 2006; Brand, Tursich, et al., 2014). Rogers subsequently added a "Trauma Index," which consists of items that traumatized individuals do not typically endorse (Rogers et al., 2010) and does not overclassify them as feigning (Brand, Tursich, et al., 2014; Rogers et al., 2009).

Forensic examiners must know the ways in which complex trauma survivors can appear to be exaggerating or feigning, and they must consider this as part of their assessment (Brand & Brown, 2023; L. S. Brown, 2009; Demakis & Elhai, 2011). Otherwise, they may draw conclusions that are not supported by research. Furthermore, they may unknowingly use measures that have questionable validity with traumatized individuals.

Chapter 3 offers guidance about process-related issues regarding assessing traumatized and potentially dissociative individuals. However, forensic examiners typically do not use the more therapeutically oriented procedures described in that chapter because of the difference in roles between clinicians and forensic assessors. If such approaches are used, they need to be thoughtfully applied and made explicit to the court, including the rationale for their use (see an example in Loewenstein, 2020).

ARE DISSOCIATIVE DISORDERS EASY TO MALINGER?

Malingering is a general concern in any forensic psychological evaluation, but particularly so in the case of trauma and severely dissociative trauma survivors. There are a multitude of reasons for this concern (Brand & Brown, 2023). Allegations of trauma are frequent in the individuals encountered in forensic contexts. Persons with a history of trauma are more likely to be the "eggshell plaintiff," that is, unusually negatively affected by allegedly tortious action (Bailey & Brown, 2020). Trauma exposure is extremely common in criminal defendants. Despite this, trauma's impact has rarely been considered during the creation of psychological tests, including tests of malingering.

Fantasy model theorists who believe that dissociation is caused by fantasy and suggestibility rather than trauma (see Chapter 2) state that it is easy for DDs to be malingered (Merckelbach & Patihis, 2018; Paris, 2019). Merckelbach and Patihis (2018) argued that malingerers tend to show "total amnesia for personal identity and past knowledge" (p. 3). This statement shows these researchers, who are not clinicians, are unfamiliar with actual presentations of DID and are not aware of the extensive research that indicates it is not easy to feign DID. Individuals with genuine DID do not tend to report *total* amnesia for identity or past knowledge (Brand et al., 2018); therefore, such reports should raise the index of suspicion of malingering DID (American Psychiatric Association, 2022).

Furthermore, although extensive research shows that many measures can distinguish genuine from malingered dissociation, there are notable exceptions, such as the Structured Interview of Malingered Symptomatology (SIMS; Smith & Burger, 1997). The SIMS does not show adequate ability to distinguish genuine from simulated DID, with a very low specificity of 0.14 (Brand, Barth, et al., 2021; see Chapter 2). The SIMS includes subscales such as amnesia and seemingly neurological symptoms that were thought to be rare but are not rare in TRD (Schiavone et al., 2018). Therefore, it is not surprising that the SIMS performed so poorly with individuals with TRD. This is important to recognize because fantasy model theorists have often used the SIMS in research claiming to show that dissociative individuals are prone to exaggeration.

Chapter 4 presents the research on measures and methods that are useful in assessing genuine versus malingered TRD. To avoid redundancy, only citations of the studies that used TRD samples and their utility scores are provided here in Tables 5.1 and 5.2. Researchers have found false-negative rates (the proportion of feigners misclassified as having genuine DID) that are similar to the false-negative rates for other disorders (Brand et al., 2018; Brand, Frewen, et al., 2021). For example, a review found the false-negative rate for the gold standard interview for diagnosing dissociative disorders, the Structured Clinical Interview for Dissociative Disorders (SCID-D and SCID-D-R; Steinberg, 1994b) was approximately zero and 22% for the Test of Memory Malingering (TOMM; Brand et al., 2018).

In one study comparing DID with DID simulators on the Minnesota Multiphasic Personality Inventory–2 (MMPI-2), the validity scales failed to achieve a positive predictive power (PPP) higher than .66 (Brand & Chasson, 2015); see Figure 5.1. Nonetheless, a discriminant function analysis that combined validity and clinical subscale predictors yielded a sensitivity of 83.0%, specificity of 86.0%, PPP of 68.8%, and overall diagnostic power of

TABLE 5.1. Utility Statistics and Error Rates for Measures With Dissociative Disorder Samples

DID to DID feigning	Sample	Method of diagnosing DD	Measure	Sensitivity[a]	Specificity[b]	False-negative rate[c]	False positive rate[d]
Welburn et al., (2003)	DID n = 12 DID Feigners n = 10	Interviewers blind to study hypotheses and group status	SCID-D	100%	100%	0%	0%
Brand et al., (2006)	DID n = 20 DID Feigners n = 43	Outpatient or inpatient team diagnosed with DID confirmed with SCID-D	SIRS	49%	65%	51%	35%
Brand, Tursich, et al. (2014)	DID n = 49 DID Feigners n = 77	Outpatient or inpatient team diagnosed DID confirmed with SCID-D	SIRS-2 with and without TI	TI alone = .86 SIRS-2 with or without TI 56%-86%	TI alone = 80% SIRS-2 with or without TI 92%-100%	TI alone = 14% SIRS-2 with or without TI = 14%-44%	TI alone = 20% SIRS-2 with or without TI = 0%-8%
Brand & Chasson (2015)	DID n = 53 DID Feigners n = 144	Outpatient or inpatient team diagnosed DID confirmed with SCID-D	MMPI-2	Fp performed best among single validity scales = 79% but PPP still only 66% Best predictor: Composite of predictors = 83%	Fp = 85% Composite of predictors = 86%	Fp = 21% Composite of predictors = 17%	Fp = 15% Composite of predictors = 14%
Ambrose et al. (2023)	DID n = 30 Feigners n = 43	Outpatient or inpatient team initially diagnosed DID, confirmed with SCID-D	MMPI-2 F, Fb, Fp, S, VRIN, F-K, Fptsd	Sensitivity .86-1.00 (VRIN = .14)	Specificity .80-.97	8% (VRIN = 36%)	8%

Study	Sample	Diagnosis	Test				
Palermo & Brand (2019)	DID *n* = 20 DDNOS *n* = 19 DID Feigners *n* = 51	Diagnosed by inpatient treatment team after being observed for 1 week	TSI-2 Atypical Response Scale	.47–.92	.49–.77	8–53%	23–51%
Brand, Webermann, et al. (2019)	DID *n* = 31 DID Feigners *n* = 74	71% were inpatients diagnosed by treatment team after being observed	TOMM	Trial 1 = .78 Trial 2 = .64	Trial 1 = .87 Trial 2 = .97	Trial 1 = 22% Trial 2 = 36%	Trial 1 = 13% Trial 2 = 3%
Barth et al. (2023)	DID *n* = 35 DID Feigners *n* = 88	DID diagnosed by SCID-D	M-FAST	Cutoff 6 = .93 Cutoff 7 = .96	Cutoff 6 = .75 Cutoff 7 = .89	Cutoff 6 = .07 Cutoff 7 = .04	Cutoff 6 = .25 Cutoff 7 = .11
Brand, Barth, et al. (2021)	DID *n* = 63 DID Feigners *n* = 90	DID diagnosed by SCID-D	SIMS	.96	.14	.04	.86

Note. DD = dissociative disorder; DDNOS = dissociative disorder not otherwise specified; DID = dissociative identity disorder; F = Infrequency scale; Fb = Back Infrequency scale; F-K = Gough's Simulation Index; Fptsd = Infrequency-Posttraumatic Stress Disorder scale; Fp = Infrequency-Psychopathology scale; M-FAST = Miller Forensic Assessment of Symptoms Test; PPP = positive predictive power; SCID-D-R = Structured Clinical Interview for Dissociative Disorders-Revised; SIMS = Structured Inventory of Malingered Symptomatology; SIRS = Structured Interview of Reported Symptoms; TI = Trauma Index on SIRS/SIRS-2; TOMM = Test of Memory Malingering; TSI-2 = Trauma Symptom Inventory-2; S = Superlative; VRIN = Variable Response Inconsistency. Adapted from "Trauma-Related Dissociation Is No Fantasy: Addressing the Errors of Omission and Commission in Merckelbach and Patihis (2018)," by B. L. Brand, C. J. Dalenberg, P. A. Frewen, R. J. Loewenstein, H. J. Schielke, J. S. Brams, and D. Spiegel, 2018, *Psychological Injury and Law, 11*(4), p. 383 (https://doi.org/10.1007/s12207-018-9336-8). Copyright 2018 by Springer Nature. Adapted with permission.
[a]Tests ability to classify feigners correctly. [b]Tests ability to classify DID patients correctly. [c]Proportion of patients misclassified as feigners by test; 1 – sensitivity. [d]Proportion of feigners missed by test; 1 – specificity.

TABLE 5.2. Utility Statistics SCID-D/SCID-D-R With Dissociative Disorder Samples

Authors	Sample	Clinical diagnostic procedure	SCID-D/SCID-D-R procedure	Test or interview	Sensitivity[a]	Specificity[b]	Error rate
Presence vs. absence of DD							
Boon & Draijer (1993c)	45 mixed control patients, 45 DD patients (21 DID and 24 DDNOS)	Clinicians diagnosed DD patients with assistance from an independent DD expert	Random sample of 16 SCID-D interviews rated by three psychologists and three psychiatrists (one self-described as "skeptical" about DID)	SCID-D	100%	95.6%	4.4% of patients misclassified as having DID
DID vs. other disorder							
Welburn et al. (2003)	Schizophrenia n = 9 DID n = 12 Controls randomly assigned: • Healthy n = 9 • DID feigners n = 10	Psychiatrists specializing in schizophrenia or DD	Interviewers blind to study hypotheses and group status	SCID-D	100% for DID	89% DID vs. schizophrenia (one patient in latter group classified as DDNOS rather than DID)	11% of patients misclassified as having DID

Note. DD = dissociative disorder; DID = dissociative identity disorder; SCID-D/SCID-D-R = Structured Clinical Interview for Dissociative Disorders–Revised; SIRS = Structured Interview of Reported Symptoms; TI = Trauma Index on SIRS/SIRS-2; TOMM = Test of Memory Malingering; TSI-2 = Trauma Symptom Inventory-2. Adapted from "Trauma-Related Dissociation Is No Fantasy: Addressing the Errors of Omission and Commission in Merckelbach and Patihis (2018)," by B. L. Brand, C. J. Dalenberg, P. A. Frewen, R. J. Loewenstein, H. J. Schielke, J. S. Brams, and D. Spiegel, 2018, *Psychological Injury and Law, 11*(4), p. 381 (https://doi.org/10.1007/s12207-018-9336-8). Copyright 2018 by Springer Nature. Adapted with permission.
[a]Tests ability to correctly classify feigners. [b]Tests ability to correctly classify DID patients.

FIGURE 5.1. MMPI-2 Profiles Across Groups

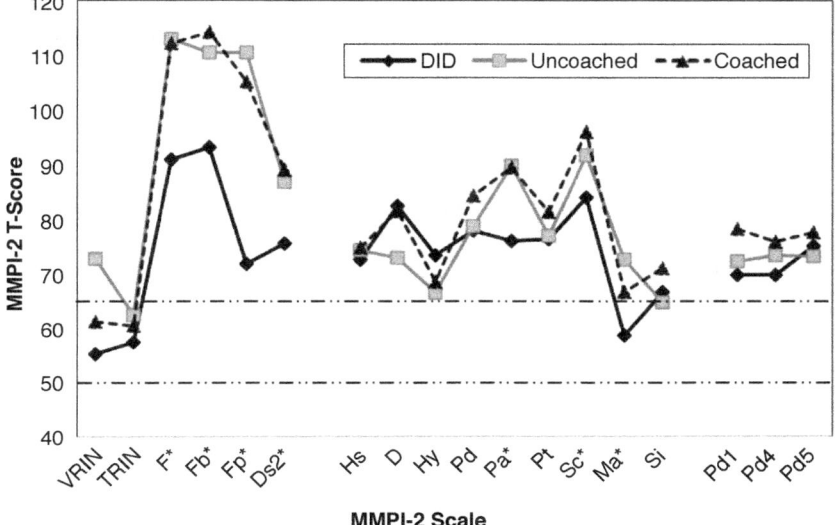

Note. MMPI-2 = Minnesota Multiphasic Personality Inventory–2. From "Distinguishing Simulated From Genuine Dissociative Identity Disorder on the MMPI-2," by B. L. Brand and G. S. Chasson, 2015, *Psychological Trauma: Theory, Research, Practice, and Policy, 7*(1), p. 97 (https://doi.org/10.1037/a0035181). Copyright 2015 by the American Psychological Association.

85.3%. The error rate using the equation was 17%. (See the published study for the classification equation with constants and coefficients that can be applied in forensic cases.)

A recent study comparing DID with DID simulators found that most of the MMPI-2's validity scales were successful in accurately distinguishing the groups in the sample of 73 White females (Ambrose et al., 2023). In this study, PPP was higher than .88 for F, Fb, Fp, S, F-K, and Fptsd. A discriminant function analysis classified correctly 72 of 73 individuals; it misclassified one feigner as a DID patient. See Chapter 4 for further discussion.

The false-positive rates (the rate at which a measure misclassifies individuals with DID as feigners) was zero with the SCID-D, between 0% and 8% with the SIRS-2, 11% with the Miller Forensic Assessment of Symptoms Test (M-FAST), 3% with the TOMM, and between 1% and 8% with the validity subscales on the MMPI-2 (Ambrose et al., 2023; Brand et al., 2018). These data indicate that it is not easy to feign DID if the measures are chosen according to research with individuals with TRD. The following studies are the sources for these data. (See Tables 5.1 and 5.2 for utility statistics.)

- MMPI-2 (Ambrose et al., 2023; Brand & Chasson, 2015; Brand, Chasson, et al., 2016; Butcher et al., 2001; see Figure 5.1)

- Personality Assessment Inventory (PAI; Morey, 1991; Stadnik et al., 2013; see Figure 5.2)

- SIRS/SIRS-2 including the Trauma Index, which significantly improves its utility (Brand, McNary, et al., 2006; Brand, Tursich, et al., 2014; Rogers et al., 2009, 2010)

- Trauma Symptom Inventory–2 (TSI-2; Briere, 2011; Palermo & Brand, 2019)

- TOMM (Brand, Webermann, et al., 2019; Tombaugh, 2003)

- M-FAST (Barth et al., 2023; Miller, 2001)

- SIMS (Brand, Barth, et al., 2021; Smith & Burger, 1997; also see Chapters 2 and 4 for information about the SIMS' lack of validity in any type of psychological assessment)

To date, the TOMM is the only symptom validity measure that has been studied with individuals high in TRD (Brand, Webermann, et al., 2019). The TOMM did not overclassify individuals diagnosed with DID as feigners. This research suggests that the memory problems associated with this disorder was not exaggerated or resulting from a lack of effort (Brand, Webermann, et al., 2019).

Individuals who feign DID have been found to overendorse symptoms in general, as is found in the general malingering literature (Rogers & Bender, 2018). Furthermore, DID feigners often endorse media-based stereotypes of DID and tend to miss the subtle, less-known symptoms and struggles such as depression, anxiety, and somatic symptoms (Ambrose et al., 2023; Brand & Chasson, 2015). Feigners strongly elevate on psychotic subscales over mood disturbance and somatic subscales of the MMPI-2, with an average of 29-point difference between these scales, compared with genuine DID individuals having comparably high scores on these symptoms with an average of 6-point difference (Ambrose et al., 2023). Feigners portray themselves as much more angry, aggressive, and sadistic toward animals and other people than do individuals with true DID. The endorsement of sadism toward animals is particularly striking because clinical experience indicates that many severely traumatized individuals, including those with DID, are able to trust animals and develop supportive, loving relationships

FIGURE 5.2. PAI Profile for DID/DDNOS Patients With T ≥ 70 Elevations Highlighted

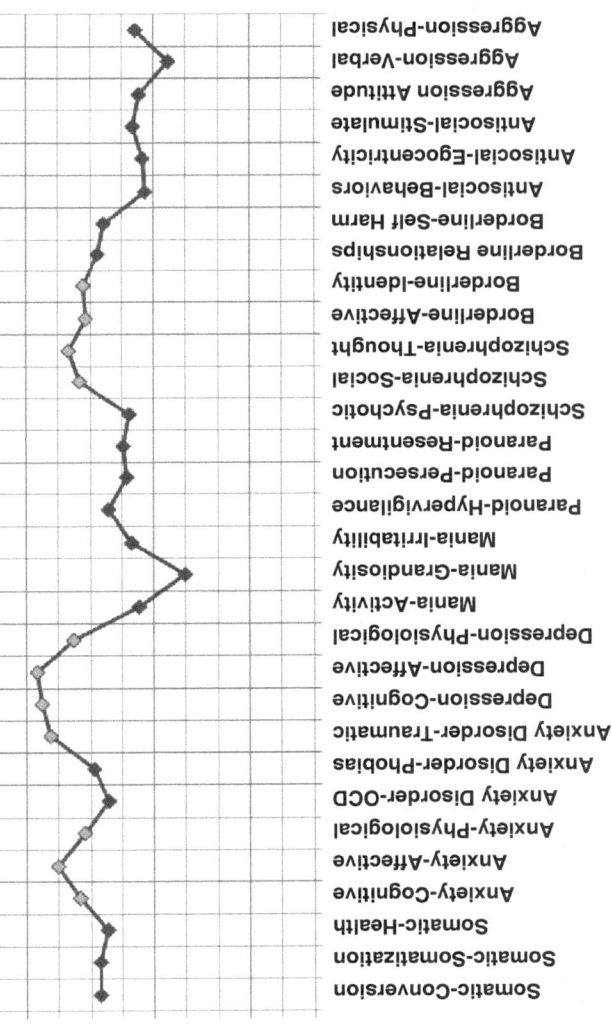

DDNOS = dissociative disorder not otherwise specified; DID = dissociative identity disorder; OCD = obsessive compulsive disorder; PAI = Personality Assessment Inventory. From "Personality Assessment Inventory Profile and Predictors of Elevations Among Dissociative Disorder Patients," by R. D. Stadnik, B. Brand, and A. Savoca, 2013, *Journal of Trauma & Dissociation, 14*(5), p. 554 (https://doi.org/10.1080/15299732.2013.792310). Copyright 2013 by Taylor & Francis. Reprinted with permission.

with pets, even when they are highly mistrustful of people. In fact, animal-assisted treatment for traumatized people has proven beneficial, according to a meta-analytic review (Hediger et al., 2021), and is associated with reductions in dissociation in traumatized children (Dietz et al., 2012). Feigned portrayals of DID suggest that stigmatizing, media-based stereotypes of DID are likely influencing the endorsement patterns of feigners. Little research has been conducted about malingering of other DDs. More research on the feigning of TRD and other DDs using well-diagnosed, genuine clinical samples and more psychological measures is urgently needed.

Social media may be contributing to more sophisticated malingered as well as factitious presentations of DDs, also referred to as "false imputation" and "imitative" DID, because access to information about DID has increased considerably with the availability of depictions and discussions of the disorder on social media and the internet (Draijer & Boon, 1999). In these cases, individuals believe they have a disorder they do not truly have. Distinguishing whether these cases are factitious, malingered, an atypical DD, or a combination of these is difficult. Their management can be quite difficult because if the clinician does not find evidence of DID, these clients often become angry and defensive and feel humiliated. Even if they do not meet criteria for DID, they may have experienced trauma and may exhibit some genuine dissociative symptoms. This is addressed in other chapters of this book. Imitative or false imputation cases of DID typically lack the complex comorbidity and the avoidance and ambivalence about dissociation. Those with imitative DID often are intrigued and seem to enjoy thinking, writing, talking, and sometimes even posting information and pictures about their "parts" on social media, which sharply contrasts the disavowal and discomfort that characterizes most individuals with DID (Kluft, 1987b; Loewenstein et al., in press). Individuals with imitative DID often report having DID with atypical features. For example, they often describe having an unusual degree of awareness of their self-states with little or no conflict among parts or little or no amnesia (or alternatively, reported "total amnesia" between "parts"; Boon & Draijer, 1993a).

SPECIAL ISSUES IN FORENSIC EVALUATION OF DISSOCIATIVE TRAUMA SURVIVORS

Some adaptations to the assessment process may allow trauma survivors to be more accurately assessed. Complex trauma survivors often require longer than other examinees to develop enough familiarity with the examiner and the assessment process to share personal details of their lives; they may also need additional time to review histories of what may be multiple traumas (Rocchio, 2020). It is important to assess a person's lifetime exposure to traumatic events, including events early in development (Bailey & Brown, 2020). Determining which, if any, traumatic experiences may have a bearing on the forensic issue at hand requires developing careful timelines of reported symptoms and life events, examining a wide range of records to determine if there is corroborating evidence, interviewing collateral individuals who may have seen signs of psychological distress, and conducting formal assessments with validated measures (preferably those which have been studied with traumatized samples). Detailed descriptions about what was occurring before, during, and after an alleged injury or crime can be especially useful in considering various hypotheses in forensic cases.

Forensic evaluations should assess the broad range of possible posttraumatic conditions. It is particularly important to assess for those symptoms "on the more complex end of the spectrum that are frequently either invisible or baffling to forensic evaluators whose training has not included this emerging area of study" (p. 109; Bailey & Brown, 2020). Severely dissociative individuals may be unable to report their symptoms and life history accurately or consistently due to amnesia; their recall can vary according to fluctuations in dissociation (Bailey et al., 2019). This can be confusing for assessors, who may mistake this for malingering, dementia, personality disorder symptoms, or substance abuse. These alternative hypotheses must also be carefully considered, particularly in forensic assessment.

The length of time needed for assessment meetings is highly case dependent. Some examinees may need many shorter appointments due to how tiring and triggering the process may be. A "trigger" is the emergence of emotions, memories, or thoughts in response to some stimulus (Briere & Scott, 2012). The individual may reexperience sensory elements of the trauma or sudden emotional distress related to the trauma. Often individuals do not recognize that their reactions, which seem to be "out of the blue," are trauma related. However, if a complex DD is present, the assessor may be more likely to observe TRD as the individual tires, even if the individual is attempting to hide or avoid dissociating. In the case of possible malingered TRD, maintaining a malingered presentation for hours is more challenging than doing so for a short period of time.

In cases of complex trauma, it is crucial to pace the interview carefully (see Chapter 3). Signs of dissociation are often subtle. Many complex trauma survivors have learned not to show their reactions because showing emotion provokes some perpetrators to be more humiliating or aggressive. It is adaptive in extremely threatening situations to disconnect from one's body, mind, and emotions, rather than experience and show emotions (see Chapter 1). It allows the victim to hold perfectly still despite being terrified, thereby possibly minimizing the risk of even more harm, as described in the tonic immobility response. Examiners need to watch carefully for signs of emotional or behavioral underarousal that may indicate dissociation because these signs are not as obvious as overt signs of distress, such as crying.

As described in Chapter 3, it is crucial to observe carefully and inquire sensitively about what the assessee is thinking and feeling (both physically and emotionally) throughout the assessment. For example, a woman was intently looking just above the examiner's head for an extended time; she seemed to be concentrating on something, although nothing other than bricks was visible. When invited to share what she was doing, the assessee explained she was counting the bricks because it helped her not "get lost." When asked about what "not getting lost" meant, it became clear that this was a grounding technique that the woman had developed in her youth to avoid dissociating. Trauma survivors frequently rely on coping techniques such as this, along with denial, avoidance, minimization, and dissociation (Dalenberg, Straus, & Carlson, 2017). Avoidance of trauma and related emotion can be subtle. The individual may repeatedly shift topics without fully answering questions, avoid revealing emotions or other reactions, or be vague in their descriptions. For example, when asked if she had ever experienced any unwanted sexual experiences, an assessee responded, "Yeah, but that happens to everyone." The examiner persisted, "Can you tell me about what happened to you?" The examinee replied, "I don't remember much about it," to which the examiner said, "Would it be OK for you to allow yourself to think about it and share as much as you can remember?"

Carefully documenting the discussions and behavioral observations is important, including recording signs of when possible over- or underarousal occurs. Some examiners record video of examinations, whereas others prefer to take extensive notes (Brand, Schielke, Brams, et al., 2017; Dalenberg, Straus, & Ardill, 2017). Many symptoms of PTSD and TRD are experiential and so must be reported rather than observed (e.g., nightmares, intrusive emotions that the individual experiences as "not mine"). However, rather than relying only on an examinee's report of symptoms, the examiner must carefully observe and document the sequence of statements; the quality, content, and organization of thought; shifts in emotion or lack thereof; defenses such as dissociation or avoidance; requests for repeating questions or directions; shifts in use of pronouns and verb tenses; and other nonverbal behaviors that provide an important source of data in a multimethod assessment. For example, in the case of Mr. Ramirez (later in the chapter), who was reluctant to acknowledge his psychological problems, including dissociation, the examiner's notes became a crucial piece of evidence because they illustrated that he avoided emotions and detailed discussions related to trauma more than a dozen times. He did not know he engaged in avoidance, and he may not have been willing to report it if he had been aware.

Examiners' notes or recordings can illustrate the changes in the complexity of language or subtle shifts in word usage. For example, traumatized individuals may briefly lose time orientation when discussing trauma, and in some cases, this may result in them feeling as if the trauma is happening now, rather than in the past (Brand, Schielke, Brams, et al., 2017). For example, in a civil case against a minister about alleged sexual abuse, an evaluee shifted verb tenses. "He made me come to the back room with him. He . . . uh . . . started . . . uh . . . sort of . . . um . . . you . . . rubbing . . . and he puts his hand over my mouth . . . and he's pushing me down." As she described the sexual abuse, the plaintiff shifted to present tense verbs and became less organized and more fragmented in her speech, consistent with research (Andrews et al., 2000; Foa et al., 1995; Harvey & Bryant, 1999; Jones et al., 2005; Malmo & Laidlaw, 2010). If severe, this shift in time orientation might indicate the individual is experiencing a flashback. Dissociative distancing from one's body may be reflected in the assessee referring to their body as "the body" or "the arm," rather than "my body" or "my arm." Individuals with DID may shift from referring to themselves as "I" or "me" to "we" or "us."

Behavioral indicators of dissociation are frequently observed in evaluations of dissociative evaluees (Brand et al., 2018). (See Chapter 3 for a list of these behaviors.) Many of these have been empirically validated, including "spacing out" and identity confusion observed by others, which are included on the validated Child Dissociative Checklist (CDC; Putnam et al., 1993). Eye flutter and eye roll are associated with dissociative as well as hypnotic states (Spiegel, 1972), with eye-roll capacity correlating 0.55 with dissociation (Torem et al., 1995).

Professionals are usually well trained in detecting common and easily observed symptoms, such as agitation and hyperventilation, but most are less knowledgeable and experienced in detecting hypoarousal and TRD (see Chapter 3). Similarly, juries, attorneys, and judges often need to be taught that an evaluee's apparent lack of emotion may be due to TRD. Experts serve an important role when they educate the courts about this possible presentation of dissociation.

Behavioral observations such as these are important data points in multi-method assessment:

> Such behavioral signs, while alone insufficient to confirm or refute diagnosis, provide either converging or diverging data supporting overall diagnostic hypotheses garnered from multiple data sources, and this approach should apply equally to dissociative disorders as any other, such as major depressive disorder. (Brand et al., 2018, p. 384)

The process of discussing trauma, as well as the process of undergoing a forensic examination, can be highly distressing or triggering. Talking about the legal case can be terribly upsetting for some people, as can be discussing traumatic experiences.

CULTURAL COMPETENCE IN FORENSIC EVALUATIONS OF TRD

Forensic examiners should be attentive to aspects of the individual's cultural background and the ways in which it impacts their exposure to traumatic events and interactions with the legal system (Rocchio, 2020). Cultural competence requires that professionals understand the meanings that stem from the individual's cultural background, contextual variables, and their intersectional identities to make each person's response to alleged trauma unique. Gender, culture, age, and other personal aspects of identity may lead to normative under- or overreporting of symptoms (Brand & Brown, 2023). For example, women from Hispanic and Caribbean backgrounds may normatively express affect in a way that others who are not from that background may perceive as "histrionic" or exaggerated (Ballou & Brown, 2002). Caution should be used in determining whether what appears to be exaggeration may be a characteristic style versus malingering. Asking the individual to describe a positive experience may provide a source of information about their characteristic style of expressing strong emotion. The client who strongly expresses positive emotion is likely to show a similar style in responding to negative emotion and life events (Brand & Brown, 2023). Alternatively, when interacting with authority figures or highly stressful situations, some trauma survivors dissociate due to this being their overlearned response to earlier trauma (see Chapter 1). This apparent lack of emotion can easily be misunderstood by individuals who do not consider cultural contexts and trauma adaptations. I have seen numerous criminal cases in which examiners, detectives, first responders, and others involved in the case misinterpreted a dissociative response as an indication of sociopathy or antisocial personality disorder.

Some aspects of identity can increase the likelihood of experiencing trauma and developing dissociative symptoms, especially if the individual identifies with a group that is disempowered within the dominant culture (Bailey & Brown, 2020). The common, low-level historical stressors known as "insidious traumatization" (Root, 1992) and "microaggressions" (Nadal, 2018) may not be considered by the current *DSM-5-TR* as PTSD Criterion A traumas, yet they can nonetheless activate the stress response system and cumulatively result in a stress and fear response that is important to recognize. Individuals from targeted groups may appear to be hypervigilant or paranoid, or they may appear to be emotionless due to TRD. Trauma survivors who have been harmed generally feel highly mistrustful of others, particularly authority figures (Ford & Courtois, 2020b; Herman, 1992b); this may include mistrust of police, attorneys, forensic examiners, and others in forensic contexts. Mistrust of the police and others may be particularly pronounced if the examinee is not White, given the frequency and severity of police violence against people of color. This pronounced mistrust may bias examiners' interpretations, especially if they are White, due to racial differences as well as the societal power imbalance in the relationship (Bailey & Brown, 2020). This power imbalance may impact the evaluee's behavior, the information they are willing to reveal, and their testing results, as in the Ramirez case that follows.

Examiners need to be culturally competent and consider the impact of trauma and examinees' potential lack of trust when they interpret test results (Brand & Brown, 2023). If examiners are not aware of these potential influences and do not sensitively follow recommendations for assessing complex trauma survivors, they may not adequately understand the individual they are assessing and may overlook or misunderstand trauma-related behaviors or symptoms (e.g., Bailey & Brown, 2020; Brand, Schielke, & Brams, 2017; Brand, Schielke, Brams, et al., 2017; Rocchio, 2020).

Individuals with complex DDs are often misdiagnosed and underserved, facing multiple assessment and treatment barriers. In many cases they have been poorly treated by clinicians as well as authority figures, such as caregivers (Nester, Hawkins, et al., 2022). Furthermore, they are an understudied, often misunderstood group and could be considered a trauma-based minoritized mental health group (Loewenstein, 2018). As such, mental health professionals, including forensic examiners, need to develop cultural competence regarding working with groups that experience layers of minoritization, stigma, and trauma, including individuals with DDs, especially individuals whose identities result in intersecting sources of disempowerment and trauma. This is critically important with Black and Latino defendants, who experience disparities in prosecution and sentencing (Kutateladze et al., 2014; Schweizer, 2013).

The Case of "Mr. Juan Ramirez"

The following case illustrates the importance of being aware of the influence of trauma, dissociation, and cultural issues in forensic assessments. It is based on a compilation of cases in my practice. "Mr. Juan Ramirez" was a defendant in a capital (death penalty) murder trial. He adamantly denied he committed the murder despite compelling DNA and other strong evidence.

During a meeting with the state's forensic examiner, Mr. Ramirez was triggered by seeing the examiner's leather belt. Afterward, he reported to his defense team that he had panicked when he saw the belt because it reminded him of the belt his father used to beat him with throughout childhood. He questioned his attorneys whether the examiner "wore that kind of belt on purpose to taunt me." His defense team had to work carefully for more than a year to gain Mr. Ramirez's trust, which they understood to still be tenuous at times, so they did not contradict his paranoid concern. After seeing the belt, Mr. Ramirez reported he had felt numb and detached from his body, a state which he reported experiencing for the remainder of the meeting. Mr. Ramirez did not tell the state's examiner that he was triggered by his belt; he did not trust him enough to share that information. Furthermore, he was highly ambivalent about recognizing and disclosing how often he dissociated. Within less than a half hour of meeting Mr. Ramirez, the state's examiner launched into questions about trauma exposure and dissociative symptoms, stating that he understood from reading the defense examiners' notes that Mr. Ramirez reported he had been beaten in childhood and that he "supposedly" had dissociative symptoms. Mr. Ramirez handled these affrontive statements in his usually avoidant way: He avoided sharing anything other than brief, summary statements about his father's beatings. He denied he dissociated except during one well-documented event as an adolescent. The forensic examiner did not ask Mr. Ramirez how he responded to the beatings, nor how he was feeling during the meeting with the examiner.

Even though it might have been helpful for his own defense to share details about the unrelenting, severe physical and emotional abuse he suffered throughout childhood, Mr. Ramirez avoided this level of disclosure due to mistrust of authority figures, particularly White men, and his ingrained pattern of avoiding talking or thinking about anything related to trauma. Instead, Mr. Ramirez simply acknowledged his father repeatedly beat him, but he stated he could not recall much other than it "happened all the time." The examiner asked about one of the violent episodes that eyewitnesses reported in which his father beat him with a hanger while telling him he wished that he had never been born. According to a reliable witness, the young boy had crawled away on the floor and curled up into a ball "like a beaten dog." Mr. Ramirez shrugged and said he did not remember that.

The state's forensic examiner did not use standardized measures of trauma exposure or dissociation, nor did he seem to recognize how often Mr. Ramirez shifted the conversation away from trauma. The state's examiner failed to ask Mr. Ramirez how he was feeling emotionally or physically at any point during any of his three examinations, which were videotaped. (See the discussion in Chapter 3 about the importance of easing into difficult material and inquiring sensitively about trauma exposure, TRD, and the examinee's reactions to the interview.) The state's examiner noticed Mr. Ramirez's lack of emotion but did not recognize that it may have been due to dissociation. The examiner concluded that Mr. Ramirez showed no affect even when discussing what would normally be upsetting topics such as trauma. He testified that Mr. Ramirez's (apparent) lack of affect was due to antisocial personality disorder, although he also diagnosed him as having PTSD. Examiners for both sides assessed for, but did not find, evidence of malingering.

In contrast, the defense's forensic experts used procedures and measures that sensitively addressed trauma-related reactions as well as the full range of possible psychological disorders. The defense team and defense experts interviewed various witnesses, including primary school teachers who recalled how Mr. Ramirez often seemed "far away," "daydreamy," and "out of it, not paying attention." One teacher who remembered him well stated she had been puzzled by his variable recall for facts he clearly knew. Another witness described Mr. Ramirez being so caught up in daydreaming when playing baseball as a boy that he got hit by a ball and simply walked away, seemingly still in a daze and not showing any pain. These experiences seemed possibly to be early signs of TRD that was developing because of his father's chronic abuse. Many witnesses corroborated that his father had been a violent alcoholic who took his rage out on Mr. Ramirez and other family members.

A mental health record showed evidence of symptoms of PTSD (e.g., nightmares, flashbacks, hypervigilance, irritability) and depression during his adolescence; there was no mention of examination for or symptoms consistent with dissociation. This was not surprising, given that clinicians in the field knew even less about the assessment of dissociation during the time when Mr. Ramirez was a child. Close family members were either dead or unwilling to speak to the defense team. Mr. Ramirez was upset by his defense team's efforts to present his trauma history and his psychological disorders as possible influences on his behavior and as mitigation factors. He almost refused to allow them to use this defense strategy and considered firing them, but ultimately agreed when they repeatedly explained that he was likely to be sentenced to death if they did not help the jury understand his development and behavior. The defense's experts diagnosed Mr. Ramirez with severe PTSD, major depressive disorder, and other specified dissociative disorder. Although the jury found him guilty of murder, they reported after the trial ended that they believed his years of being abused as a child and suffering from serious psychological disorders were mitigating factors. He was sentenced to 20 years in prison.

CRIMINAL CASES OF ALLEGED DISSOCIATIVE DISORDERS

It is not uncommon in criminal cases for defendants to allege dissociative amnesia for their behavior or, less frequently, to claim to have different personalities and that the "bad one" engaged in the criminal behavior. Assessing such reports to determine whether someone with alleged amnesia or DID is reporting genuine or exaggerated symptoms requires a rigorous approach to forensic assessment. The legal system and scholars have discussed how to respond to DID for decades (e.g., Kluft, 1987b; Loewenstein, 2020; Saks, 1994, 1995, 1997).

Extensive reports of amnesia, particularly when they are dramatic or are limited to primarily "bad" behaviors, are often suggestive of feigned amnesia or feigned DID (Coons & Milstein, 1994; Draijer & Boon, 1999). Individuals with borderline personality disorder reported higher levels of amnesia than did the DD group in one study, despite the DD individuals having higher levels of amnesia, according to the SCID-D-R (Şar, Alioğlu, Akyüz, et al., 2014). The authors interpreted this to mean that individuals with borderline personality disorder may be more aware of amnesia and less distressed about reporting it than the DD group.

Individuals with genuine DID typically show shifts in knowledge that are circumscribed, fluctuate over time, and cause shame and distress (Draijer & Boon, 1999; Spiegel et al., 2011). Individuals with DID do not typically enjoy discussing their dissociative self-states, amnesia, or other symptoms (Draijer & Boon, 1999; Steinberg, 2000), although this may be changing due to the influence of social media encouraging more open displays and discussions of a wide range of psychological problems. Individuals with DID are usually anxious about dissociative symptoms and attempt not to recognize or talk about these symptoms even in many criminal cases, as shown in the case of Mr. Ramirez. An absence of dissociation during examinations accompanied by a sense of pride or excitement about dissociative states or other symptoms is suggestive of possible factitious and malingered DID, rather than genuine DID (Draijer & Boon, 1999). Behavioral signs of dissociation, and ambivalence and discomfort in revealing information about dissociative symptoms, is characteristic of genuine DID (Draijer & Boon, 1999; Steinberg, 1994a).

Individuals malingering DID fail to report the lesser known comorbid conditions such as depression, somatoform disorders, and PTSD (Brand, Chasson, et al., 2016; Loewenstein, 2020). Instead, they emphasize stereotypic, media-hyped symptoms: unrealistically severe, lengthy periods of amnesia along with dramatic presentation and focus on personality states. Individuals malingering DID are prone to emphasize amnesia repeatedly for the alleged criminal behavior, often failing to realize at least some amnesia should occur throughout the lifespan of someone with DID and certainly should not occur for the first time at the time of the alleged criminal behavior (American Psychiatric Association, 2022). Feigners do not show the avoidance, shame, and hiding of dissociation that is characteristic among individuals with genuine DD, as illustrated by the Ramirez case.

Less than 5% of individuals with DID dramatically call attention to their parts and the process of switching, nor do the vast majority of individuals with DID readily know all about and disclose their dissociative states' "names" and "functions" (Kluft, 1991; Loewenstein, 2020). However, awareness of parts and their roles may be a focus of treatment for DID, so treatment history and the nature of the work done in treatment needs to be considered. Individuals with malingered DID do not usually endorse the passive influence intrusions (e.g., experiencing intrusive, puzzling emotions that are alien and "not mine"; thought insertion) that characterize genuine DID (see Chapter 1). Feigners rarely report the lifelong history of symptoms suggestive of PTSD and TRD. However, in genuine DID, symptoms such as nightmares, prolonged bedwetting, frequent trancelike states, or imaginary friends that continued well beyond the normative age may have been noticed by some friends, teachers, or family members in childhood and adolescence. Nonetheless, these signs were rarely recognized or treated as signs of possible trauma.

In cases of malingered DID that I have evaluated, malingerers show a desire to be diagnosed with DID, rather than demonstrating the more classic ambivalence or even reluctance to be diagnosed with a DD (see Chapter 4). For example, a middle-aged man who reported having DID asked at the end of an assessment for psychiatric disability, "Don't you need to see me switch to diagnose DID?" This assessment occurred when the *DSM*'s DID criteria required the clinician to observe a switch of self-states, which is no longer a requirement in the *DSM-5-TR*. His question suggested he had researched the criteria for DID. The man was well-groomed and well-dressed in a suit, indicating no obvious difficulty with hygiene and dressing, unlike many severely depressed and dissociative individuals. He showed no obvious symptoms or signs of distress or dissociation throughout a 7-hour assessment. He planned to use some of the disability money to take an extended vacation due to being "exhausted" by his "DID." Individuals with DID are typically more impaired than this man, although some function well until they become highly stressed or triggered by events such as an anniversary date of a trauma, the serious illness or death of an abuser, being retraumatized in adulthood, or a child they love reaching the age at which they were abused (American Psychiatric Association, 2022).

In another case, a young man presented dressed in the clothing, gloves, pill hat, and jewelry that were common among women in the 1950s. Despite how DID is portrayed in the media, I have never seen an individual with DID present in such a flagrantly dramatic, theatrical style. He gave a woman's name as his own name and indicated that he was one of "Jim's parts." This is highly atypical. Furthermore, this man denied a history of child abuse. He did not profess to have PTSD or any other psychological disorders. He was missing other key features and comorbidities associated with DID, including a history of amnesia and dissociation predating the alleged crime. Neither of these individuals' psychological testing was consistent with the assessment literature on DID. The man in the first case scored above the cutoffs on the M-FAST and SIRS, suggesting possible malingering. In the second case, there was no need to go beyond preliminary testing because "Jim" was clearly feigning DID.

The most challenging differential diagnostic cases entail apparently genuine trauma-based symptoms intermingled with exaggeration or malingering. Loewenstein (2020) described serving as an examiner in such a criminal case. The state's experts had sharply contrasting views of the defendant's competency to stand trial, her sanity, and whether she was malingering. Loewenstein was hired as an expert in DDs to address all three forensic issues. After completing a forensic assessment, Loewenstein diagnosed "Ms. Neely" with DID, PTSD, major depressive disorder without psychotic features, conversion disorder, somatoform pain disorder, and personality disorder not otherwise specified with severe antisocial, paranoid, and avoidant features. However, he also concluded that Ms. Neely was malingering some of her symptoms of DID (particularly her inability to control switching and the extent of amnesia), amnestic disorder, and somatic and somatoform symptoms. The defendant had a history of destruction of property, including vandalizing a former therapist's car and garage and stalking that therapist after she ended treatment with Ms. Neely. The current charges included two counts of arson and burglary, one of which was witnessed and the other of which took place in the home of a second therapist who had recently ended Ms. Neely's treatment. The defendant evaded questioning about the fires by suddenly beginning to switch chaotically to self-states that engaged in self-harm, causing the premature termination of the interview. Ms. Neely had a prior conviction for shoplifting which she had mostly evaded by claiming that dissociation "caused" the crime. Loewenstein's collateral interviews of her husband and son and his review of medical records suggested Ms. Neely had malingered some of her medical symptoms. Ms. Neely took an excessively long time to complete the SIRS. She also left so many questions unanswered that several tests (e.g., TSI-2) could not be interpreted. The totality of her behavior and history suggested conscious manipulation of the interviews and an attempt to interfere with the data collection. Importantly, when she was motivated to remember events and control her behavior, she could do so.

Loewenstein described Ms. Neely as acting unusually chaotic during the assessment. He assessed Ms. Neely's self-states directly to determine competency and sanity. Due to her level of apparently severe switching and dyscontrol, Loewenstein determined that it was necessary to use hypnotic containment techniques, with the goals of decreasing the intrusiveness of traumatic material, reducing overwhelming emotion, and decreasing switching so that Ms. Neely could complete the examination. Loewenstein articulated his rationale for using these techniques, which are typically reserved for treatment. He made it clear that he used containment techniques because the woman's chaotic switching and dyscontrol would have otherwise precluded a full forensic assessment. After using these techniques, her chaotic switching stopped, and she discussed the events related to the crimes. Loewenstein concluded that Ms. Neely had been aware of what she was doing and in sufficient control of her behavior when she entered her ex-therapist's home and set fire to objects in it. He opined that she was both competent and sane and that she had more control of her manipulative behavior than she led clinicians and forensic examiners to believe. Ms. Neely pled no contest to all charges and was sentenced to 5 to 15 years in prison with all but 5 years suspended. Lowenstein (2020) advised, "Clinical and forensic evaluation always should assess DID in terms of the individual self-states, the self-state-system, and the mind as a whole" (p. 219).

Notwithstanding Ms. Neely's case, experts in TRD sometimes conclude that individuals with DID are incompetent to stand trial or that they meet the standard for being legally insane. For example, Armstrong (2001) described the case of Mr. Woods, a man she diagnosed with DID whom she opined was so impaired by his dissociative and comorbid psychosis that he was not competent or sane. I, too, have seen some cases in which individuals with DID (typically with comorbid psychosis) were not sufficiently able to appreciate the criminality of their conduct or conform their behavior to the requirements of law (i.e., the standard for not guilty by reason of insanity, which varies slightly between states). If the court agrees that the individual was insane at the time of the criminal action, the individual may be sent to a forensic psychiatric hospital. Sometimes after reading forensic reports detailing the presence of well-corroborated chronic childhood trauma and the presence of severe psychiatric disorders including DDs (usually DID or other specified DD), prosecuting attorneys have agreed to stop pursuing capital punishment in exchange for the defendant admitting guilt and receiving a shorter sentence.

DISSOCIATION AND DAUBERT CRITERIA

Forensic experts may be permitted to offer testimony if their opinion is substantively and methodologically consistent with scientific procedures. Space constraints limit a full discussion about recovered memory and dissociative amnesia. For more information, see (Dalenberg, 2006; Dalenberg et al., 2012; Loewenstein et al., in press). Dalenberg (2006) reviewed the most rigorous studies of traumatic amnesia and recovered memories. Traumatic amnesia has been documented in adult rape survivors, child victims of physical and sexual abuse, victims of car accidents, war refugees, victims of traumatic loss, and survivors of natural disasters. Surveys of psychologists and published statements from professional organizations indicate that the concept of recovered memory is generally accepted in the scientific community.

Dalenberg's (2006) review found evidence for two paths to developing traumatic amnesia. First, dissociative detachment can contribute to a loss of emotional content, which can lead to the loss of factual content. Second, dissociative compartmentalization can interfere with the integration of emotion, sensory experience, and memory. Avoiding thinking about the trauma and state dependency are mechanisms that may contribute to dissociative compartmentalization. State dependency occurs when memories encoded in an emotional state, such as terror, are less accessible while the individual is not in that state. Dalenberg (2006) concluded, "Research during the past two decades has firmly established the reliability of the phenomenon of recovered memory" (p. 274).

Experts may be questioned about the scientific foundation supporting their testimony, referred to as the Daubert criteria (*Daubert v. Merrell Dow Pharmaceuticals*, 1993): whether their theory or technique can and has been tested, whether it has been subjected to peer review and publication, its known or potential error rate, and whether it has been generally accepted within the relevant scientific community. To succeed during Daubert questioning, experts must be able to support their opinions by showing that they followed scientifically supported procedures and used empirically validated tests. They need to be able to explain clearly that their opinion was derived from the scientific method. One method for conducting a forensic assessment that follows the scientific method involves looking for support or refutation of three possibilities: (a) This is a valid posttrauma presentation,

(b) this is a malingered presentation, or (c) there is a combination of both present. Experts should use tests and techniques that have known rates of error. For cases involving recovered memory, Dalenberg (2006) suggested extracting error rates from research such as from a prospective study (Williams, 1994, 1995) of recovered memory. In cases of possible DID, examiners can use tests and interviews that have been studied with DID samples and refer to their error rates (see Tables 5.1 and 5.2).

CONCLUSION

TRD is a common response to trauma that needs to be considered and assessed in many forensic contexts. Few mental health professionals receive systematic research-based training in TRD. That lack of training can contribute to misunderstanding and misdiagnosis, sometimes leading to injustices in forensic settings. This chapter advocates for using multimethod assessment consisting of measures and interviews that have been validated and peer reviewed to meet Daubert standards of admissibility when TRD may be part of the presentation. Developing knowledge, training, and experience with TRD and related research permits forensic examiners to be better prepared to understand TRD and knowledgeably differentiate genuine TRD from partially or wholly malingered dissociative conditions.

6

ASSESSING CHILD AND ADOLESCENT DISSOCIATIVE DISORDERS AND WHY IT MATTERS

AMIE MYRICK AND JOYANNA SILBERG

Note from Bethany Brand: The assessment and treatment of dissociative youth is overlooked and understudied, even more so than for dissociative adults. Many dissociative disorders begin to develop in childhood due to child maltreatment. There are often early signs of dissociation in traumatized youth, but few clinicians have adequate training and knowledge in dissociation, particularly developmental presentations of it. This chapter on assessing child and adolescent dissociative disorders is written by two experts in childhood trauma and dissociation, Amie Myrick and Joyanna Silberg.

The roots of most dissociative disorders (DDs) develop in the earliest years of childhood (Dutra et al., 2009; Kluft, 1984; Liotti, 2006; Putnam, 1997), yet clinical attention to childhood manifestations of DDs has been marginalized. As of 2022, there were only a handful of books about child treatment of DDs (Shirar, 1996; Silberg, 1998, 2022; Sinason & Marks, 2021; Struik, 2014; Waters, 2016; Wieland, 2015) and fewer still on theoretical aspects of child dissociation (Kluft, 1984; Putnam, 1997; Silberg, 2022; Sinason & Marks, 2021; Waters, 2016). Although some textbooks on trauma and psychopathology have begun to include chapters on child dissociation (Ford & Courtois, 2013;

https://doi.org/10.1037/0000386-006
The Concise Guide to the Assessment and Treatment of Trauma-Related Dissociation, by B. L. Brand

Gold, 2017; Lewis & Rudolph, 2014), there is still too little emphasis on this younger population in the dissociation literature.

MAKING THE CASE FOR ASSESSING DISSOCIATION IN YOUTH

Dissociation in youth is a robust clinical symptom and has powerful predictive validity for clinical risk and negative childhood outcome. One study found that a single item assessing dissociation predicted symptom severity, disrupted placements, hospitalizations, and risk-taking behaviors such as fire-setting for children involved with the child welfare system (Kisiel et al., 2020).[1] The fact that this single item had such strong predictive validity highlights the importance of paying attention to dissociative symptoms and disorders in the younger population. Yet often, little attempt is made to screen for or conceptualize childhood trauma-related dissociative symptomatology. The real-world results of failing to screen for dissociation, conceptualize symptoms as trauma-related dissociation (TRD), or understand the best ways to treat dissociative youth can be devastating. In one case, a 12-year-old girl diagnosed with dissociative identity disorder (DID) by three psychiatrists, languished in a juvenile detention center in Indiana after being refused entrance by 16 treatment facilities because all felt ill-equipped to handle her (Salinger, 2015). This sad scenario repeats itself as experts in child dissociation are flooded with calls nationwide from those seeking appropriate treatment for dissociative youth but who have few appropriate resources for referral. When overlooked, misdiagnosed, and/or misunderstood in treatment, unresolved dissociative symptoms can contribute to prolonged treatment and suffering for the child and their family and may continue into a chronic, disabling DD in adulthood.

DIAGNOSTIC CONSIDERATIONS

The *Diagnostic and Statistical Manual of Mental Disorders* (5th ed.; *DSM-5*; American Psychiatric Association, 2013) provides five categories of DDs, including otherwise specified DD, dissociative identity disorder, dissociative

---

[1]The item was a part of the Illinois Department of Children and Family Services' Child and Adolescent Needs and Strengths Comprehensive tool (CANS; Lyons et al., 2005). The 105-item Illinois version of the CANS catalogues a child's symptoms, needs, and strengths based on comprehensive provider information in collaboration with caregiver's observations on a 4-point scale ranging from 0 to 3. The clinical descriptions that accompany scores on the dissociation item can be found in Table 6.3.

amnesia (with or without dissociative fugue), depersonalization/derealization disorder, and otherwise specified dissociative disorder. Because children and teens are growing and can change presentations rapidly, relying on the otherwise specified DD category is useful for children not fitting into other stricter criteria.[2]

A diagnosis of posttraumatic stress disorder (PTSD) may also be appropriate when a child evidences both dissociative and posttraumatic symptoms. For young children, the diagnosis of preschool PTSD includes specific descriptors of dissociative symptoms such as "complete loss of awareness of present surroundings" and "emotional numbing." The dissociative subtype of PTSD (DPTSD) was introduced in the *DSM-5* and includes symptoms of derealization, depersonalization, or both. A recent meta-analysis found that DPTSD was highly prevalent in youth—significantly more so than in adults (White et al., 2022), and it may be a good diagnostic fit for many youths' complex presentations. However, the *DSM-5* definitions of dissociation in both DDs and PTSD are limited, particularly when it comes to diagnosing children, and more research, particularly about DPTSD in youth, is needed. We recommend collecting comprehensive clinical information over simply relying on the *DSM* categorizations of dissociation when planning for treatment.

A combination of comprehensive clinical case descriptions (Silberg, 2022; Waters, 2016; Wieland, 2015) and research findings (e.g., Cintron et al., 2018; Hébert et al., 2017; Putnam et al., 1996) help construct a picture of the manifestations of dissociative children through the lifespan. These descriptions can provide clinical "guideposts" to focus diagnostic attention on a child or teen for whom a DD is suspected. Clinicians are encouraged to defer to the diagnosis that best encompasses the complete picture of symptoms presented and reported.

DISSOCIATIVE PROCESSES AND PRESENTATIONS IN YOUTH BY AGE GROUPS

Preschool Children

Clinicians working with young children impacted by trauma must be attuned to typical development and understand how trauma disrupts attainment of developmental milestones, rather than looking for dissociative symptoms commonly seen in adults. Unlike adults who may show several discrete dissociative

---

[2]The not otherwise specified DD diagnosis is used when there is little information available and is not discussed here as a diagnosis in and of itself.

self-states, young children's dissociated aspects of the self may not have an elaborate sense of autonomy. It is common for feelings, thoughts, impulses, or traits that the child rejects to be projected onto stuffed animals, body parts, fantasy playmates, cartoon characters, or even animals (Silberg, 1998).

Transitional Identities

The term *transitional identities* refers to the self-states, voices, or internal identities of children who are showing the beginnings of a dissociative process (Silberg, 2022). Transitional identities are a method of projecting and containing unintegrated emotions, memories, or other unacceptable mental contents and do not yet have enduring patterns of relating to the world, as is the case with self-states found in DID. Clear-cut childhood DID is uncommon in very young children but can occur. A documented case of a 3-year-old with two "personalities" appeared to represent adaptive reactions to two discrete environments (Riley & Mead, 1988).

Transitional identities describe a developmental transition between imaginary friends (or other normative fantasy phenomena) and dissociative self-states. There are several significant differences between the transitional identities found in dissociative children and imaginary friends that appear in nondissociative children (see Table 6.1). Unlike normal imaginary friends, transitional identities are usually accompanied by intense posttraumatic symptomatology, such as fearfulness, night terrors, or intrusive traumatic thoughts. Children describe a feeling of being compelled to follow directions of these transitional identities against their perceived will; some describe it as a form of "internal warfare." The clinician should assess whether the child believes that the identities that they see or feel internally are "real." Finally, whereas

TABLE 6.1. Considerations for Imaginary Friend Versus Transitional Identity

	Imaginary friend	Transitional identity
Experiencing fearfulness, night terrors, intrusive traumatic thoughts	No	Yes
Feeling compelled to follow directions against perceived will	No	Yes
Believing friend is "real"	No	Yes
Experiencing friend while happy or excited	Yes	No
Experiencing friend while angry	No	Yes
Amnesia for actions while experiencing identity's anger	No	Yes
Feeling multiple imaginary friends in conflict with one another	No	Yes

nondissociative children experience the presence of imaginary friends while feeling happy or excited, the dominant emotion reported when the transitional identities are activated is anger (Silberg, 2022). Amnesia for actions engaged in while the child experienced anger from a transitional identity and other memory problems are common.

Dissociative Symptomatology and Assessment Considerations

During dissociative episodes, preschool children may appear to be in a trance, have a faraway look in their eyes, or fail to recognize familiar places or people, even beloved caregivers (Putnam et al., 1993; Silberg, 2022; Waters, 2016; Young, 2022). Sometimes during these dissociative states, the children may appear to reenact traumatic scenarios with shouts of "no" and body movements that simulate a violent or sexual assault (Cintron et al., 2018; Silberg, 2022). A particularly salient symptom involves a child having no memory for recent positive events, such as birthday parties or accomplishments (Hornstein, 1996; Silberg, 2022). Not acknowledging oppositional or destructive behaviors may also represent amnesia rather than simply denial of responsibility as one might see with oppositional disorder. It may be helpful to consider whether the child experiences amnesia in other areas, not just when trying to avoid taking responsibility for negative behavior. A child stating they "forgot" only in situations they are in trouble may be more indicative of denying responsibility, whereas forgetfulness across settings is more likely to indicate a dissociative experience. Denial accompanied by a sense of being perplexed and confused may suggest amnesia.

Psychosomatic manifestations of dissociation are common among young children, including enuresis or encopresis, headaches and stomachaches, pain at the sites of previous injuries or sexual intrusion, insensitivity to pain, or distortions in body image (e.g., looking fat or big to oneself in the mirror, despite being slight in build; Silberg, 2022; Waters, 2016). Young dissociative children may also display shifting conversion symptoms, such as an intermittent inability to walk, read, or understand academic work (Silberg, 2022).

Young dissociative children often engage in lengthy and intense tantrums that seem to "come out of nowhere" (Cintron et al., 2018). Regressive behavior is frequently present, such as sudden baby talk, or clinginess, which may be detected more readily by the parent than the clinician. Dissociative preschool children may also display sleep disorders (Hébert et al., 2017), including difficulty sleeping alone; resisting sleep; suffering from nightmares; insomnia; talking, walking, or crying during sleep; waking frequently; or being constantly overtired (Silberg, 2022).

These issues are often discounted as attention-seeking or oppositional, especially when a child is "acting like a baby" or is resistant to go to sleep at bedtime. It is our experience that sleep issues and regressive behaviors are almost always indicative of a more complex issue for the child, albeit not always dissociation. Like the other symptoms discussed in this chapter, sleep and regressive issues are only one part of the diagnostic puzzle. A complete assessment and understanding of attachment relationships, psychosocial stressors, trauma history, and medical history can assist with ruling out other possibilities. For example, sleep problems and issues with low energy can also be indicative of internalizing problems (e.g., anxiety, depression, mood disorder), externalizing problems (e.g., attention-deficit/hyperactivity disorder), or medical issues (e.g., thyroid dysfunction). In general, any behavior that seems outside of typical child behavior should be taken seriously and discussed with a pediatrician or other provider.

School-Age Children

With age, the frequency of DID-like symptoms in highly dissociative children typically increases (Putnam et al., 1996). School-age children may present with more differentiated transitional identities, which may continue to be projected onto stuffed animals or toys (McElroy, 1992). Identity fluctuations are more readily discernable as children age because regressive states become more differentiated. For example, a child who has mastered speaking fluently, may suddenly talk in two-word sentences or "baby talk." Children may have variations in cognitive skill or behavior that can become frustrating in school settings, where the behavior may be interpreted as willful or avoidant (Yehuda, 2011).

Dissociative school-age children may forget autobiographical information such as their birthdays or other recent events. Trance-like behavior may span from vacant staring and "blanking-out" to profound states of dissociation in which children are unresponsive to their surroundings for hours (Perry et al., 1995; Silberg, 2022). Dissociative children have difficulty remembering what they did while angry and aggressive. They may also complain of changes in their sense of identity—feeling as though, when angry or upset, it is not really them. Some dissociative children have difficulty awakening from sleep and may display changes in self-state (e.g., waking up in a regressed state; Silberg, 2022).

Adolescents

During adolescence, dissociative symptoms more closely parallel those of adults (Ruths et al., 2002) and can include shifting patterns of relatedness, such as alternating between regression and severe mistrust. Adolescent dissociation is strongly correlated with self-harm (Černis et al., 2019; Hoyos et al., 2019; Kisiel & Lyons, 2001) and may allow the adolescent to identify with abusive caregivers, punish the self, call attention to pain, and potentially release internal opioids that reinforce the self-harm (Ferentz, 2012). Sometimes the purpose of self-harm, such as banging or hitting one's head, may be to silence inner voices (Silberg, 2013, 2022). Self-harm may be conducted outside of the adolescent's consciousness. For example, Ratnamohan and colleagues (2018) described a teenage boy who engaged in self-harm with a knife while in dissociated sleep states.

Assessment Considerations
Assessing adolescents can be complicated because comorbid, nondissociative symptoms, which tend to increase during adolescence, may be the primary complaint. The teen may present with conduct problems, sexual acting out, mood disorders, eating disorders, self-mutilation, substance abuse, obsessive-compulsive disorders, and suicidal ideation or attempts (Silberg et al., 1997; Waters, 2016).

Substance use can complicate assessment and diagnosis of depersonalization/derealization disorder among adolescents (Simeon & Abugel, 2006). However, sometimes sudden onset of depersonalization/derealization after an experience with substances can begin a process of long-term dissociation in teens. The most common age for the onset of depersonalization/derealization disorder is around 16 (Simeon, 2004).

Some dissociative adolescents report auditory hallucinations and may be diagnosed as having a psychotic disorder (Altman et al., 1997). Sometimes psychogenic nonepileptic seizures (PNES) may be the first presentation of a DD. Some teens may have a form of traumatic flashbacks that present as grand mal seizures yet have normal EEG results (Bowman, 2006).

Self-Diagnosis of DID
Another complicating factor in the assessment of DD among adolescents is the recent increase in teens who are diagnosing themselves as having DID. Social media sites including TikTok and YouTube feature videos about individuals with DID. Online groups are available that may provide accepting and approving environments for individuals who are facing identity challenges and experiencing multiple senses of self. Given the critical developmental task of identity development in adolescence, teens may be particularly susceptible to these types of groups. Online support groups may normalize the experience of having multiple selves and promote equal rights for all

self-parts. These groups may serve as a validating means of self-acceptance and self-understanding among teens struggling with shifting moods or gender confusion. This philosophical emphasis on individual rights also encourages the sense of dividedness rather than integration of multiple but connected parts of oneself and may compete with therapeutic goals.

The number of online dissociative symptoms/disorder support groups has increased over the past decade, and an online community of "plurals" has emerged (Christensen, 2022; Rettew, 2022). Plurals is a term generated by the online community for those who identify as either having DID or view their sense of plurality as a nontraumagenic lifestyle choice. This heterogenous group of individuals includes those who employ a form of self-soothing through a rich fantasy life called "maladaptive daydreaming" (Theodor-Katz et al., 2022). This fantasy life may include internal introjects taken from popular media called *fictives*. Fictives can include comic book, video game, and movie characters and are popular among gaming enthusiasts and those involved in anime. Over time, fictives can become internalized as an integral part of the individual's internal landscape.

Gaming platforms are another avenue through which individuals can further develop this notion of multiple selves. Individuals can create multiple avatars to represent different characters who may be male or female, represent aliens or other nonhuman entities, and who prefer to play different games and have different regular online gaming partners. These different avatars or online self-representations can become more and more real to the individual's sense of identity over time. Multiplicity may be reinforced through multiple online relationships unique to each avatar.

The increased isolation during the COVID-19 pandemic has contributed to higher rates of online activity, less face-to-face interaction with peers, and greater reliance on and identification with these online communities among teens (e.g., Zhang et al., 2021). Individuals with gender dysphoria, autism spectrum disorders, or histories of other psychiatric issues such as bipolar disorder and social anxiety may be particularly vulnerable to the online encouragement of dissociation.

From evaluating a series of teenagers who were influenced by social media in this way, it is our clinical experience that some of these teens do have significant dissociative tendencies that predated their online involvement. The second author has evaluated a series of teenagers influenced by online communities, finding that many of them have had dissociative features without full-fledged DID before media exposure, but the social encouragement online may have helped to shape their dissociation into more discrete self-state shifts. Christensen (2022) termed these presentations of multiplicity that are facilitated by online media as *sociogenic* (a result of social influence) versus *traumagenic* (resulting from trauma influences).

Rather than distinguishing the presentations in this way, it may be more clinically useful to see these presentations as occurring on a continuum. DID evolves from both traumatic elements (Dalenberg et al., 2012) and interpersonal elements (Dutra et al., 2009). Within the "plural" community, the type and quality of both traumatic and interpersonal influences may differ but may still produce dissociative functioning. Understanding where on the continuum teens fall with respect to trauma history and interpersonal variables may assist clinicians in determining diagnosis and type of treatment needed. Some teens may present self-state shifts and memory loss as seen with conventional DID. As with DID, there are generally angry, depressed, fearful, and regressive parts of self, which hold different feelings. Teens with these presentations typically experience considerable dysfunction associated with their dissociative symptoms. However, teens whose self-states have coalesced from online influence have fewer symptoms of posttraumatic stress, less frequent symptoms of nightmares and flashbacks, and less morbid intrusive ideation, and they generally demonstrate fewer difficulties in functioning. Although some trauma may have been experienced such as a sexual assault, a history of early attachment disruption, or extreme peer bullying, there tends to be less intense early, interpersonal, complex trauma common among DID clients heavily influenced by social media, as well as fewer trauma-related symptoms. These clients experience less shame and hiding associated with the state shifts, and in general, the condition appears to be more cohesive and less disruptive to daily functioning. Even with initial memory "fuzziness," it is often easy to establish coconsciousness with the other parts of self for these clients.

These teenagers have come to our attention during the pandemic and have responded well to therapy that supports the discrete states as important parts of the self that need integration. These parts have a specific role to play in holding feelings of the whole self. Containment and safety interventions may not be as prolonged with this subset of clients, although the rest of the basic treatment model of DID treatment for youth is the same. This can be a legitimate pathway for the development of DDs among vulnerable youth, and it is important not to negate their experience. For example, it is generally not therapeutic to challenge their sense of themselves by telling them they do not have "real DID." Instead, it can be helpful to support the client's reliance on this kind of self-conception as a method to portray identity conflict and help the teen work on the conflict with internal contracts, bargaining, and other traditional DID techniques. In general, we have found that it is better not to get overly constrained by debating differences in diagnoses but to accept teens however they present themselves and work on integration and self-acceptance through well-known techniques in the trauma and dissociation field.

KEY DIMENSIONS OF DIAGNOSTIC ASSESSMENT

Clinicians use diagnostic assessment to try to gather as much information to inform diagnosis and treatment planning as possible. It can be difficult to know which topics to prioritize, particularly for clinicians who may not have a lot of experience assessing dissociation. We consider the following to be particularly key dimensions of any clinical assessment of youth presenting with dissociative symptoms:

- normal developmental trajectory
- severity and level of disruption of symptoms
- child strengths
- family strengths and vulnerabilities
- flexible approach

Developmental Trajectory

It is important to understand where the child is developmentally and how far off the trajectory of typical development they are. For example, when assessing "voices," one can use the Imaginary Friends Questionnaire (Silberg, 2022) in combination with the clinical interview to determine how similar or dissimilar a child's transitional identities are to imaginary friends and if they are still developmentally appropriate. Depending on where the child presents developmentally, the therapist may identify socialization, peer engagement, and specific skills training as treatment targets.

Severity and Level of Disruption of Symptoms

Another key component to learn from assessment is which symptoms are the most severe and which have the highest risk, potential lethality, or disruptive effects. For example, how much does the child suffer from intrusive voices? How severe is the amnesia? These are pieces of information that can be gleaned from both self-report measures and through interviews with the child and family. It is important to prioritize symptoms that put the child at the most risk and are currently causing the most disruption. Sometimes this may mean putting another set of challenges aside for the time being to establish safety and provide some symptomatic relief for the child and family. Amnesia for recent events, particularly school or interaction with peers, is one example of a symptom that may cause chaos in the lives of children and is often something they are motivated to resolve. Switching that the child cannot control is another symptom that creates extreme disruption to everyday life.

Child Strengths

In addition to the importance of understanding risk factors, difficult symptoms, and barriers to healing, clinical assessment should always include and be guided by an assessment of the client's strengths. The Healthy Outcomes from Positive Experiences (HOPE) model places value on positive childhood experiences and encourages the skilled weaving of hope with concern in its interactions with families (Sege, 2021). This is especially relevant when working with youth who may have experienced trauma. Skills in sports, arts, and community involvement, for example, can facilitate a sense of belonging, provide opportunities to practice emotion regulation skills, and encourage integrative functioning. Self-awareness, motivation for change, availability of some supportive adults, or a strong peer group are all beneficial to treatment and prognosis.

Flexible and Ongoing Approach to Assessment

A diagnostic approach to children with dissociative symptoms must emphasize flexibility. The assessment of a child's trauma history is unlikely to be settled in your initial assessment. Parents are often unaware of the extent of trauma that their child may have experienced, and negative interactions with peers, assaults, or maltreatment at previous foster homes or out-of-home placements may only reveal themselves later once a relationship has been established. Uncovering new sources of trauma throughout treatment is typical; significant child or family secrets about traumatic events may not be discovered until years into treatment.

New symptoms, newly identified self-states, or transitional identities may emerge, and what may first be seen as the central issue may fade as treatment progresses. Diagnostic assessment provides an initial road map for intervention, but symptoms may change, life may provide new challenges and opportunities, and past traumatic influences become more apparent. The most successful clinicians begin treatment with a thorough assessment but continue to modify initial perceptions as treatment progresses.

CLINICAL INTERVIEW

The measures reviewed here are invaluable sources of information but should never replace the clinical interview in the assessment of dissociation in youth. Clinical interviews assist the clinician in learning about symptoms, understanding the phenomenology of the youth's view of self, assessing the severity of amnesia and the level of self-destructive or antisocial tendencies and allows for carefully watching for possible behavioral indicators of dissociation. The clinician's goal during the interview should be creating a psychologically safe environment such that the child can acknowledge memories and symptoms without fear or shame. The information gathered during a clinical interview can also help the clinician understand the symptoms that are the most disruptive and prioritize treatment interventions.

Dissociative experiences are just one part of a comprehensive clinical interview. The clinician should always assess for risky behaviors, internalizing, externalizing, and developmental disabilities as with any other clients. When assessing for dissociation, we recommend asking questions about the youth's experiences across five primary domains (Silberg, 2022):

1. alterations in consciousness
2. hallucinations
3. fluctuations in behavior and affect
4 memory impairment
5. somatic symptoms

Alterations in Consciousness

To gain a better understanding of symptoms in this domain, consider asking about

- times the child finds themself "blanking out" or not paying attention, including what the child is thinking, feeling, hearing, seeing, and doing during those times

- imaginary places the child likes to go in their mind

- behaviors surrounding sleep (e.g., being told they act differently or strangely after sleep, trouble waking in the morning, feeling different after going into a deep sleep)

- depersonalization or feeling like they are not really there or watching themself from a distance

- derealization or feeling like they are watching the world through a fog or camera

When observing a child dissociating during the session (e.g., seems to be daydreaming, does not seem to remember what was happening just a few moments before, rapid regression in behaviors or speech, begins referring to self in third person), consider asking the child what they were doing or thinking/feeling right before. Direct, specific questions can be helpful for children who have a hard time describing what is going on during "blank" moments, for example, "Were you thinking about when this interview would be over?"

Hallucinations

Hearing voices is more common than once thought, particularly in children and adults who have been impacted by trauma (see Chapter 1). When assessing for hallucinations, it can be helpful to first normalize the experience for children by saying, "Many times, children who have lost someone special to them still hear them talking to them in their mind. Does this ever happen to you?" Additional questions might assess topics such as

- feeling like their brain is fighting with itself
- mean words stuck in their head
- feeling someone made them do something they didn't want to do
- imaginary or invisible friends
- inanimate objects that can talk to them

Fluctuations in Behavior and Affect

For this section, we suggest focusing on what children, rather than parents or teachers, find surprising. Areas that may provide clinicians with some important information include the following:

- fluctuating abilities (i.e., able to do something one day but not the next)
- reactions to mood changes
- tastes or interests changing from day to day
- changing feelings about family members
- out-of-context behaviors that do not match up with what is going on around the child
- animal-like behaviors

Memory Impairment

Memory impairment can be difficult to assess in youth with dissociative symptoms, especially because many children and teens use "I forgot" as an avoidance technique. Saying, "I forgot" can be a way to try to avoid consequences for behavior and is not always indicative of actual memory gaps. However, it can also signal possible dissociative memory impairment. Refrain from arguing with the child about what they can remember and offer positive incentives for participating in the interview. Some ways to assess memory impairment with children include asking about

- forgetting pleasant events such as birthdays, activities with friends, or vacations
- forgetting behaviors that occurred when they are angry
- family and friends noticing the child doing things that the child does not remember

Somatic Symptoms

Clinical interviews should include a discussion about the child's relationship to their body, including skin picking, nail biting or tearing, or other self-injurious behaviors. Many children who have experienced trauma are proud to share that they do not feel pain. Discussing this as a strength rather than a pathology can open the dialogue about dissociation as a means of coping. Children may also share strengths and weaknesses that change, feelings of disconnection from their bodies, movements that feel out of their control, or pain that has no organic cause. Topics to discuss include the following:

- experiencing pain differently from other children (e.g., more intense, less intense)
- frequent injury and feelings related to injuries
- unusual strengths or weaknesses at different times
- feeling as if their body is not theirs
- depersonalization (described earlier)
- derealization (described earlier)

FAMILY ASSESSMENT

No full diagnostic assessment of a child or teen is complete without an assessment of the family system within which the child resides. Families need to be engaged as allies in treatment, continuing the essential work of validation of feelings and establishing attachment at home (Waters, 2016). The family's ability and readiness to serve in this collaborative relationship needs to be assessed. James (1994) outlined the multiple skills necessary for a family to parent a severely traumatized child successfully. These skills include an ability to collaborate with the treatment team, ability to recognize one's own trauma reactions and contribution to disruptive behavior, knowledge about dissociation and trauma, intervention skills, a life outside of the child, and commitment to the child's need to process a traumatic past. Diagnostic assessment should yield information relevant to the family's ability to provide this supportive environment to the child. Many factors can interfere with parents' participation in the process, including dissociative processes in the parents, a history of ongoing family trauma, a parent's unresolved trauma or attachment history, a parent's mental illness or substance abuse, or parental conflict. As needed, clinicians can refer parents for other therapy to assist in stabilizing their own mental health and increasing their capacity to serve in the needed collaborative, supportive role for their child.

ASSESSMENT TOOLS FOR CONSIDERATION

Dissociation in childhood and adolescence can present as perplexing forgetfulness, fluctuations, shifts in identity, trancelike states, unusual somatic experiences, and hallucinatory phenomena. Careful assessment is needed to provide appropriate diagnosis and establish treatment to prevent higher levels of symptomatology and resistance to treatment as youth age. Assessment involves carefully teasing out comorbid conditions and diagnoses and engaging in a full analysis of all the social, interpersonal, and traumagenic factors that may lead to DDs and symptoms in young people. Additionally, early recognition and treatment of DDs may prevent greater levels of impairment and treatment difficulties for clients as they get older. Indeed, the Treatment of Patients with Dissociative Disorders study revealed that although young adults diagnosed with DD were more impaired at the beginning of treatment, they tended to stabilize more quickly than older adults, with decreasing destructive behaviors and symptoms (Myrick et al., 2012).

The clinician treating child and adolescent clients has the benefit of several initial screening tools; guidelines for comprehensive clinical interviewing; and comprehensive self-rating, psychological testing, and clinician rating tools. We recommend that all youth be screened for trauma exposure, and measures that assess for dissociation (see Table 6.2) can easily be included in standard assessment protocols so that youth with high risk for significant long-term morbidity can be identified and symptoms can be addressed. Table 6.2 includes a column that describes the type of dissociative symptoms addressed in each measure.

Children and adolescents who show indications of trauma exposure or disruptions to attachment figures should be carefully assessed for dissociation,

TABLE 6.2. Dissociation Assessment Tools for Children and Adolescents

Name of test/ interview	Author(s)/ source	Age range	Type of assessment	No. of items	Reporting period	Symptomatic area(s) assessed	Validity data available
			Diagnostic clinical interviews				
Semi-Structured Clinical Interview for Dissociative Symptoms and Disorders (SCID-D)	Steinberg, 1994b	Adults but has been used with adolescents as young as 14	Youth/adult client	277	Not specified	AC, H, FBA, MI, SS	Cronbach's alpha = 0.72-.96) (For a review, see Mychailyszyn et al., 2021)
			Published measures with validity				
Adolescent Dissociative Experiences Scale (A-DES)	Armstrong et al., 1997	Ages 11+	Self-report	30	Not specified	AC, H, FBA, MI, SS	Cronbach's alpha = 0.93 (Armstrong et al., 1997)
Adolescent Multi-dimensional Inventory of Dissociation (A-MID)	Dell, 2006a[a]	Adolescence	Self-report	218	Not specified	AC, H, FBA, MI, SS	
Child Dissociative Checklist (CDC)	Putnam et al., 1993	Not specified	Observational	20	12 months	AC, H, FBA, MI, SS	Cronbach's alpha = 0.86 (Putnam et al., 1993; Putnam & Peterson, 1994)
Child and Adolescent Needs and Strengths (CANS) Dissociation Item	The John Praed Foundation, n.d.[b]	6-17	Observational	105 items (one related to dissociation)	Past 30 days	AC, FBA, MI	Scores 1-3 are indicative of dissociative symptomatology (Anderson et al., 2003; Lyons et al., 2004)

Measure	Source	Age	Format	Items	Time frame	Codes	Reliability
Somatoform Dissociation Questionnaire (SDQ-20)	Nijenhuis et al., 1996	Adults and youth aged 14-17	Self-report	20	Past year	SS	Cronbach's alpha = 0.95 (Nijenhuis et al., 1996) Swedish version with adolescents, alpha = 0.84 (Nilsson et al., 2015)
Trauma Symptom Checklist for Children (TSCC)	Briere, 1996	8-16	Self-report	54 (2 dissociation subscales)	Not specified	AC, FBA, MI, SS	Cronbach's alpha = 0.77 (Briere, 1996; Briere & Lanktree, 1995)
Trauma Symptom Checklist for Young Children (TSCYC)	Briere et al., 2001	3-12	Self-report	90	Last month	AC, FBA	Cronbach's alpha = .81 to 9.3; average 0.87 (Briere et al., 2001; Gilbert, 2004)
Additional emerging measures							
Brief Dissociative Experiences Scale (DES-B)	Dalenberg & Carlson, 2010	11-17	Self-report	8	7 days	AC, FBA, MI, SS	Not available[c]
Children's Dissociative Experiences Scale & Posttraumatic Symptom Inventory (CDES-PSI)	Stolbach, 1997	7-17	Self-report	37	Not specified	AC, H, FBA, MI, SS	Stolbach, 1997

(continues)

TABLE 6.2. Dissociation Assessment Tools for Children and Adolescents (*Continued*)

Name of test/ interview	Author(s)/ source	Age range	Type of assessment	No. of items	Reporting period	Symptomatic area(s) assessed	Validity data available
Children's Perceptual Alteration Scale (CPAS)	Evers-Szostak & Sanders, 1992	8–12	Self-report	28	Not specified	AC, H, FBA, MI	Split-half reliability, $r = 0.82$ for clinical group (Evers-Szostak & Sanders, 1992)
Imaginary Friends Questionnaire	Available in Silberg, 2022	Not indicated	Self-report	15	Not specified	H	Items 1, 3, 4, 5, 7, 10, and 14 are more characteristic of children who have been diagnosed with dissociative symptoms and disorders (Silberg, 2022)
Measure in development							
Checklist for Indicators of Trauma and Dissociation in Youth (CIT-DY)	Available online[d]	3–19 (caregiver version) 7–19 (youth version)	Both observational and self-report available	35	12 months	AC, H, FBA, MI, SS	Not available[e]

Note. AC = alterations in consciousness; H = hallucinations; FBA = fluctuations in behavior and affect; MI = memory impairment; SS = somatic symptoms.
[a]See also https://www.mid-assessment.com/mid/. [b]See also https://praedfoundation.org/tcom/tcom-tools/the-child-and-adolescent-needs-and-strengths-cans/. [c]All information about the DES-B measure can be found at https://www.psychiatry.org/File%20Library/Psychiatrists/Practice/DSM/APA_DSM5_Severity-of-Dissociative-Symptoms-Adult.pdf. [d]See https://www.waterscounselingandtraining.com. [e]All information about the CIT-DY measure can be found at https://www.waterscounselingandtraining.com/check-list-for-trauma-assessment.

preferably using multiple methods of assessment including careful behavioral observations by the clinician, self-report measures for youth 12 or older, assessment measures completed by caregivers, and interviewing by a clinician familiar with the signs and symptoms of trauma and dissociation in youth.

Validated Measures of Dissociation for Youth

The measures described in this section are validated assessments for dissociation in youth. It is important to add that none of the following measures should be the sole basis for diagnosis, particularly in the case of parent- or self-report measures. The data they provide should always be followed up on by the clinician to ensure that the parent or client (a) understood what the question is asking and (b) can give examples that provide more context to their responses to the measure. We have worked with parents who have over- or underreported their children's symptoms for reasons ranging from fear of social services involvement to denial of their children's challenges.

Adolescent Dissociative Experiences Scale

The Adolescent Dissociative Experiences Scale (A-DES; Armstrong et al., 1997) is a free measure that adapted items from the adult Dissociative Experiences Scale (DES; Bernstein & Putnam, 1986) to make them applicable to those aged 11 years and older. Dissociative experiences are scores on a 10-point scale and include items such as "feeling like there are different people inside me" and "I get back tests or homework that I don't remember doing." Scores that average 4 or higher suggest significant dissociation. This measure can be particularly helpful in discussing symptoms with adolescents who are new to treatment. The A-DES is also frequently used in research, and versions of it have been validated for several languages and cultures (e.g., Martínez-Taboas et al., 2004; Nilsson & Svedin, 2006).

Sample items:

- When I am somewhere I don't want to be, I can go away in my mind.
- I look at the clock and realize that time has gone by and I can't remember what has happened.

Adolescent Multidimensional Inventory of Dissociation

The Multidimensional Inventory of Dissociation (MID; Dell, 2006a) is a free comprehensive tool that can be used to assess dissociation in adults and adolescents. The adolescent version contains 218 items that are consistent with experiences unique to the adolescent population and asks adolescents to rate items on a 0-to-10 scale. The adolescent MID uses less formal language than the adult MID, and some of the items are modified to be more age-appropriate (Dell, 2006a). The items aim to capture the same information as the MID for adults and have been used to assess the prevalence of dissociative symptoms among adolescent psychiatric inpatients (Goffinet & Beine, 2018). Preliminary research shows that adolescent patients clinically diagnosed with DID closely mirror adults with DID in their MID responses (Ruths et al., 2002). Although lengthy, this tool can provide a comprehensive picture of the adolescent's symptom profile (Ruths et al., 2002), and the author provides resources to assist clinicians with interpretation and application of the results (Dell, 2006a). A French version of the measure has demonstrated a high correlation between the Adolescent MID and the A-DES in identification of dissociative teens (Goffinet & Beine, 2018).

Sample items:

- More than one part of you has been reacting to these questions.
- Your thoughts and feelings are so changeable that you don't understand yourself.

Child Dissociative Checklist

The Child Dissociative Checklist (CDC; Putnam & Peterson, 1994) is a free, 20-item tool that many clinicians use to evaluate dissociative symptoms in children between ages 5 and 16. The CDC is completed by a caregiver or someone else who knows the child well. Items are rated on a scale from 0 to 2 and assess symptoms such as children referring to themselves by other names, having vivid imaginary friends, avoiding talking about traumatic events, nightmares, and sleep problems. Putnam (1997) considers scores above 12 to indicate a need for further assessment and scores above 19 to be strongly associated with dissociation in young children. The CDC has been found to reliably differentiate young dissociative children from controls (Putnam et al., 1993).

Sample items:

- Child goes into a daze or trance-like state at times or often appears "spaced-out." Teachers may report that he or she "daydreams" frequently in school.

- Child frequently talks to him or herself, may use a different voice, or argue with self at times.

Child and Adolescent Needs and Strengths

The Child and Adolescent Needs and Strengths (CANS; Lyons et al., 2005) is a free, multipurpose tool developed to assist providers in assessing and supporting youth through all levels of care by linking assessment and treatment planning. It includes six core domains and 50 core items that represent strengths and needs. The core domains include Behavioral/Emotional Needs, Caregiver Needs & Resources, Cultural Factors, Life Functioning, and Risk Behaviors. There are also optional, individualized assessment modules which include Trauma (includes traumatic/adverse childhood experiences and traumatic stress symptoms), Substance Use Disorder, Violence, Developmental Needs, Juvenile Justice, and Runaway. Each strength and need is rated at four levels; needs range from *no evidence of a need* to *immediate/intensive action needed*, and strengths range from *centerpiece strength* to *no strength identified*. This tool has demonstrated interrater reliability and predictive validity (Lyons et al., 2004), is appropriate for children aged 6 to 20, and can be beneficial in planning clinical interventions (Anderson et al., 2003).

One CANS item specifically addresses dissociation, with ratings ranging from *no evidence of dissociation* to *severe dissociative disturbance*. The item content provided in Table 6.3 is outlined in the measure's 2021 reference guide (Lyons & Fernando, 2021, p. 56). The descriptors provide a shorthand way for clinicians to capture the impact of dissociation in children and adolescents. The manual and CANS forms are available online at the John Praed Foundation (n.d.) website. This item has a high level of predictive validity for mental health symptom severity, disrupted placements, hospitalizations, and risk-taking behaviors in youth (Kisiel et al., 2020).

Somatoform Dissociation Questionnaire

The Somatoform Dissociation Questionnaire (SDQ-20; Nijenhuis et al., 1996) is a free, self-report measure that assesses the presence of somatic symptoms that may accompany dissociation. Clients are asked to identify the extent to which each statement feels applicable using a 5-point rating scale. For each item, there is also a question about whether any physical reason for the symptom is known. The SDQ-20 has demonstrated internal, convergent, and discriminant validity. It has been translated into several languages (e.g., González-Vázquez et al., 2017; Pietkiewicz et al., 2019; Şar et al., 2001) and can be administered to adolescents beginning at age 14.

Semi-Structured Clinical Interview for Dissociative Symptoms and Disorders

The Semi-Structured Clinical Interview for Dissociative Symptoms and Disorders (SCID-D; Steinberg, 2023), and its predecessors, the SCID-D (Steinberg et al., 1990) and the SCID-D-R (Steinberg, 1994a), are interviews for diagnosing dissociative disorders. The SCID-D is the *DSM-5* version (Steinberg, 2023) and is for use by trained clinicians. The interview typically takes between 1 and 3 hours to complete and is considered the gold standard for diagnosing

TABLE 6.3. Child and Adolescent Needs and Strengths Dissociation Item

Dissociation: Symptoms included in this item are daydreaming, spacing or blanking out, forgetfulness, detachment, and rapid changes in personality often associated with traumatic experiences.

Questions to consider:

- Does the child/youth ever enter a dissociative state?
- Does the child/youth often become confused about who or where they are?
- Has the child/youth been diagnosed with a dissociative disorder?

Rating	Description of rating
0	No evidence of dissociation
1	Child/youth has history or evidence of dissociative problems, including some emotional numbing, avoidance or detachment, and some difficulty with forgetfulness, daydreaming, spacing or blanking out.
2	Child/youth exhibits dissociative problems that interfere with functioning in at least one life domain. This can include amnesia for traumatic experiences or inconsistent memory for trauma (e.g., remembers in one context but not another), more persistent or perplexing difficulties with forgetfulness (e.g., loses things easily, forgets basic information), frequent daydreaming or trance-like behavior, depersonalization and/or derealization. This rating would be used for someone who meets criteria for dissociative disorders or another diagnosis that is specified "with dissociative features."
3	Child/youth exhibits dangerous and/or debilitating dissociative symptoms. This can include significant memory difficulties associated with trauma that also impede day-to-day functioning. Child/youth is frequently forgetful or confused about things they should know about (e.g., no memory for activities or whereabouts of previous day or hours). Child/youth shows rapid changes in personality or evidence of distinct personalities. Child/youth who meets criteria for dissociative identity disorder or a more severe level of a dissociative disorder would be rated here.

DDs in adults. The SCID-D measures the presence and severity of amnesia, depersonalization, derealization, identity confusion, and identity alteration. Research has also demonstrated effectiveness in using the SCID-D with adolescents (Carrion & Steiner, 2000; Şar, Önder, et al., 2014; Steinberg, 1996; Steinberg & Steinberg, 1995). In particular, the measure has items that can be particularly helpful in distinguishing between developmentally appropriate identity issues in adolescents and dissociative symptoms. A validated Turkish version of the SCID-D for adolescents is also available (Kundakçi et al., 2014).

Sample Item:

- Sometimes a lot of adolescents feel confused about who they are. Do you know if your confusion is similar to your friends', or is it different? (Steinberg & Steinberg, 1995).

Trauma Symptom Checklist for Children or the Trauma Symptom Checklist for Young Children

These measures assess trauma-related symptoms, including dissociation, in children. The Trauma Symptom Checklist for Children (TSCC; Briere, 1996) is a 54-item, self-report scale that assesses symptoms across six clinical scales (anxiety, depression, posttraumatic stress, sexual concerns, dissociation, and anger) using a rating scale of 0 to 3. Children aged 8 to 16 report how often they experience a range of symptoms, including 10 items that assess dissociative symptoms (e.g., feeling like one's mind goes blank, feeling like one is in a fog). The TSCC can be readministered in a short time and has two validity scales to indicate over- or underreporting of symptoms.

The Trauma Symptom Checklist for Young Children (TSCYC; Briere et al., 2001) is a 90-item caretaker-report measure developed to assess trauma-related symptoms in children aged 3 to 12. This measure also assesses dissociation with nine items as well as symptoms commonly seen in young children who have experienced trauma, such as types of hypo- and hyperarousal (e.g., startling in response to loud noises, avoidance behaviors). It can be particularly useful when working with nonverbal children. The TSCC and TSCYC can both be purchased at https://www.parinc.com.

Additional Emerging Measures

These measures can assist with and enhance clinical decision making; they have preliminary information available regarding their validation yet may not be as commonly used as some of those already described. We encourage readers to consider using these tools to allow for the sharing of additional information about the measures' utility in both clinical- and research-based capacities. Researchers are encouraged to consider further validation studies of these measures.

Brief Dissociative Experiences Scale

The Brief Dissociative Experiences Scale (DES-B; Dalenberg & Carlson, 2010) is a free, eight-item, self-report measure that assesses eight dissociative symptoms based on *DSM-5* criteria. The client is asked to agree or disagree using a 5-point rating scale. Symptoms include staring into space, feeling that the world is unreal, talking to self, ignoring pain, changing behaviors, feeling the world is in a fog, acting like different people, and changing abilities or skills. This measure was developed for research and is applicable for children aged 11 to 17.

Children's Dissociative Experiences Scale & Posttraumatic Symptom Inventory

The Children's Dissociative Experiences Scale & Posttraumatic Symptom Inventory (CDES-PSI; Stolbach, 1997) is a free, 37-item, self-report measure designed for children aged 7 to 12, although it can also be used with adolescents. Youth are provided with two fictional characters with different likes, dislikes, and behaviors and asked to identify which one they are like. An example item is "When Michael gets to school, he sometimes doesn't remember getting there" and "Kevin, when he gets to school, remembers how he got there and what happened on the way." The child chooses a response ranging from "I'm a lot like Michael" to "I'm a lot like Kevin." The CDES-PSI has three scales: dissociative experiences, posttraumatic symptoms, and faking.

Children's Perceptual Alteration Scale

The Children's Perceptual Alteration Scale (CPAS; Evers-Szostak & Sanders, 1992) is a free, self-report measure of dissociation for children 8 to 12 years old. It contains 28 items scored on a 4-point scale ranging from *never happening* to *happening all the time*. The CPAS was derived from the Perceptual Alteration Scale for adults (Sanders, 1986).

Imaginary Friends Questionnaire

The Imaginary Friends Questionnaire (Frost et al., 1996; Silberg, 2022) is a 15-item self-report measure developed to assess imaginary friends among children. The measure was originally developed for use with preschool children and inquiries about typical imaginary friends (e.g., My imaginary friend gives good advice) and those that are more characteristic of children who may be experiencing dissociative symptoms (e.g., My imaginary friend[s] is more than just a pretend friend). It is recommended for any youth who describes having internal companions or imaginary friends that may be difficult to distinguish from dissociation. Although some older, preteen children keep imaginary friends without dissociative features, this is somewhat rare.

Measures in Development

Checklist for Indicators of Trauma and Dissociation in Youth

The Checklist for Indicators of Trauma and Dissociation in Youth (CIT-DY) is a new assessment tool that was developed by Frances Waters for caregivers, adolescents, or clinicians to rate the presence and severity of traumatic events, treatment episodes, medications, diagnoses, and dissociative symptoms among youth with histories of complex trauma. This measure is applicable for children aged 3 to 18, is available free of charge, and is currently undergoing preliminary validation studies.

STANDARD PSYCHOLOGICAL TESTING

Silberg (1998) found that dissociative children could be distinguished from nondissociative inpatients on projective testing by unique elements in their testing protocols. Dissociative children demonstrated behaviors during testing such as staring, inattentiveness, stating they forgot, not recognizing their previous answers, and repetitive motor movement. In addition, their responses included distinguishing features such as characters who were described as forgetting, pretending or sleeping to solve a problem, having multiple body parts (e.g., on the Rorschach describing a character with multiple heads), undergoing magical transformation (e.g., a person shifting into an animal), and confusing emotions (e.g., calling "happy" "sad"). The children also struggled to remember storytelling tasks or directions (Silberg, 1998). If a child shows these signs during testing, additional assessment for possible dissociation is recommended.

RELATIONAL IMPACT OF DIAGNOSTIC ASSESSMENT

> Diagnosis can be seen as a mutually agreed on narrative, an abbreviated story that distills the essence of the problem. (Silberg, 2001, p. 4)

A mutually agreed-on view of diagnosis enriches the therapeutic relationship. When the therapist and clients have a shared view of "what is wrong," it can have significant impacts on the course and success of treatment. Thus, building an alliance with the child is of key importance from the beginning and should be one of the goals of assessment. For example, while sharing with the child what has been learned from the assessment, the clinician explains what the child is experiencing through empathic psychoeducation. Children can learn about the importance of neural connections and some basic ways in which trauma interrupts or alters connections within the brain. The child or teen can also learn that dissociation involves difficulty with emotional awareness when feelings are overwhelming and makes it harder to experience and express emotions. Such education serves several purposes. First, it gives children words to understand what they are experiencing, which can serve to decrease anxiety. Making trauma-based symptoms understandable and something that can be articulated may provide some containment of anxiety and traumatic material and decrease phobic avoidance. Second, by accepting the child's experiences nonjudgmentally, the clinician begins building the framework for an accepting, collaborative relationship. Third, it provides direction for treatment, where the child and clinician aim to work together to find ways to connect feelings, self-states, memories, and other mental contents. This supports improved integration of the child's experiences and self-states.

Similarly, it is essential to ensure that parents have an accurate understanding of dissociation. Parents may initially misunderstand treatment as an attempt to extinguish angry or acting out self-states, rather than moving toward unification and acceptance of all aspects of the child. Other practitioners may have rejected the idea of dissociation in previous consultations. Explaining your careful diagnostic process and the critical role you see the parent playing in treatment can help build credibility, decrease defensiveness, and facilitate engagement. It can help parents understand that a healthy parent–child relationship will be essential to assisting in supporting and healing their child's changing dissociative landscape. Perhaps most important, a diagnosis of dissociation in a child or teen should always be accompanied with a message of hope. Be sure that parents understand that these young clients are highly treatable and able to return to a path of more normal functioning as they age (Silberg, 2022; Waters, 2016; Wieland, 2015).

CASE STUDY

Anita[3] was an 11-year-old who was born biologically female and identified as female, preferring the pronouns "she/her." She was being discharged from a local inpatient eating disorder program after a month with no improvement. Anita stated that she heard a voice in her mind saying, "Don't eat, throw up," and she felt compelled to listen to the voice and throw up after meals. While she appeared to be compliant at the hospital, the treatment team's approach involved encouraging her to talk back to the voice and tell it to be quiet. Anita continued vomiting each morning and evening, did not feel vomiting was within her control, and did not gain weight during her 30-day stay. Anita was becoming dangerously underweight and had also begun hitting her head with her fist to try to quiet the voice. Someone at the

---

[3]All case study material in this chapter is fictional, uses composites, or has been altered by changing names and removing identifying information to preserve client confidentiality.

treatment program suggested she may have a DD, and the mother, hopeful that another approach might work, made an outpatient appointment at the second author's clinic.

Anita had wispy blonde hair and a strange, awkward smile. She looked younger than her 11-year-old age and, due to her low weight, looked frail sitting in her chair during the intake appointment. Her eyes frequently darted back and forth during the interview as though she was tracking something internally, and she often asked the therapist to repeat questions, saying "What?" as if she just noticed the therapist was talking. The therapist conducted the interview patiently, aware Anita may have little trust in professionals after her lack of success at the previous treatment program. Throughout the interview, the therapist gently focused on the onset of Anita's current symptoms—namely, her nausea and the voices telling her not to eat—and learned that Anita had begun to hear the voice shortly after starting sixth grade at her new middle school. This school was coed, which meant she would be attending school with boys for the first time. The therapist also had learned that Anita's parents were scheduled for family court to work out a new visitation agreement, and Anita would have to sleep at her father's house for the first time in 2 years. Her parents had separated when she was 5, and Anita's father was in recovery from substance abuse. He had only recently regained visitation. Anita told the therapist that the voice started in her new school, and the first thing she heard was, "You are fat." At first, she thought it had come from a boy in the class but soon realized it came from her own mind. Anita said she'd had a male imaginary friend when she was younger, "Adam," and the voice sounded like him.

In asking about other dissociative symptoms, the therapist learned that Anita sometimes had no memory for the vomiting that occurred in the hospital, even though she saw the evidence and felt a bad taste in her mouth. Anita also shared that she sometimes heard a baby crying, reported frequent headaches and nausea, and said, with embarrassment, that she felt surprised about how big she looked in the mirror. Anita appeared happiest when talking about schoolwork and proudly reported she was an A student. She didn't like boys because their talking made it difficult for her to concentrate. When asked about the expected reunion with her father, Anita expressed fear that she would not get her homework done at his house because he liked to watch TV. Anita denied significant trauma in her earlier years.

In the interview with mother, however, the therapist learned that Anita had been sexually abused at the ages of 4 and 5 at a local preschool. The case had received significant publicity after the teacher perpetrator was found guilty and sentenced to prison. Anita received short-term treatment for the sexual abuse, in part because she had not remembered much of what happened. At the time, the therapist's approach had been to avoid "stirring up" memories that might upset Anita.

Anita had not testified in the perpetrator's trial, and her family did not talk about the abuse or share any information about the case with her. Her parents' conflicts over Anita's trauma contributed to their divorce and, her mother believed, to the onset of Anita's father's substance abuse issues. Anita's mother was currently the sole custodian. She presented as sincere, motivated, and highly committed to finding the right treatment program for her daughter. Anita's father was not present for the clinical interview. Anita also had a younger sister who was in third grade and appeared to be doing well.

The therapist's clinical impression was that Anita showed many signs of dissociation, including hearing voices, inattentiveness, amnestic episodes, somatic concerns, depersonalization (not recognizing herself in the mirror), and a clear history of trauma and recent stressors—school change and reunification with an absent father. Anita's mother completed the CDC during the interview, and Anita completed the Adolescent DES. The therapist also administered the Imaginary Friends Questionnaire due to Anita's recollection of vivid imaginary friends when younger and her hearing "Adam's" voice.

Anita's mother's responses on the CDC yielded a score of 17. Specifically, she acknowledged Anita's denial of a history of trauma, somatic symptoms, hearing voices, and regressive behaviors. This score is above the cutoff of 12 for significant dissociation according to Putnam's (1997) original validation sample.

On the Adolescent DES, Anita scored a 3.8, which is suggestive of a DD but not as high as published samples of dissociative adolescents (average of 4). Endorsed items included "I have walls in my mind" and the items that involve doing things against one's perceived will, such as "Something inside makes me do things that I don't want to do," and items tapping amnesia, such as "People tell me I do or say things that I did not remember doing or saying." The answers allowed the therapist to inquire more about the way Anita felt when she vomited. Anita described it was "as if it is someone else" who had a different memory than she did engaged in vomiting. Her answers to the inquiry strongly suggested a dissociative process.

On the Imaginary Friends Questionnaire, all the dissociation suggestive items were positive. Again, key information was learned by inquiring into these responses. Anita acknowledged having more than one "imaginary friend and they disagree." When asked about this, she stated she sometimes hears the "crying baby in her mind" say "You will be hungry." This sound got drowned out by the voice of "Adam," who told Anita not to eat. Anita perceived her imaginary friends as "bossing her" and did not see them as helping with loneliness or fear. She perceived her imaginary friends as taking over and making her do things she did not want to do. Anita's answers were more typical of a child with transitional identities or self-states rather than developmentally appropriate imaginary friends.

As a result of the clinical interview with the mother, the assessment tools, follow-up and clinical interview with Anita, the therapist diagnosed Anita with otherwise specified dissociative disorder, concluding that "Adam" was a self-state who might hold traumatic memories and was contributing to her disordered eating behaviors and vomiting. Anita's earlier history of abuse, having not been processed at the time, was hypothesized as finding expression in this dissociative presentation. Having learned that Anita's mother perceived Anita as displaying regressive behaviors at times, in addition to hearing about the "crying baby" voice, the therapist suspected that traumatic memories from Anita's earlier abuse might also be sequestered in a younger child self-state. The key to her treatment would be accessing these previously hidden states. Rather than encouraging her to fight against the voice telling her not to eat as the previous treatment team had done, the therapist believed it would be important to understand the feelings held in these self-states to release her from the current self-destructive cycle of behavior.

Anita progressed well in a dissociative treatment following the EDUCATE model as detailed in (Silberg, 2022). EDUCATE is an acronym that represents sequential treatment stages and related tasks (see Table 6.4). The first stage of treatment, E, involves education ("Educate") about how self-states benefit from working together and how the different senses of self who have helped during challenging times in life can be one's own feelings "talking" to oneself. Once Anita understood that her "imaginary friends" could have come to help her when she was in a difficult situation, she began drawing pictures of things her "friends" recalled from the past, despite not understanding what she was drawing at first. The second stage of the EDUCATE model, D, involves a discussion about the motivation behind dissociation (i.e., "Dissociation Motivation"). Anita's need to keep the past at a distance was assessed and discussed. Specifically, forgetting the past allowed her to move forward with positive aspects of life. By dissociating these memories instead of working through them and healing, the memories were not resolved and therefore could come back and disrupt her current life. During the "U" ("Understand") stage of the model, Anita learned to understand how the voices she heard held important messages about fearful experiences she had suffered (i.e., the ones that were expressed in her drawings). During the "C" stage she was encouraged to "Claim" those fearful experiences as part of

TABLE 6.4. The EDUCATE Model

Acronym	Step of model	Description of model	Sample tasks
E	Educate	Educate about dissociation and traumatic processes	• Behaviors and symptoms have meaning or purpose • Trauma can cause disconnection in the mind • The whole self must work together
D	Dissociation Motivation	Address and analyze the factors that keep the client tied to dissociative strategies	• Confront the need for dissociation • Consider pros and cons • Encourage central responsibility
U	Understand Unravel	Understand what is hidden Unravel automatically activated affect, identity, or behaviors	• Encourage expression through art, symbolic play, and music • Encourage the child to "listen in" • Gently confront "unremembering"
C	Claim	Claim hidden aspects of the self as one's own	• Make bargains with hidden parts of the self • Highlight feelings with role-play • Imagine together to fill in blanks in autobiographical, not traumatic, memory
A	Arousal Affect Regulation Attachment	Learn to regulate arousal and feelings in the context of loving relationships	• Reinforce safety • Practice breathing and calming imagery • Reward awareness and connection
T	Triggers Trauma	Identify precursors to automatic, trauma-based responding Process traumatic materials	• Process traumatic meaning of events and develop alternate view • Encourage mastery of experiences both in life and symbolically
E	End	End treatment	• Reinforce differences between "then" and "now" • Use symbols and metaphors to reinforce integration

Note. For a more complete list of tasks associated with each step in the EDUCATE model, see Silberg (2022).

herself and her memories. During the "A" stage she was taught how to modulate her "Arousal" using breathing and imagery to tolerate the feelings that came to her when she thought about these imaginary friends and looked at the drawings. Anita also created a "toolbox" that she took to school to help her with difficult feelings that came up during the day that assisted her with "Affect regulation" (another part of the A stage of treatment). This box was specially decorated and included pictures, items to touch, self-soothing statements, and a special scent. She learned that "Adam" told her not to eat because it was during the "lunch bunch" break at her preschool that the abuse happened. By being nauseous, she could go to the nurse's office and miss the lunch time. Sometimes she had been allowed to leave school early, so the nausea became associated with soothing and connection with her mother. During the period where she was being abused, Anita had felt abandoned by her mother and terrified, and this "Attachment" rupture was also addressed as part of the "A" stage in therapy. Anita's mother reassured her daughter that, had she known what was happening, she would have immediately rescued her. They also used play to reenact the experience of rescue to counter Anita's feelings of abandonment. Anita learned how to process the "Traumatic memories" during the "T" stage of treatment and came to understand how "Triggers" at school and home reminded her of trauma from the past. The therapist helped "Adam" understand that it was a different time now and that the "bad person" who had hurt him was no longer a threat. Over time, Anita felt more confident in her ability to manage the "imaginary friends" who tried to "help her" deal with stressful situations.

As Anita began to stabilize and understand the inside "friends" that came to help her during her difficult time, she remembered feelings, sensations, and thoughts associated with the events that had happened at the preschool. These were processed in therapy. She came to understand that some of the cognitions she had come to believe about herself such as "I am ugly and fat," were a result of the sexual, physical, and emotional abuse she had suffered and were not true.

The many strengths in this family allowed treatment to progress smoothly. The level of attachment predating the trauma was secure with her mother, although Anita described being somewhat suspicious and fearful of her father's temper. The family participated in various stages of parent–child work and parenting work to repair ruptures that occurred because of the family's missing the early signs of the abuse and not rescuing Anita sooner. "Adam" learned that her mother was truly committed and loved "him" as well as Anita. Anita's father lessened his demand for custodial time so that Anita became accustomed to time with him slowly and decided herself when she was ready for "sleep over" time. During one joint session, Anita explained how she tried to give her parents clues about the abuse (i.e., drawings left around the house), but they had not understood her subtle messages. Over time, both parents showed Anita a new level of attention and concern about the past. They apologized for not getting her more help earlier and for not being there in time to save her. The therapist worked with all of them to recognize that they were not to blame for the abuse.

Anita's parents advocated to keep her in school, even during some of the most stressful parts of treatment. They believed, and the therapist agreed, that it was important to keep Anita in school to continue along the developmental path of her peers, as much as possible, but there were some challenges at times. For example, Anita learned that her new school was on the same street as her preschool, which felt triggering and scary. With the support of her school, Anita was permitted stress relieving tools at school such as her "toolbox," and the administration worked with the therapist and parents to structure classes in a way that was manageable for Anita. Despite her strong negative feelings toward "boys," Anita learned the traumatic source of some of these feelings and was willing to give the new school a chance. The family also followed through on recommendations to work with Anita's pediatrician. Anita was helped by an antinausea medication that allowed her to eat without reflexive vomiting.

As the dissociative symptoms became less prominent, they reached the "E" or "Ending" stage of therapy, where Anita worked with the therapist to manage more typical concerns for her age, including balancing social time with academic demands and sexuality, which was complicated by her early history. When asked 3 years later about the "imaginary friends," Anita said "Adam" was like a "weird feeling in her stomach that something bad might happen." She explained that she didn't mind the feeling because she could use it to figure out what she was scared about. She no longer thought much about the abuse, even though she still sometimes struggled with nightmares. She felt her relationship with both parents had improved, and she became fascinated with psychology and wanted to be a "brain scientist."

Having the correct diagnosis was key to the successful treatment and resolution of this case. The eating disorder treatment program that focused only on the negative cognitions and trying to "defeat the voice" were unable to get to the root of the issues. Anita's first treatment episode that did not address her sexual abuse unfortunately allowed the traumatic memories to become increasingly sequestered from her awareness. By understanding dissociative symptoms, what the transitional identities were trying to communicate about the early trauma, and how they were trying to help, Anita was able to free herself from the past and find new strength as an emerging adolescent. Of note, Anita's perpetrator was not a family member, and he was in jail. This was helpful for Anita and reinforced her need for a sense of universal justice. Unfortunately, few perpetrators are caught and imprisoned, so many children must manage feelings of unfairness and anxiety that their perpetrator may resurface in their lives.

Although the course of treatment may not be as seamless for many young people diagnosed with DD as it was for Anita, careful, intentional clinical interviewing, use of self-report measures, and consideration of diagnostic criteria are key to determining the best next steps on the path to healing. Arriving at the correct diagnosis and determining a treatment plan that considers parents' and children's strengths and vulnerabilities makes it possible to navigate challenging symptom presentations most successfully. More information about treatment is available (Silberg, 2022; Sinason & Marks, 2021; Waters, 2016; Wieland, 2015).

CONCLUSION

Dissociation in youth is an important clinical symptom; its presence can be predictive of a complex treatment trajectory. When overlooked or not attended to in treatment, dissociative symptoms can also contribute to unnecessarily prolonged treatment and suffering for the child. For clinicians to recognize, conceptualize, and treat trauma in youth, they must be prepared to assess for dissociation adequately and understand the various ways dissociation presents in different stages of development. A thorough clinical interview, together with data from validated assessment tools, combined with a family assessment, can provide crucial treatment-relevant information about a child's symptomology and the family's readiness for treatment. It can also guide treatment planning such as when serious risks (e.g., suicidality) or severe dissociative symptoms (e.g., amnesia for self-harm) need to be addressed immediately. The interview assists clinicians in learning about symptoms, understanding the youth's view of self, and assessing the severity of symptoms, both dissociative and nondissociative. Finding the exact diagnosis should not be the primary focus, as research is still relatively limited on DD and DPTSD diagnoses in youth. Rather, clinicians should focus on the symptoms that are most severe or causing the most difficulty, rule out other common childhood disorders, and consider the role of social media influences on symptoms. Above all, clinicians should be prepared to take a nimble, ongoing approach to assessment because both youth and families often reveal more as they feel more comfortable in the therapeutic relationship.

7 TAILORING TREATMENT FOR TRAUMA-RELATED DISSOCIATION

Traumatized clients are most likely to be able to tolerate and benefit from treatment if assessment informs treatment planning. Treatment differs according to the type and severity of the client's presenting problems, such as trauma-related dissociation (TRD). Assessment should be conducted at the beginning of treatment as well as episodically throughout treatment, even if only informally. This chapter provides a brief overview of the treatment of TRD that is consistent with best practices for treating complex trauma, with an emphasis on chronic, complex dissociative symptoms and dissociative disorders (DDs). The chapter addresses the limitations of current treatment guidelines for posttraumatic stress disorder (PTSD) and complex PTSD as they relate to TRD. Space limitations allow only limited citations of the excellent clinical resources addressing the treatment of TRD (see Appendix C).

Treatment studies of individuals with various psychiatric disorders generally find that patients with TRD tend to have more severe symptoms, worse outcomes, and higher dropout rates (e.g., Chlebowski & Gregory, 2012; Hagenaars et al., 2010; Jaycox et al., 1998; Kleindienst et al., 2011; Michelson

https://doi.org/10.1037/0000386-007
The Concise Guide to the Assessment and Treatment of Trauma-Related Dissociation,
by B. L. Brand

et al., 1998; Rufer et al., 2006; Speckens et al., 2006; Spitzer et al., 2007; Tamar-Gurol et al., 2008; Taylor, 2003; Yen et al., 2009; but see also Hagenaars et al., 2010; Halvorsen et al., 2014). In some PTSD studies, patients with dissociation have shown slower response, lack of response, lower effect size, or, in some cases, deterioration, if standard prolonged exposure or cognitive behavioral treatment for PTSD is used, despite these being evidence-based treatments for PTSD (e.g., Cloitre et al., 2010; D'Andrea & Pole, 2012; International Society for the Study of Trauma and Dissociation [ISSTD], 2011).

Individuals with high TRD also have high levels of comorbid, severe symptoms that require more intensive treatment than other diagnostic groups. For example, a study in *The New England Journal of Medicine* found that individuals with dissociative symptoms and DDs require the most therapy sessions compared with 17 other psychiatric disorders, including mood, anxiety, and substance abuse disorders (Mansfield et al., 2010). Dissociation can also be challenging to treat due to its association with high rates of suicidal ideation, suicidal behavior, nonsuicidal self-injurious (NSSI) behavior, and multiple hospitalizations (Brand, Classen, Lanius, et al., 2009; Brand, McNary, et al., 2013; Foote et al., 2008). There is often a tremendous personal burden for individuals with TRD as well as high socioeconomic costs (Langeland et al., 2020). There have been calls for clinicians to assess and specifically target dissociation in treatment for all clients, not just traumatized individuals (Ellickson-Larew, Stasik-O'Brien, et al., 2020; Lyssenko et al., 2018; Vonderlin et al., 2018). Together, these data illustrate that many highly dissociative individuals require intensive inpatient and outpatient treatment.

The core problems that require treatment in complex trauma include affect, behavioral, and somatic dysregulation; dissociation; impaired self-concept; insecure, unhealthy relational patterns; and a lack of existential or spiritual meaning or purpose (e.g., Ford & Courtois, 2020b). The conceptualization of treatment for TRD is built on assessing trauma-related deficits and adaptations, vulnerabilities (e.g., medical conditions, ongoing interpersonal violence, living in a high-violence community), and strengths (e.g., social support). The client's current knowledge and use (or lack thereof) of self-regulation and symptom management techniques is a critical area for both initial and ongoing assessment. Even after learning techniques for self-regulation and symptom management, many trauma survivors do not consistently follow through with using them. Discussing and resolving the underlying beliefs and roadblocks related to not caring for oneself (e.g., "I don't deserve to be treated well") is essential to successfully treating TRD.

Treatment should focus on developing or restoring self-regulation capacity; a cohesive, more stable identity; a sense of connection and meaning; and secure attachment that allows for engagement and maintenance of healthy relationships. Developing skills in self-regulation includes enhancing the ability to recognize, allow oneself to experience, and manage emotions and body sensations without engaging in excessive avoidance. Avoidance of feelings and trauma often underlies dissociation, substance use, risky and unhealthy or unsafe behaviors, frequent crises, and reenactments of trauma (Brand, 2001; Nester, Boi, et al., 2022). Many survivors of developmental trauma also need guidance in developing basic self-care such as healthy patterns of eating; hydrating; sleeping; balancing relaxation, work, and caring for self versus others; and realistic goal-setting and management. Developing a sense of identity requires working toward resolving shame and other trauma-related emotions and beliefs, conflicted patterns of attachment, and overcoming the tendency to disown or compartmentalize aspects of self. In individuals with complex DDs, developing a more cohesive sense of self is also supported by gradually reflecting on traumatic experiences and developing a coherent trauma narrative (discussed later in the chapter). Treatment fosters developing a sense of self as competent, worthy, and capable of managing daily life, including stressors and problem solving, as well as reflecting and being present to experience one's own and others' experiences (i.e., mentalizing).

INDIVIDUALIZING TREATMENT TO THE NEEDS AND PREFERENCES OF THE PATIENT

Treatment needs to be individualized to be consistent with the individual's presenting symptoms, deficits, and resiliencies, as well as their treatment preferences and aspects of their identity and to fit with their sociocultural context. It should be tailored to address and respect culture-specific manifestations of trauma and modes of help-seeking that are viewed as culturally acceptable. These variables should be considered when clinicians discuss treatment options. For example, some trauma survivors do not want to engage in retelling and reexperiencing the emotions and sensations that occurred during trauma. Some survivors cannot tolerate engaging in such an intensive treatment without becoming extremely overwhelmed and at risk for NSSI, substance abuse, or other poor outcomes. On the other hand, avoidance of trauma can paradoxically create more traumatic intrusions and contribute to unrecognized reenactments and vulnerability to destabilization.

If a clinician attempts to convince a client to participate in a treatment intervention that they do not want, this could be a reenactment of trauma in that an authority figure is controlling and limiting the independence of a survivor. Research shows that patients who are given the treatment that they prefer, such as exposure versus medication for PTSD, show better adherence to the treatment and greater improvement of symptoms of PTSD, depression, and anxiety (Zoellner et al., 2019).

Another example illustrates the importance of respecting a client's identity and autonomy: Although eventual fusion or integration of self-states into one integrated identity is possible with many DID patients, some individuals prefer to work toward increased awareness, collaboration, and cooperative functioning among self-states without integration. However, higher levels of integration are associated with less severe levels of dissociation, PTSD, and depression, as well as greater ability to recognize emotions (Lebois et al., 2020). Individuals with DID who prefer to retain young self-states may be more vulnerable to trauma-related difficulties. Ideally, clinicians should be aware of and present the range of possible treatment options, including each option's potential risks, benefits, relevant treatment research, and clinical or expert practice guidelines so that clients can make informed choices about their treatment options.

Clinicians should be well-trained in assessing dissociation as well as emotion regulation and the presence and management of risky and potentially dangerous impulses and behaviors, among others (see Chapters 3 and 4), to determine the extent to which treatment should address stabilization of safety and emotion regulation. Clinicians informed about the assessment of trauma exposure and reactions to trauma, including dissociation, can individualize treatment to include assistance stabilizing safety, regulating emotions, and managing dissociation or other trauma-related symptoms. Clinicians also need to be able to assess progress accurately throughout treatment and therefore must be skilled in conducting ongoing assessment of symptoms and functional capacities to pace treatment appropriately (see later in this chapter and Chapter 4).

If clinicians do not understand how complex and severe the client's dissociative symptoms are, they may mistakenly believe that the client is able to tolerate trauma processing without first developing foundational skills such as regulation and management of suicidal thoughts and urges and emotion regulation. Discussing trauma almost inevitably brings up shame and other intense emotions, often with the client feeling a concomitant need to escape or avoid the memories and emotions. This need often triggers dissociation or unhealthy coping such as NSSI, substance use, and suicide attempts. Although long-term avoidance of dealing with trauma prevents healing, focusing too early, frequently, or intensely on trauma also prevents healing. Therefore, the foundation of healing from complex trauma starts with an assessment of traumatized individuals' symptoms, adaptations, and resiliencies, which then informs treatment planning including the timing and pacing of present- versus past-focused work (see Chapters 1 and 3, this volume; Briere & Scott, 2015; Ford & Courtois, 2020b; Frewen & Lanius, 2015). Well-developed distress tolerance and emotional engagement are necessary components of successfully processing traumatic memories in psychotherapy. If the client cannot stay grounded in the present moment, it will be impossible for them to attend to, learn, and remember new ways of thinking about themselves, others, and traumatic experiences (Price et al., 2014). If they are so dissociated in session that they cannot feel emotions, they will not be able to experience the relief and therapeutic repair that can come from sharing and processing traumatic experiences with an empathic, attuned therapist.

If assessment indicates acute flooding of PTSD, severe dissociation that is disrupting daily life (e.g., amnesia for events at work or while parenting), or recent trauma or overwhelming stressors, treatment should focus on stabilization such as providing support, reducing the level of nervous system activation and environmental stimulation, grounding, and ensuring that safe shelter, food, and other necessities are available. Medication consultation may be indicated. If NSSI has become severe enough to require medical attention, suicidal ideation has increased above the client's typical baseline level, or there are risk factors that increase risk of suicide attempts (e.g., active substance abuse, little social support), hospitalization may be indicated.

TREATMENT OF COMPLEX TRAUMA

Judith Herman (1992b) conceptualized the impact and treatment of complex trauma in her landmark book *Trauma and Recovery*. Elaborating on the work of early trauma pioneers such as Pierre Janet, Herman described the treatment of complex trauma as occurring in three stages. This staged approach has been supported in expert consensus guidelines for decades as well as research about complex TRD (Cloitre, Courtois, et al., 2012; ISSTD, 2011; Kezelman & Stavropoulos, 2019). Similarly, the treatment of DDs requires a trauma-informed, staged approach to treatment that typically involves long-term psychotherapy and psychotropic medications. Space constraints limit the depth of this discussion, but detailed descriptions of the treatment of complex DDs are available (see Appendix C).

First Stage

In the first stage, following assessment, treatment emphasizes a "here-and-now-focus" in contrast to a past-focused, intensive exploration of trauma. This first stage emphasizes the *stabilization of safety* (particularly suicidality and severe NSSI, as well as other high-risk behaviors), development of healthy emotion regulation (including reducing over- and underactivation—that is, "feeling too much or too little"), establishment of an initial level of a therapeutic alliance, psychoeducation about trauma and its impact, and the stabilization of treatment-interfering comorbid conditions including depression, eating disorders, and substance abuse.

Even in the stabilization stage, trauma is addressed from an educational perspective. This preliminary trauma-informed work is essential to the success of the treatment. Learning about trauma's impact can foster self-compassion and enhance motivation to change. For example, shame and self-blame about having been sexually abused as a child can be reduced by teaching about the prevalence and impact of sexual abuse, along with the neurobiological and behavioral adaptations (e.g., dissociation and NSSI) that allow individuals to survive it. Reduced shame and self-blame make the challenging work of processing trauma in Stage 2 less distressing, thereby reducing the client's avoidance and the risk for becoming overwhelmed or dropping out of treatment. Learning that adaptations such as dissociation and NSSI may have been crucially beneficial in the past but, once the trauma has ended, interfere with healing motivates clients to do the work necessary to heal from complex trauma.

Stabilizing safety involves developing an understanding of the client's triggers and functions of NSSI and dissociation. This approach to stabilizing safety is beneficial to clients with complex DDs, according to the Treatment of Patients With Dissociative Disorders (TOP DD) studies (discussed later in the chapter; Brand, Schielke, et al., 2019; Brand et al., 2022; Schielke et al., 2022). The alliance is strengthened as clients begin to understand themselves and recognize that the therapist is helping them achieve progress in healing. Many clients become more determined to find ways of regulating themselves that foster recovery rather than avoidance (e.g., grounding) and that use here-and-now resources, rather than the more limited resources they had while being traumatized.

The stages of treatment should not be considered as discrete periods because the focus may shift according to changes in health, social support, stressors, and response to therapy. Flexibility and individualizing the treatment, including how much stabilization a client needs, is necessary to successfully resolve complex trauma. Many trauma survivors drop out of treatment, including from evidence-based treatments, before benefiting from it. For example, in a study comparing exposure therapy to treatment with sertraline, approximately one third of the patients dropped out of exposure therapy, most typically by Session 5 (Rauch et al., 2019). Clients who receive the trauma treatment they prefer drop out of treatment less frequently and show better response to treatment (Zoellner et al., 2019). Improving treatment so that trauma survivors can tolerate it, along with carefully pacing treatment to avoid overwhelm, and routinely assessing for therapeutic ruptures and repairing the alliance, is crucial. Some clients can move quickly through the first stage, but many, particularly the most severely dissociative, need years to stabilize, and some never attain the ability to safely tolerate trauma processing (Kluft, 1994c).

Second Stage

Before beginning the second stage, which focuses on *trauma processing*, the patient's safety must be stable. Furthermore, the relationship with the therapist must be strong, and the patient must be able to manage emotions and symptoms without relying on dissociation, NSSI, substances, or other high-risk behaviors and forms of excessive avoidance (Cloitre, Courtois, et al., 2012; ISSTD, 2011; Kezelman & Stavropoulos, 2012). Without this foundation, trauma-focused work can be overwhelming and even retraumatizing (discussed subsequently). The high rates of dropout or symptom worsening found in some of the evidence-based treatments may be due in part to not providing stabilization before trauma processing among those with complex trauma and high TRD (D'Andrea & Pole, 2012).

Stage 2 involves reflection and exploring traumatic memories with the therapist, while staying grounded in the present. Patients process trauma-related memories, emotions, beliefs, and physical sensations that may have been avoided, with the goal of gradually integrating dissociated memory fragments into a coherent narrative that places events into the context of the individual's life. Individuals with numerous traumas typically begin processing the most easily tolerated traumas. Trauma processing leads to a shift in beliefs rooted in trauma (e.g., "I am permanently damaged"; "no one can be trusted") to recovery-based beliefs (e.g., "I am a worthwhile person capable and deserving of good things"). The survivor gains a sense of mastery over their traumas as the fragmented elements of the trauma (e.g., intense emotions, horrifying images and sensory experiences) gradually cease to be intrusive and disruptive.

Individuals with complex DDs are prone to shifting frequently into dissociative states and autohypnotic states, including when processing trauma

(Butler et al., 1996; Dell, 2017). Kluft and other experts recommend using complex DD individuals' innate hypnotic skills to "fractionate" trauma processing—that is, break into tolerable chunks various aspects of the trauma (ISSTD, 2011; Kluft, 1982, 2013). This is an important aspect of pacing and makes the trauma processing more manageable.

Third Stage

In the third stage, the tasks of *integration and reconnection* are emphasized (Herman, 1992b). This stage fosters connections and integration within the individual (including more connection with their body and self-states, if present) as well as beyond into their communities. The survivor's social connections are expanded, and their identity, career, sense of meaning in life, and engagement with meaningful activities are further developed. Relationships deepen as survivors develop greater awareness of their needs, boundaries, and communication skills. Some survivors chose to develop or enhance sexual intimacy. There is less focus on trauma, although many survivors become engaged in helping prevent and heal trauma in their communities and society. Herman (2023) speculated that this step, developing a "survivor mission," may be considered a fourth stage of healing from trauma.

A number of specific treatments for complex trauma survivors have been developed (for examples, see the review by Ford & Courtois, 2020b). There are key commonalities across the treatments (Herman, 2020). First, most treatment approaches emphasize a staged model, as just outlined. Second, survivors developing a collaborative relationship with the therapist is essential, although this is challenging with individuals who have been subjected to manipulation, coercion, and violence. As a result, survivors frequently perceive people in the present as acting "just like" past abusers and nonprotective caregivers. Thus, clinicians need to be able to tolerate being seen as untrustworthy and harmful and able to process these perceptions nondefensively with clients (as discussed later in the chapter). Third, a recognition and appreciation of the survivor's strengths is crucial. This recognition supports the client's developing sense of competence and the alliance between the client and therapist, which contributes to improved treatment response for clients, including those with DDs (Cronin et al., 2014). Fourth, processing relational dynamics including reenactments is a powerful opportunity for survivors to learn how to observe, communicate, and collaborate in relationships and contributes to developing the capacity for observing themselves and others (Ford & Courtois, 2020b)—that is, the capacity to "mentalize" (Fonagy et al., 2002).

TARGETS IN TREATMENT OF TRD

Treatment of highly dissociative individuals requires targeting dissociation and emotion regulation, teaching grounding, stabilizing safety, and working with self-states in the patients who have them. Attending to each of these targets is essential for treatment to be beneficial.

Dissociation, Grounding, and Emotional Regulation

Dissociation can become a habitual method of coping with emotion, conflicts, and stress. Many have a phobia of emotion, so dissociation becomes their primary method of regulating or, more accurately, avoiding emotion (Steele et al., 2005). It is important to target dissociation because it appears to contribute directly to severe comorbid symptoms and dysfunction (Boyd et al., 2018). For example, among patients hospitalized for PTSD treatment, dissociation mediated the relationship between PTSD and alcohol-related problems (Patel et al., 2022). Greater PTSD severity was associated with higher dissociative symptoms, which in turn were associated with greater alcohol-related problems. Dissociation had a unique mechanistic role contributing to worse alcohol-related problems. This supports the self-medication hypothesis—that is, individuals use substances to cope with psychiatric symptoms (Khantzian, 1985). Therefore, targeting dissociation in treatment may improve treatment outcome among those with TRD.

Another consideration for treatment planning is the *timing* of dissociation. Lanius et al. (2012) hypothesized that dissociation occurring *during* treatment sessions might particularly interfere with the learning that takes place. For example, dissociation during trauma-processing could prevent the extinction of trauma-based fear and shame. In support of this, dissociation at the onset of treatment was the only variable that predicted treatment response in individuals presenting to an emergency department after having been acutely traumatized (Price et al., 2014). Many clients with chronic TRD have grown so accustomed to being dissociated that they prefer being dissociated over being grounded. They are unlikely to report being quite dissociated in session because they do not fully recognize it or do not realize that it impedes their ability to respond to treatment. This suggests that clinicians should frequently assess for level of dissociation during sessions. Further, they should teach and practice grounding techniques in session to improve full awareness of the present moment and enhance learning. More information about the range of grounding techniques and how to teach them to clients is available (Brand et al., 2022; Schielke et al., 2022).

Clients may believe in "rules" about emotions, including that having emotions is unsafe, wrong, or a sign of weakness; showing emotions will lead to punishment, violence, or abandonment; and engaging in unsafe behaviors or dissociation are the only ways that "work" to manage strong emotions (Brand et al., 2022). Emotion regulation skills are a crucial component of treatment for individuals with TRD, as dissociation may be a primary method that they developed to avoid emotional overwhelm. In a meta-analysis, Cavicchioli and colleagues (2021) found moderate to large effect sizes showing that dissociation was associated with maladaptive domains of emotional regulation, including disengagement (behavioral and experiential avoidance, emotion and thought suppression) and aversive cognitive perseveration (rumination, worry, nonacceptance). Emotion dysregulation is addressed further later in the chapter.

Working With Self-States

If assessment indicates the client struggles with identity alteration and fragmentation or ongoing amnesia, particularly if they cannot recall risky behaviors such as NSSI or substance use, further assessment for a DD is strongly indicated. If the client suffers from a complex DD (dissociative identity disorder [DID] or other specified DD-1 [OSDD01]), treatment will need to be adapted. The foci addressed in complex trauma treatment—safety, grounding, and containment of trauma—are likely to require much more time and attention. Furthermore, the client will need to learn gradually about their self-states, which typically requires learning the function of each self-state (e.g., learning which state(s) assists by compartmentalizing various traumas and related affect, which state(s) assists by maintaining daily functioning, and which state(s) are responsible for acting on NSSI and suicidal ideation; Brand et al., 2022; Steele et al., 2005; van der Hart et al., 2006). Self-states often have very different recollections of childhood attachment relationships and memories about trauma, which can lead to considerable conflict—and at times, suicidal ideation and NSSI. Furthermore, due to discrepant patterns of dealing with emotion, relationships, and conflict, there is often intense disagreement about managing daily matters, sometimes leading clients to be caught up in inner "wars" among self-states. Thus, developing an understanding and gradual acceptance of self-states and capacity to work cooperatively is a crucially important, yet time-intensive, task (ISSTD, 2011). Healthy emotion regulation will need to be considerably strengthened before exploring trauma, as well as ensuring that no self-state is adamantly against discussing trauma in therapy. The treatment should follow the expert consensus guidelines developed by international experts in the treatment of complex DDs. Guidelines for working with youth and adults with complex DDs are available without charge from the ISSTD (https://www.isst-d.org/resources/).

Treating individuals with DID/OSDD-1 requires additional training, supervision, and consultation. Many resources and trainings are available at https://www.isst-d.org/resources/ and in Appendix C. The Finding Solid Ground program is a research-informed and supported educational program that is beneficial for dissociative clients as well as therapists (discussed subsequently and in Brand, Schielke, et al., 2019; Brand et al., 2022; Schielke et al., 2022). Therapists who participated in the program reported that they learned many new ways of working to stabilize symptoms and enhance the client's motivation to do the work needed to recover. Clinicians have told me that the program is a "game changer" when they use it as part of their treatment with dissociative adults as well as motivated and insightful older youth.

Stabilizing Safety Problems

Clients with complex PTSD (CPTSD), the dissociative subtype of PTSD (DPTSD), and complex DDs frequently engage in NSSI. Preliminary data from the randomized controlled trial of the TOP DD studies illustrate the importance of this treatment focus. (At the time of writing this book, this study was still underway.) Specifically, 82% of the individuals with DID or OSDD-1 had a lifetime NSSI history compared with 52% of those with CPTSD or DPTSD. In the 6 months before starting the study, 46.63% of the DDs group engaged in NSSI compared with 26.92% of the PTSD group, a statistically significant difference (Brand, 2023). Clearly, clinicians need to understand and be competent at treating NSSI in clients with TRD. The need for evidence-supported methods for stabilizing NSSI was one of the primary reasons the TOP DD research team developed a program (i.e., the Finding Solid Ground program) aimed specifically at establishing safety, among other foci, for individuals with TRD.

Individuals with complex trauma histories often engage in behavioral reenactments and/or unhealthy, risky, or unsafe behaviors. These behaviors are attempts to manage the emotions that may have felt, and may continue to feel, to be life-threatening. Furthermore, the behaviors can serve to regulate body sensations and symptoms of PTSD and dissociation. For example, some trauma survivors hurt themselves to stop terrifying images of trauma or body sensations associated with trauma. As such, NSSI and other risky or unhealthy behaviors are *adaptations* to trauma. What clinicians and researchers, myself included, refer to as "symptoms" and "pathology" need to be recognized as attempts to survive what may have been otherwise beyond survival. Thus, dissociation is both an essential adaptation and survival mechanism while the trauma was ongoing, yet also a symptom that causes dysfunction after the trauma is over. As noted by Brand and colleagues (2022),

> The notion of "getting safe" can feel entirely unconceivable because they may have never known safety. What is unknown is unpredictable to trauma survivors, and therefore is a trigger signaling danger. Getting safer can seem like a trick, a way the therapist or other supportive people may be attempting to reduce the patient's defenses in order to humiliate or harm them. (p. 65)

Directly acknowledging that these behaviors likely helped them survive or are the best strategies they have discovered so far is important, as is offering hope that they can learn new ways of managing overwhelming emotion that help them heal from trauma. It takes tremendous work and courage to gradually relinquish reliance on dissociation and unsafe behaviors and begin to develop other, often less rapid and only somewhat helpful, ways of coping.

Almost all individuals with complex DDs (92.31%) are at least partially unaware of what contributes to their urges to hurt themselves (Nester, Boi, et al., 2022), according to the findings from the TOP DD studies. Thus, clients need to discover the triggers and multiple functions NSSI may serve, which can vary over time and situations. Nester, Boi, and colleagues (2022) found that the most common reasons DD patients engaged in NSSI were, in order of frequency, as follows: trauma-related cues, emotion dysregulation, overwhelming stressors (e.g., financial concerns or social disappointments), psychiatric and physical health symptoms, dissociative experiences (e.g., conflict among self-states), and ineffective coping (e.g., neglecting self-care or failing to use grounding techniques). Trauma-related cues included situations that were reminiscent of trauma such as interactions with angry people and anniversary dates associated with traumatic experiences. Other trauma-related triggers included intrusive symptoms such as flashbacks and hyperarousal. NSSI was used to manage emotional dysregulation, particularly in response to feeling anger, shame, or being overwhelmed. Some participants described using NSSI to shift from feeling emotional to physical pain. One person described using NSSI to "feel real pain." Many of the individuals used NSSI to punish themselves, often related to trauma-based beliefs they were "bad" or had somehow caused their childhood abuse. Understanding these reasons for self-harm for each patient enables clinicians to identify what areas to focus on in treatment to stabilize that patient's NSSI. If a client's NSSI is primarily triggered by trauma-related cues, treatment should focus on grounding in present reality, distinguishing past from present, and containment of traumatic intrusions (descriptions of methods to do this are available in Brand et al., 2022, and Schielke et al., 2022). Another client's NSSI may primarily occur when they believe they "need to be punished"; therefore, exploring and working through this belief is indicated. A third client's NSSI may primarily occur in response to a self-state demanding self-harm. This suggests that it is necessary to work with this self-state (and possibly other self-states) to learn why they urge self-harm and then resolve that conflict or belief to help stabilize safety.

In another study of individuals with high TRD, NSSI was linked to poor emotion regulation, stress, and difficulty dealing with psychiatric or physical health symptoms (Nester, Brand, et al., 2022). Participants also engaged in NSSI related to dissociative issues (e.g., a self-state urged NSSI as self-punishment or young self-states were triggered). These studies underscore the importance of improving emotion regulation, PTSD symptom management, grounding skills, and exploring and resolving the trauma-related belief that one deserves to be punished.

Individuals with complex trauma and high dissociation reduced their reliance on dissociation when treated in a stage model that taught emotion regulation and healthy relationship skills before focusing on trauma processing (Cloitre, Petkova, et al., 2012). Furthermore, they continued to show improvements in PTSD symptoms at follow-up, whereas those with high dissociation who did not receive skills training but instead only trauma processing showed worsening PTSD symptoms.

THE IMPORTANCE OF MATCHING TREATMENT TO PATIENTS' NEEDS

Clinicians working on inpatient trauma units find that a substantial subgroup of the patients require hospitalization due to worsening symptoms, often in response to not matching the pace or the focus of treatment to the patient's skills and symptoms (Brand, 2001). Richard J. Loewenstein, MD, directed an inpatient and outpatient treatment program for highly traumatized adults for 28 years, during which he directly treated, supervised, or consulted on the treatment of approximately 4,000 individuals with TRD. He estimated that approximately one third of the patients needing hospitalization had decompensated in response to too much or too rapid trauma processing without sufficient stabilization, particularly in recent years due to inappropriate use of eye movement desensitization and reprocessing (EMDR) in nonstabilized individuals (R. J. Loewenstein, personal communication, February 9, 2022). He described typical decompensations as including increased NSSI; suicidal behavior; increased and highly dysregulated PTSD and dissociative symptoms; and worsening of mood, eating, substance use, and other comorbid disorders.

My inpatient and outpatient consultations are consistent with Loewenstein's observations. For example, clients with self-states may have profound conflict regarding whether they should reveal trauma. If treatment is focused on revealing trauma, some self-states may attempt to prevent "secrets" from being told by escalating NSSI, attempting suicide, or causing other forms of interference with treatment. Dissociation experts have cautioned about carefully pacing trauma processing and adapting it so that it is titrated and manageable (Chu, 1988; Kluft, 1992, 1997, 2013). Also, individuals with DID may be in conflict about whether the trauma memories are accurate. Accordingly, premature exposure work may increase the rate of confabulated memory retrieval.

Dissociative clients can become extremely overwhelmed, even when evidence-based treatments are used, if they are applied without careful attention to their capacity to tolerate exposure-based interventions. Highly respected experts in exposure types of therapy have sought referrals or consultation from me for their dissociative clients who have not made progress despite treatment with evidence-based treatments. If a clinician does not know how severe a client's dissociation is or does not know how to help clients develop skill in recognizing and decreasing dissociation via grounding, they cannot adequately pace treatment to match the client's dissociative complexity and ability to manage emotions, unsafe impulses, and symptoms.

I share an example so readers can understand that the risk to clients is real. I was consulted about a client who had been intubated in the local emergency department over a dozen times in a single year due to repeated, sudden onset of an inability to breathe. The clinician had been conducting prolonged exposure sessions as she had been trained to do according to the protocol. She was alarmed that the patient had gotten much worse, with an escalation of NSSI, suicidal ideation, and increased PTSD and dissociative symptoms, including a voice telling her to kill herself. The client had undiagnosed (but suspected) DID and lacked skills in grounding, self-soothing, or containment. She frequently shifted into childlike states and had experienced more frequent flashbacks since starting exposure therapy. She lost awareness of present reality and was flooded with traumatic intrusions. Sleep was fragmented due to nightmares from which she would wake up screaming. To prevent nightmares, she avoided sleeping at night and could only sleep on the couch in the daytime.

In the process of several consultation sessions, it became clear that some self-states believed her abusers were still raping her—that is, she was confusing flashbacks as what was happening in the present reality. We learned that flashbacks precipitated her difficulty in breathing. Additionally, a dissociative self-state revealed that she was causing some of the flashbacks because she was terrified of the retaliation that would come from abusers for "telling secrets." I advised the clinician to stop focusing on trauma immediately and instead work with the client to stabilize safety, develop ways of grounding and improving orientation to the present, teach containment to reduce the flood of traumatic material, and begin to create communication and cooperation among self-states. This approach to working with individuals with DID is consistent with expert consensus guidelines and in research has been linked to improvements in safety, PTSD and dissociative symptoms, and enhanced emotion regulation and daily functioning (Brand, Classen, McNary, et al., 2009; Brand, McNary, et al., 2013; Brand, Schielke, et al., 2019; ISSTD, 2011). In the subsequent year, the patient stabilized and had just one intubation following an unanticipated encounter with an abuser from childhood.

Although this case was particularly severe, it exemplifies why and how patients are at risk of becoming more dissociative or symptomatic in treatment if TRD is not carefully assessed and addressed in treatment. It is essential for clinicians to be mindful of clients' tendency toward dissociation; to be aware of clients' ability to tolerate distress, emotions, and traumatic material; and to assess them repeatedly throughout treatment.

ASSESSING PROGRESS IN TREATMENT

Progress in treatment should be periodically assessed, even if only informally, so that adjustments based on the individual's current symptoms, resources, and situational variables can be taken into consideration. Informal assessment should be conducted at each session according to the struggles and needs of each client. Areas of particular importance include urges and behaviors related to NSSI, suicidal behavior, substance use and other risky behaviors; recent crises or stressors; quality of sleep; and engagement with recovery-focused coping and social interactions. Many clinicians would be surprised to learn how infrequently clients use crucial skills such as grounding, containment, and internal communication (for those with self-states). Ongoing assessments, as well as the clinician's decision-making related to changes in the treatment plan, should be documented in the patient's chart.

In addition to informal assessments, it is valuable to obtain systematic assessment periodically using validated measures such as the Progress in Treatment Questionnaire—patient (PITQ-p; see Chapter 4 and Appendix B, this volume; Schielke et al., 2017). The PITQ-p ascertains the client's perception of their ability to be aware of and manage emotions, trauma-related thoughts and symptoms, urges to be unsafe, and dissociative self-states (if present). The PITQ-p also assesses their perception of the degree to which they can collaborate with the therapist, experience meaning in life, and view themselves and others in a generally positive manner. In the TOP DD studies, the PITQ-p was the most sensitive measure for capturing change during treatment for TRD (Brand, Schielke, et al., 2019). An additional measure to assess progress in treatment for individuals with TRD, the Dimensions of Therapeutic Movement Instrument, is promising but requires validation (Kluft, 1994a).

TREATMENT OF THE NONCOMPLEX DISSOCIATIVE DISORDERS

Next, I review treatment recommendations and research for the dissociative disorders. Recent research is illuminating much about the treatment of the complex DDs, although research is urgently needed about all these disorders.

Dissociative Amnesia

The treatment literature on dissociative amnesia consists mostly of case studies. Some of the cases who were thought to have dissociative amnesia show many of the symptoms and history associated with DID, so the amnesia may have been due to unrecognized DID with the acute presentation of amnesia stemming from an amnestic self-state (Loewenstein et al., in press; Staniloiu & Markowitsch, 2014; Staniloiu et al., 2018). Dissociative amnesia can be conceptualized as a response to overwhelming stress or trauma (American Psychiatric Association, 2022). Thus, it can often be treated with the three-stage trauma-informed approach described earlier in the chapter. In individuals with a classic presentation of acute dissociative amnesia in response to a single severe stressor or trauma, improving physical and emotional safety by reducing the impact of the stressful situation or preventing additional trauma may be sufficient to produce a spontaneous or rapid recovery (Loewenstein et al., in press). In patients with a more prolonged course and with ongoing trauma, it is typically necessary to address the full range of symptoms that accompany complex trauma and issues of mistrust and harm related to betrayal by caregivers (Fung et al., 2022;

Loewenstein et al., in press). In some cases, amnesia becomes chronic, and the patient cannot tolerate recalling the stressors or trauma that precipitated the onset of amnesia. These chronic dissociative amnesia patients may remain severely disabled. Experts advise that hypnosis may be used cautiously to enhance containment, or, in some cases, integration of previously dissociated traumatic material (Loewenstein et al., in press). Pharmacologic approaches do not appear to produce meaningful improvement in dissociative amnesia, although medications targeting comorbid anxiety and depression can be useful (Loewenstein et al., in press).

Depersonalization/Derealization Disorder

Depersonalization/derealization disorder usually begins in adolescence or early adulthood and is associated with impairments in attention and cognitive function. This disorder is often accompanied by intense emotional distress including anxiety, depression, and obsessive self-monitoring for symptoms of depersonalization and derealization. A range of variables have been proposed to account for its development including chemical triggers (e.g., illicit drug use); childhood maltreatment; severe life stressors, including life transitions; genetics; and episodes of severe mental illness (reviewed in Loewenstein et al., in press). Approximately two thirds of these patients will have a chronic course, and although the disorder is associated with mood and anxiety symptoms, it does not generally respond well to standard treatments for depression and anxiety.

Somer and colleagues (2013) reviewed the treatment literature for depersonalization/derealization disorder. A small, open-label trial of naltrexone showed improvement in symptoms in 33% of patients (Simeon & Knutelska, 2005). Transcranial magnetic stimulation showed some promise in reducing symptoms in a small, uncontrolled trial (Mantovani et al., 2011). An open trial of manualized individual cognitive behavioral therapy consisting of psychoeducation, interventions targeting anxiety and avoidance behavior, and symptom monitoring was linked to improvements in dissociation, depersonalization, anxiety, and depression (Hunter et al., 2005). There have been four randomized controlled trials (RCTs) including two lamotrigine studies, one fluoxetine study, and one biofeedback study. One study found evidence for the efficacy of lamotrigine although the other study did not. Fluoxetine and biofeedback were not more effective than a control condition, although there was a trend for fluoxetine to be more efficacious for patients with comorbid anxiety disorder. Somer and colleagues concluded that RCT studies demonstrate inconsistent evidence for the efficacy of lamotrigine and no efficacy for other interventions. Additional treatment research on this disorder is clearly needed.

TREATMENT OF COMPLEX DISSOCIATIVE DISORDERS

As discussed earlier, the expert consensus guidelines (ISSTD, 2011) and research support the effectiveness of using a staged treatment model for complex DDs. A meta-analysis of eight DID outcome studies found that despite the methodological limitations of the studies, DID treatment that is consistent with expert guidelines was associated with improvements across a range of symptoms and comorbidities (Brand, Classen, McNary, et al., 2009). Patients showed reductions in diagnoses of comorbid disorders, as well as decreased levels of dissociation, depression, anxiety, suicidality, substance abuse, and general psychiatric distress. Effect sizes based on within patient pre–post assessments were in the medium to large range. The improvements in trauma-related symptoms persisted for 2 years following inpatient treatment for DDs and trauma (Ellason & Ross, 1997). Preliminary new research suggests that inpatient treatment for complex DDs is associated with reduction in dissociation as well as beneficial changes in brain network functioning related to improved emotional regulation (Schlumpf et al., 2019).

A survey of 36 international DD experts inquired about the interventions they recommended for most frequent use with complex DD patients across the stages of treatment (Brand, Myrick, et al., 2012). The experts' recommendations were consistent with ISSTD expert consensus guidelines (2011). Table 7.1 lists the most frequently recommended interventions for complex DD patients in the stabilization and trauma-processing stage. Experts recommended that patients in both stages work on stabilizing safety, along with learning and practicing grounding, PTSD containment, emotion regulation, and stabilizing from crises. In the trauma-processing stage, those areas were again emphasized with experts also recommending assisting clients in learning to cooperate and communicate with self-states and developing awareness of body sensations. Notably, even though Stage 2 is the trauma-processing stage, intensive, highly emotional processing of trauma was not recommended as one of the top 10 interventions to frequently use. Instead, experts emphasized careful titration of trauma processing with continued, frequent emphasis on safety, grounding, and regulation even while processing trauma. This recommendation runs counter to the way some evidence-based exposure treatments are conducted. The reason for this adaptation is that individuals with complex DDs cannot tolerate intense

TABLE 7.1. "Top 10" Expert Recommendations for Treatment of Complex Dissociative Disorders in Stages 1 and 2

Intervention	Stage 1 Stabilization and safety	Stage 2 Trauma processing
Establish safety	Yes	Yes
Establish/repair alliance	Yes	Yes
Teach/practice grounding	Yes	Yes
Educate about disorders and treatment options	Yes	
Diagnose comorbid disorders	Yes	
Teach/practice self-care	Yes	
Develop healthy relationships	Yes	
Develop affect tolerance and impulse control	Yes	Yes
Stabilize from current stressors and crises	Yes	Yes
Teach/practice containment	Yes	Yes
Teach cooperation with self-states		Yes
CBT focus on cognitive distortions		Yes
Identify/work with self-states		Yes
Develop awareness of body sensations		Yes

Note. CBT = cognitive behavior therapy. Intervention recommendations based on survey of 36 dissociative disorder experts in Brand, Myrick, et al. (2012).

exploration of trauma, week after week. The experts strongly advise that treatment needs to be more carefully paced and individualized for these patients (Brand, Myrick, et al., 2012; ISSTD, 2011).

Two research teams have developed studies that have substantial methodological improvements over the early studies that were included in the DD meta-analysis. One of these studies was led by Ellen Jepsen in Norway (Jepsen et al., 2013, 2014). Jepsen and colleagues compared the outcomes of women with and without complex DDs who received inpatient treatment for childhood sexual abuse. Patients with complex DDs showed reductions in PTSD symptoms and some types of dissociation, although the symptoms indicative of self-states (e.g., amnesia and identity fragmentation) did not improve. Furthermore, the patients who did not have complex DDs showed larger decreases in dissociation ($d = .69$) than did the complex DD group ($d = .25$). Although the treatment was generally consistent with best practices for complex trauma, it did not directly address dissociative self-states. The authors suggested that treatment may need to target amnesia directly and identity fragmentation to impact those symptoms. The other series of studies that have been methodologically improved—that is, the TOP DD studies—are described next.

The TOP DD Studies and the Finding Solid Ground Program

A series of prospective, international studies of treatment of patients with complex DDs, called the TOP DD studies, have been informative to the trauma field. A notable strength of the TOP DD studies is that all complex DD patients in treatment with a clinician who was also willing to participate were enrolled, even if they presented with severe NSSI, suicidal ideation or behavior, current substance abuse or dependence, hallucinations, or recent hospitalization(s). In contrast, patients with these severe symptoms are almost always excluded from RCTs. Thus, the results of the TOP DD studies generalize to the highly dissociative clients treated by clinicians in the community.

The first TOP DD study, that is, the "naturalistic study," used a naturalistic design meaning there was no change made in the treatment that patients were already receiving. The researchers collected assessment data from 280 individuals across 19 countries diagnosed with DID or DDNOS over the course of 30 months of treatment. Additionally, 292 therapists reported on their DD patients' progress. The acuity of the sample was sobering: Almost one quarter of the patients (23%) had required between one and three hospitalizations in the 6 months before enrolling in the study.

Patients in the first stage of treatment were highly impaired. They had higher levels of dissociation, PTSD, and NSSI and more hospitalizations, with lower levels of functioning, than those in the last stage (Brand, Classen, Lanius, et al., 2009). Longitudinal within-patient analyses showed that, as treatment progressed, patients showed reductions in dissociation, PTSD, depression, suicide attempts, NSSI, drug use, physical pain, and hospitalizations, as well as improvements in daily functioning (Brand, McNary, et al., 2013). Patients were more often volunteering or attending school, feeling good, and socializing over the course of 30 months of treatment. Even the individuals with the most severe depression and dissociation showed improvements (Engelberg & Brand, 2012). At a 6-year follow-up, the patients continued to show improvement according to their therapists; they had fewer stressors, revictimizations, and hospitalizations as well as improved daily functioning (Myrick, Webermann, Loewenstein, et al., 2017). Only 1.6% of the patients had required hospitalization in the 6 months before the 6-year follow-up. Therapists reported that patients experienced less internal conflict among self-states, which is important because ongoing conflict among self-states is associated with poor prognosis (Kluft, 1994c). The authors concluded that, despite severe, chronic impairment at the start of the study, patients made substantial improvements in treatment that directly addressed their DDs and trauma history.

The TOP DD team also estimated the costs of outpatient and inpatient treatment for each patient in the naturalistic study (Myrick, Webermann, Langeland, et al., 2017). The data showed that estimated treatment costs decreased over time. This was likely due to a decrease in days spent hospitalized as well as a decrease in outpatient sessions.

The next TOP DD study was the online educational program called the TOP DD Network study. The TOP DD Network study assessed the outcome of therapists and DD patients participating in an educational program that aimed to help patients stabilize their safety, improve emotion regulation, and reduce their dissociative symptoms. The educational program was an adjunct to individual psychotherapy and focused primarily on Stage 1 interventions, as per the DD expert survey results (Brand, Myrick, et al., 2012). The content and pacing of the program were informed by research, participants' feedback, feedback from a panel of individuals with lived experience, and a pilot of the program conducted in a group format with hospitalized complex trauma patients conducted by the co-primary investigator of the TOP DD studies, Dr. Hugo Schielke.

Next, I review some of the key research that informed the development of the educational program, which, as noted earlier, is called the Finding Solid Ground program (Brand et al., 2022; Schielke et al., 2022). Research from the TOP DD studies showed that individuals with DDs have higher levels of emotion dysregulation and NSSI than most psychiatric patients, even higher than those with PTSD (Nester, Boi, et al., 2022). NSSI was linked to emotion dysregulation as well as dissociation. This vulnerability to emotional dysregulation appeared to contribute to the alarmingly high rates of NSSI and suicide attempts among individuals with DDs (Foote et al., 2008; Nester, Boi, et al., 2022; Nester, Brand, et al., 2022; Nester, Pierorazio, et al., 2023). We found that DD individuals have considerable difficulty with awareness, acceptance, and cognitively processing emotions; furthermore, they tend to act less impulsively on emotions compared with individuals with borderline personality disorder (Nester, Boi, et al., 2022). Their difficulty being aware of, accepting, and processing emotions is consistent with the theoretical understanding of TRD being a method of compartmentalizing and distancing from overwhelming trauma-related emotions and intrusions. This research illustrates that complex DDs are not identical to borderline personality disorder.

The rich clinical and theoretical research literature on TRD and complex DDs, expert guidelines, discussion with the TOP DD collaborators,[1] and our decades of clinical experience informed the development of the educational program (Boon et al., 2011; Kluft, 1993a, 1993b, 2007; Loewenstein, 1991a, 1993, 2006, 2022; Mendelsohn et al., 2011). We anticipated that learning symptoms and adaptations were common among trauma survivors and linked to trauma-related neurobiological changes (which they could help heal by practicing the skills taught in the program) would foster the development of self-acceptance and self-compassion. We anticipated that these changes would increase participants' motivation to do the hard, daily work of developing healthy emotion regulation, grounding, and containment skills, as well as, for those with self-states, greater self-awareness and acceptance of disowned parts of self. We hypothesized that participating in the program would increase both patients' and therapists' knowledge of the patient's specific triggers for NSSI and guide them in developing and using alternative methods for meeting the needs (e.g., regulation of shame) that had previously been met through NSSI.

We were thrilled when the data showed that the program met these goals. Specifically, patients showed reductions in dissociation, PTSD, and NSSI, as well as improved emotion regulation and higher adaptive capacities (Brand, Schielke, et al., 2019). Although the whole sample showed benefit, those with the highest level of dissociation showed greater and faster improvement compared with those with moderate dissociation (i.e., $|d|s =$ 0.54–1.04 vs. $|d|s =$ 0.24–0.75, respectively). There were particularly striking improvements in NSSI among the individuals who had most often engaged in NSSI before enrolling in the study. Therapists reported that the patients who had engaged in NSSI approximately 100, 125, and 150 times in the 6 months before enrolling in the study had reduced self-harm to 0, 10, and 10 times, respectively, by the end of the 2-year study. Furthermore, on average, patients had required approximately 23 days of hospitalization in the 6 months before the study compared with 11.5 days in the last 6 months of the study. Although the change in hospitalization was not statistically significant, it was clearly in the direction indicating stabilization.

The TOP DD Network findings and feedback from participants led to further refinement of the educational program. The refined version is called the Finding Solid Ground program, which is described at length in

---

[1]The TOP DD team of collaborators include Bethany L. Brand, Hugo J. Schielke, Frank W. Putnam, Richard J. Loewenstein, Amie Myrick, Karen Putnam, Ellen K.K. Jepsen, Willemien Langeland, Clare Pain, Kathy Steele, Suzette Boon, Paul A. Frewen, and Ruth A. Lanius.

two books about the program (Brand et al., 2022; Schielke et al., 2022), one of which is geared toward therapists and one for individuals with TRD. The patient workbook includes the program's factual information sheets, journaling, and behavioral practice exercises. At the time of writing this book, the TOP DD team is conducting an RCT to determine if participants with CPTSD, DPTSD, and complex DDs who participate in the Finding Solid Ground program will show improvement compared with those on a waitlist who participate in individual psychotherapy before participating in the program.

The results of the TOP DD studies and other DD studies strongly challenge the myth promulgated by the fantasy model theorists claiming that treating DID or attending to dissociation makes it worse (Lilienfeld, 2007).

Insights From the TOP DD Network Study About Treating TRD

The TOP DD Network study provided rich insights about treating TRD. The majority of TRD patients who participated in the TOP DD Network study reported that they often had little idea what they were feeling and that they very often felt out of control of their emotions. However, therapists were generally unaware of how overwhelming and out of control these patients felt about their emotions. A lack of awareness about patients' difficulty with emotions could easily contribute to clinicians moving more quickly in treatment than patients can manage. This could lead to patients feeling overwhelmed and possibly not benefiting or dropping out of treatment.

The study provided additional insight into the importance of pacing treatment for TRD patients. The research team thought it would be manageable for clients to work through 45 modules of psychoeducation in 1 year. The second year of the study was planned to be a follow-up during which participants would no longer have access to the educational materials. However, therapists and patients informed us that they could not move through the materials quickly enough to finish the program in 1 year, and they did not want to miss out on part of the program. We adjusted the study to allow participants to work through the program for the entire 2 years. Although this change resulted in not having follow-up data, it was much more important to honor the need for moving slowly so that participants could learn, practice, and internalize the skills. The patients also advised us to "focus on emotions only after we have developed a lot of skill in grounding." Similarly, we learned that real progress in improving safety could only come after patients had developed facility in—and a willingness to use—grounding skills.

Although many of the clinicians in the study had taught similar skills to those in the Finding Solid Ground program, patients often experienced this information as "new" or felt the study presented it in an easily learned manner. We may have been perceived as "safer" in that we could not have direct contact with the patients so we could not hurt them (see the Traumatic Transference and Countertransference section later in the chapter). Furthermore, *they* were in control: They could choose when and how often to view and use the materials.

The TOP DD Network study and other DD treatment studies showed that although individuals with complex DDs have a wide range of very serious, chronic symptoms that require extensive stage-oriented treatment, when they are provided with individual psychotherapy and psychoeducation about trauma and TRD, they can ultimately improve many facets of their lives. The consistency of expert recommendations and research documenting the effectiveness of treatment in alignment with the expert consensus guidelines indicates that a standard of care is emerging for the treatment of complex DDs (Brand, Loewenstein, & Lanius, 2014; Loewenstein et al., in press).

CAUTIONS ABOUT TREATMENT GUIDELINES AND ULTRA BRIEF "CURES" FOR COMPLEX DDs

Many professional organizations have developed clinical practice guidelines regarding the treatment of PTSD. The treatment guidelines strongly recommend three first-line treatments for adults with PTSD: prolonged exposure, cognitive processing therapy, and cognitive therapy (reviewed in Ford & Courtois, 2020b). These treatments emphasize focusing on trauma processing, sometimes at every session, with trauma-focused work as homework between sessions. These approaches imply that a stabilization stage is unnecessary. Four additional treatment approaches are also recommended: EMDR, narrative exposure therapy, brief eclectic psychotherapy for PTSD, and some types of pharmacotherapy (reviewed in Ford & Courtois, 2020b). Unfortunately, most of the guidelines for PTSD treatment do not adequately address dissociation or DDs, as indicated by how rarely dissociation and dissociative disorders are mentioned in the guidelines, with some notable exceptions (see Table 7.2). Boyd et al. (2020) warned,

> Emotion regulation difficulties and dissociative symptoms are not directly targeted in current first-line interventions for PTSD. This is critical, given that functional impairment persists following treatment for PTSD, suggesting that current treatments do not adequately address this aspect of recovery. (p. 740)

Most practice guidelines rely on research with individuals with classic PTSD, rather than individuals with complex PTSD, TRD, and DDs, and

TABLE 7.2. References to Dissociation in Clinical Practice Guidelines, Expert Consensus Guidelines, and Position Papers

Guideline	Publication date	No. of pages	No. of mentions of "dissociation"	No. of mentions of "dissociative disorders"
Guidelines for PTSD				
Australian Guidelines for the Treatment of Adults with Acute Stress Disorder and Post-Traumatic Stress Disorder[a]	2007	13	0	0
United Kingdom's NICE Guideline for Post-traumatic Stress Disorder[b]	2018	54	4	0
American Psychological Association Clinical Practice Guidelines for the Treatment of Posttraumatic Stress Disorder[c]	2017	139	4	1
Appendices[d]		556	1	0
U.S. Veterans Administration/Department of Defense Clinical Practice Guidelines for the Management of Posttraumatic Stress Disorder and Acute Stress Disorder[e]	2017	200	8	0
Guidelines for complex PTSD, chronic PTSD and dissociative identity disorder				
ISTSS Expert Consensus Guidelines for Complex PTSD[f]	2012	21	13	0
ISTSS Guidelines Position Paper on Complex PTSD in Adults[g]	No date	7	1	0
Blue Knot Foundation Practice Guidelines for Clinical Treatment of Complex Trauma[h]	2019	270	727	174

(continues)

TABLE 7.2. References to Dissociation in Clinical Practice Guidelines, Expert Consensus Guidelines, and Position Papers (*Continued*)

Guideline	Publication date	No. of pages	No. of mentions of "dissociation"	No. of mentions of "dissociative disorders"
International Society for the Study of Trauma and Dissociation Guidelines for Treating Dissociative Identity Disorder in Adults[i]	2011	74	242	97
Cochrane Review Psychological Therapies for Chronic Post-traumatic Stress Disorder (Adults) Review[j]	2013	167	1	0

Note. ISTSS = International Society for the Study of Traumatic Stress; NICE = U.K. National Institute for Health and Care Excellence; PTSD = posttraumatic stress disorder.
[a]https://pubmed.ncbi.nlm.nih.gov/17620160 [b]https://www.nice.org.uk/guidance/ng116 [c]https://www.apa.org/ptsd-guideline [d]https://www.apa.org/ptsd-guideline/appendices.pdf [e]https://www.healthquality.va.gov/guidelines/MH/ptsd/VADoDPTSDCPGFinal012418.pdf [f]https://istss.org/ISTSS_Main/media/Documents/ComplexPTSD.pdf [g]https://istss.org/getattachment/Treating-Trauma/New-ISTSS-Prevention-and-Treatment-Guidelines/ISTSS_CPTSD-Position-Paper-(Adults)_FNL.pdf.aspx [h]https://aztrauma.org/wp-content/uploads/2020/11/BlueKnot_Practice_Guidelines_2019.pdf [i]https://www.isst-d.org/resources/adult-treatment-guidelines/ [j]https://www.cochranelibrary.com/cdsr/doi/10.1002/14651858.CD003388.pub4/epdf/full

they prioritize research from RCTs (Ford & Courtois, 2020b). As noted in Chapter 1, those with classic PTSD typically have less severe symptoms, fewer comorbid disorders, better functioning, and less severe or chronic trauma histories. RCT studies are often considered the most rigorous evidence of treatment benefit. (In non-RCT studies, all the participants receive the treatment under investigation, and the symptoms before and after treatment are compared; in RCTs, the symptoms in the waitlist group or alternative treatment group are compared with those in the treatment under investigation group.) Treatments shown to be effective in RCT studies are designated "evidence based." Treatments that have shown benefit using non-RCT designs are labeled "evidence (or research) informed" or "evidence (or research) supported." The strength of RCT studies is that this design allows researchers to conclude definitively that treatment caused improvements (or worsening), rather than changes in symptoms being caused by other factors, such as the passage of time.

In RCT PTSD treatment studies, patients are often excluded if they have current suicidal ideation, severe NSSI, serious eating disorders, DID or other

DD diagnoses, active substance abuse or dependence, and/or psychotic symptoms. These criteria would exclude most patients with histories of childhood trauma and TRD. For example, childhood trauma survivors commonly experience multimodal hallucinations, due to autohypnotic, dissociative, and posttraumatic factors; these hallucinations may be interpreted by researchers as evidence of psychosis. Other exclusion criteria may include recent psychiatric hospitalization, current involvement in a violent relationship, or taking or changing psychiatric medications. These exclusion criteria are ubiquitous in complex trauma and TRD patients and are the norm among patients seen in many community clinics and outpatient programs. Furthermore, RCT treatments are usually brief, lasting only 4 to 5 months and consisting of, at most, 12 to 20 sessions. Such brief treatment is unlikely to offer much benefit to the most impaired and symptomatic trauma survivors, especially those with these active comorbidities and long-term psychosocial problems. Also, there may be problems in scalability of the RCT-based PTSD treatments in real-world community settings because these models require frequent and often lengthy psychotherapy sessions (90–120 minutes several times per week), detailed homework assignments, and strict adherence to the protocols (Kaysen et al., 2019).

These research limitations have led to challenges about the applicability of RCT studies and some trauma treatment guidelines to "real-life" complex trauma patients, particularly those with severe TRD (Brand, Classen, Lanius, et al., 2009; Courtois & Brown, 2019; Ford & Courtois, 2020b; Westen et al., 2004). Ford and Courtois (2020b) argued that many of the guidelines imply or explicitly state that patients with PTSD should receive one of the RCT "evidence-based treatments" that *do not use a staged approach* to address comorbid disorders and struggles with safety that logically would have to be prioritized before undertaking trauma-focused psychotherapy. Many PTSD guidelines recommend treatments that immediately focus on in-depth trauma processing, regardless of symptom complexity, level of trauma exposure, multiple comorbidities, or client preference. This suggestion starkly contrasts with the staged model for treating complex trauma and severe TRD, which prioritizes stabilizing safety and symptoms and enhancing emotional regulation before trauma processing (Cloitre, Courtois, et al., 2012; ISSTD, 2011; Kezelman & Stavropoulos, 2012). In well-designed non-RCT studies, this staged model has been associated with many benefits for individuals with DDs, including in studies that had virtually none of the usual exclusion criteria of the RCT studies (Brand, Classen, Lanius, et al., 2009; Brand, McNary, et al., 2013; Brand, Schielke, et al., 2019).

There is an ongoing debate among researchers about whether individuals with high TRD need a staged treatment approach to benefit from evidence-based treatments. To determine whether stabilization was needed for dissociative clients, researchers conducted a meta-analysis to examine whether dissociation impacted treatment outcome for PTSD. They examined the studies for levels of dissociation pre- and post-PTSD treatment and concluded that dissociation did not impact treatment outcome (Hoeboer et al., 2020). If this conclusion is accurate, it would imply that those who had high dissociation did not do worse than those without dissociation when given standard, mostly RCT treatments. However, the average dissociation scores (as measured by the Dissociative Experiences Scale [DES]), in 10 of the 13 studies were below the average score for PTSD (i.e., score of 28.6; Lyssenko et al., 2018). Only three of the studies had average dissociation scores that were at or above the score typical for PTSD. Essentially, most of these studies involved individuals with low levels of dissociation. Furthermore, only one study in the Hoeboer et al. (2020) meta-analysis had dissociation scores at or above the average score typical for DDs (i.e., 38.9; Lyssenko et al., 2018). Hence, in the meta-analysis that sought to assess whether dissociation impacts treatment outcome, dissociation scores were relatively *low* in the majority of the studies. In addition, almost all the studies excluded participants with active suicidality, substance abuse, and the other exclusion criteria commonly found in individuals with high TRD. The original studies in the meta-analysis excluded the most complex, highly dissociative patients. This means that the most symptomatic and impaired dissociative individuals that might require additional destabilization were excluded.

In short, a meta-analysis cannot inform treatment decisions about patients that were not included in the studies it analyzes. Accordingly, it is premature to conclude that high levels of TRD do not impact PTSD treatment outcome.

Some researchers argue that staged treatment is not needed. Some go so far as to say that delaying trauma processing by having a stabilizing stage could cause iatrogenic harm by delaying recovery or conveying a sense of hopelessness to clients about the severity of their symptoms (De Jongh et al., 2016). Note that no research has shown that providing stabilization to highly complex, TRD patients causes harm. In fact, the opposite is true, as discussed earlier.

Some researchers are attempting to provide ultra-short, extremely intensive treatment, even to patients with complex DDs and PTSD related to childhood trauma (Bongaerts et al., 2021; Van Woudenberg et al., 2018; Voorendonk et al., 2020). These treatments immediately start with hours of intensive exposure and EMDR for 4 to 8 days. These studies typically have short follow-up periods that fail to assess long enough to detect recurrence of symptoms. Some of these ultra-brief treatments may have considerable iatrogenic effects for individuals with severe TRD. For example, the authors of a case report claimed to cure DID in 8 days by providing daily double sessions of EMDR and exposure therapy, after which they prompted the patient to "wave goodbye" to her dissociative self-states as they are "no longer needed" (van Minnen & Tibben, 2021). According to the published report, the patient's PTSD and dissociative symptoms improved, including at follow-up. However, there are serious problems with this report. Although the authors claimed the patient did not need or receive stabilization-focused treatment before engaging in their treatment, the report states that the patient had already undergone substantial stabilizing for substance abuse, eating disorders, and NSSI, as well as prior EMDR treatment. The authors opined that these prior treatments did not reduce the patient's dissociation, although they did not provide data to support this conclusion. Furthermore, the patient had already achieved sobriety for 15 months. The authors do not seem to realize that substance abuse treatment is, in fact, part of the stabilization provided in the first stage focused on stabilizing complex trauma disorder and TRD patients. Thus, it is inaccurate to claim that stabilizing treatment was not needed or beneficial. There is an additional problem: The patient's DES score dropped from 61.0 to 1.0 at a 3-month follow-up, the former being quite high and the latter being extremely low (even among nontraumatized individuals). Such unusual scores suggest the possibility that the client was unconsciously or consciously exaggerating and minimizing symptoms, respectively (Lyssenko et al., 2018). The extremely low posttreatment score suggests probable symptom minimization or the possibility that the patient felt compelled to give the researchers the result they wanted. Demand characteristics and response bias may have resulted in artificially low scores that may underestimate the true extent of dissociation.

In summary, most PTSD treatment studies and PTSD clinical practice guidelines generally apply to less severely traumatized and less severely dissociative clients. Thus, clinicians working with survivors of complex trauma, particularly trauma that occurred throughout different developmental eras, and those who are truly high in dissociation, may find useful guidance for working with these clients in expert consensus guidelines for complex trauma and DDs. Additionally, clinicians should rely on research conducted with participants with high levels of TRD to guide and inform their treatment of individuals with TRD.

PROGNOSIS

At this point, validated prognostic indicators of treatment response in individuals with TRD have not been studied, although measures have been developed to assess prognosis (Baars et al., 2011; Kluft, 1994a). According to a consensus survey of experts in CPTSD and DDs, variables that negatively impact prognosis include lack of motivation, lack of healthy relationships, lack of healthy therapeutic relationships, lack of other internal and external resources, serious comorbidity, poor attachment, and self-destructive behavior (Baars et al., 2011).

CHALLENGES IN TREATING TRD

The TRD clinical literature describes a multitude of beliefs, fears, and reenactments that may present roadblocks in treatment (e.g., Brand et al., 2022; Chefetz, 2015; Chu, 1988; Dalenberg, 2004; Herman, 1992b; Kluft, 1992). Trauma-based beliefs such as "I don't deserve to feel better" or "If I get better, it means I wasn't really hurt" may lead to a lack of progress or clients being reluctant or inconsistent in their use of recovery-focused skills. Often attachment-based fears contribute to the lack of progress, such as "If I get better, I will lose you (therapist)," or "You will stop caring for me if I'm doing okay." Identity-based fears can also often undermine progress, such as "I've been dysfunctional and sick all my life; I don't know who I will be if I get better" and "One of my parts thinks you are trying to take away his/her power and control, so is creating more symptoms."

Pragmatic concerns also hinder progress; for example, a client might think, "If I get better, I will lose disability payments and won't be able to afford treatment, but I can't manage working without treatment" or "Who other than chronically mentally ill people will be friends with me if I get off of disability after all these years of not working?" Open, compassionate explorations of roadblocks to treatment are essential to overcoming, very gradually, these fears and establishing healthier relationships so that the clinician is not the patient's primary support. Developing a sense of identity that is built on more than having experienced trauma and dissociation, and that includes a sense of oneself as a person worthy of positive experiences and good self-care, is also crucial.

Although most patients in outpatient treatment for DDs show progress over time when treated by a clinician trained in trauma and dissociation, a small subgroup may develop brief worsening of symptoms. In the naturalistic TOP DD study, between 9% and 14% of the sample showed temporary sudden symptomatic worsening during the prior 6 months of treatment (Myrick et al., 2013). The patients who showed worsening had higher rates of recent sexual revictimization, higher resource-related stressors (e.g., financial difficulties), higher stressors overall, and/or more difficulty establishing a trusting relationship with their treatment team. This rate of worsening is similar to the rate of worsening found in treatment studies for depression and anxiety (e.g., 8.7% in Hansen et al., 2002) and lower than that found in some studies of chronic PTSD (e.g., 25% in Tarrier et al., 1999). This similar rate of worsening is notable, given that the TOP DD study did not exclude patients who were misusing substances, engaged in NSSI or suicidal behaviors, or diagnosed with comorbid psychiatric disorders.

TRAUMATIC TRANSFERENCE AND COUNTERTRANSFERENCE

Treating individuals with TRD can be personally challenging and result in countertransference that is difficult to acknowledge and manage (Chefetz, 1997b; Dalenberg, 2000; Kluft, 1994b; Loewenstein, 1993). Self-awareness, self-regulation, self-care, seeking consultations with colleagues, and perhaps engaging in one's own psychotherapy are particularly important when treating individuals with TRD (Saakvitne, 2017). These individuals often have strong trauma-based transference reactions to clinicians, most of which are rooted in their experiences of having been tricked, manipulated, neglected, or abused by important people, including caregivers. Openly discussing and processing these reactions is a powerful vehicle of change for complex trauma survivors (Kinsler, 2018). Excellent resources are available about addressing and managing lack of progress in treatment and trauma-based transference and countertransference (Brand et al., 2022; Chu, 1988; Dalenberg, 2000; Kluft, 1992; Myrick et al., 2013).

ADJUNCTIVE INTERVENTIONS FOR TREATING TRD

Adjunctive interventions are often highly useful in treating TRD. Clinicians are recommended to seek additional training in their use with complex trauma survivors.

Hypnosis

Patients with DID are almost always highly hypnotizable and frequently engage in self-hypnotic phenomena (Dell, 2017). Hypnosis will likely be a part of DID treatment, regardless of whether the clinician is aware of it or facilitates it. For the trained clinician, it can be a highly useful technique for containment of traumatic material (e.g., imagery of putting traumas "away" into a bank vault until the client is ready and willing to process them) and emotion regulation (e.g., safer place imagery, healing stream imagery, feelings dials that "dial down" emotions), rather than for uncovering trauma (Hammond, 1990; Kluft, 1982, 1989). Hypnosis is not a treatment in and of itself but rather a set of techniques within the context of the patient's existing psychotherapy (Brand, Loewenstein, & Lanius, 2014). Hypnosis should only be used if the clinician has been trained in using it with TRD patients and obtains informed consent from patients.

Psychopharmacology

Space limitations restrict this discussion. The management of medications with highly dissociative individuals requires thoughtful consideration and discussion of many issues, including trauma-based beliefs and traumatic transferential issues, particularly among those with DID. For a review, see Loewenstein (2005, 2016). Rather than being "curative," a reasonable goal for medication should be a conservative regimen that acts as a "shock absorber" for some of the emotional distress (Brand, Loewenstein, & Lanius, 2014).

Naltrexone decreases dissociative symptoms and flashbacks in patients with borderline personality disorder; however, double-blind trials showed a small, insignificant effect (Bohus et al., 1999; Schmahl et al., 2012). Although there is little research to guide psychopharmacological interventions with complex DDs, the majority of these individuals do receive psychiatric medication, especially in the early stages of treatment. For example, 80% in the TOP DD participants were taking psychiatric medication (Brand, Classen, Lanius, et al., 2009). As symptoms stabilize, it may be possible to reduce medications (ISSTD, 2011; Loewenstein, 2005).

Body-Focused Interventions

Trauma-based reactions are experienced in the mind as well as the body, so it is important to address and heal somatic reactions such as chronic startle reactions, which often do not fully respond to top-down treatment approaches (Lanius, Paulsen, & Corrigan, 2014; Ogden et al., 2006; van der Kolk, 2014). One approach that is currently showing promise in Ruth Lanius's research lab is "deep brain reorienting" (Corrigan & Christie-Sands, 2020; Kearney et al., 2023). In deep brain reorienting, the client is guided to access the orienting tension that preceded the emotions related to a traumatic experience, then slowly proceed through memory processing. This intervention has shown clinical utility with individuals with TRD without being destabilizing (Frank Corrigan, MD, personal communication, September 1, 2022). As with all types of trauma processing, caution, careful pacing, and client readiness are essential to this adjunctive intervention being beneficial.

CONCLUSION

Current treatment research indicates that if TRD is diagnosed and treated in accordance with expert consensus guidelines for dissociation, symptoms can be significantly reduced and functioning greatly improved, even among patients with severe and chronic TRD. Much needs to be learned about dissociation's impact on treatment outcome. We need to learn more about how the timing (i.e., dissociation at intake into a study vs. during therapy sessions), chronicity (i.e., peritraumatic dissociation vs. chronic trait-like dissociation), severity (i.e., mild vs. moderate vs. severe), and type of dissociation experienced (e.g., absorption vs. numbing vs. depersonalization/derealization vs. amnesia vs. identity fragmentation) impact the course of trauma treatment. More research is needed on the treatment of dissociative amnesia and derealization/depersonalization disorder, as well as the complex DDs. To ensure generalizability to individuals with complex trauma, patients with high levels of dissociation and comorbid conditions, including suicidal behaviors and NSSI, must be included in treatment studies. Innovative treatments that ease these patients' suffering and improve their quality of life are urgently needed, as is widely available clinician training in the identification and treatment of TRD.

Appendix A

DIAGNOSTIC INTERVIEW OUTLINE

BETHANY L. BRAND AND NICHOLAS A. PIERORAZIO

PRELIMINARY SUGGESTIONS FOR THE DIAGNOSTIC INTERVIEW:

Responding to Trauma:

You do not want to flood a client with traumatic flashbacks- avoid talking in a lot of detail about trauma for now. Disclosures about trauma should be immediately followed by empathic statements by the interviewer. It is important to be empathic, not overwhelming. Assess for an approximate history of trauma so as to determine its severity and possible impact. Roughly speaking, it is helpful to know approximately what age(s) the client was during periods of trauma and the type of relationship with the abuser (e.g., parent, babysitter, peer). Only inquire about these details if the client can manage without getting overwhelmed and have been informed regarding duty to report.

Be aware of your jurisdiction's laws about duty to report child abuse and abuse of vulnerable adults. Most clinicians have information about confidentiality and their legal and ethical requirement to break confidentiality in their informed consent form that clients read before they do an initial diagnostic interview. In some states, clinicians must report all reported and suspected cases of child abuse, even if the abuser is dead or the abuse happened many years ago.

While it is important to assess for trauma history and trauma symptoms, it is important to not ask for too much detail before the therapeutic relationship has been established and before the clinician knows how well the client can manage emotions, safety, and their symptoms. If the client begins to talk about trauma in detail, the clinician may say:

"I'm sorry to interrupt but I want to be sure we do not overwhelm you by talking in detail about trauma right away because that can sometimes cause a person to have more anxiety, nightmares, or other problems later. It is very important for me to know about experiences like this, though. Could you tell me about them at the "headline level" like in a newspaper or blog (Loewenstein, 2006), and we can get into the details at another time when we have gotten to know each other better?"

If the client begins to look either very anxious or dissociated, gently ask how they are feeling. Give them permission to return to the topic of trauma at another time. If they are struggling, remind them to look around the room, move a bit, and get grounded.

Mirror their Language:

In the initial diagnostic interview, it is important to mirror the client's language, especially as it relates to trauma. Do not use "rape" if they don't use the word, or "sexual abuse" unless that is what they call it. It is also important to mirror the client's language in terms of symptoms; for example, a dissociative client may use a term such as "a part of me" instead of "dissociated self-states."

Assessing Safety:

Assessing safety is of the utmost importance in the diagnostic interview. The clinician *must* assess self-harm, violence toward others, suicidal ideation, and homicidal ideation. The clinician will need to continue to monitor safety in subsequent sessions.

Interview Structure:

The proposed structure begins with "free speech" from the client and becomes more directive as the interview progresses in order to control the timing of the later interview. The intended length of the interview is 50 minutes although in some cases it is not possible to cover all these topics in one session. It is important to note other potential problems that were not thoroughly explored in the initial interview, as these may be explored in subsequent sessions.

Client Name: _____

Age: _____

Pronouns:

How they prefer to be called:

Chief Complaint: What problem brings you in for therapy? What was going on in your life when these problems started? Why are you seeking help *now*? (Listen for duration and severity. Allow approximately five minutes- remember to use empathy! Listen for a statement that conveys the client's main concern.)

> After allowing the client approximately 5 minutes of free speech, summarize their main concern(s) in a sentence, and use that to segue to asking directive questions about vegetative symptoms. Example: "The break up with your partner has been incredibly painful for you. How has your sleep been since the breakup?"

> Nightmares may be trauma sequelae. Nightmares may not only contain direct traumatic material and intrusions, but also other elements of trauma, such as related emotions.

Vegetative Symptoms:

Hours of sleep per night: _____

Nightmares? ☐ Yes ☐ No

Do you feel rested when you wake up? ☐ Yes ☐ No

Have you ever gone without sleep or with very little sleep and <u>not</u> felt tired?
☐ Yes ☐ No

Energy: ☐ Normal ☐ High ☐ Low

Ever so much energy you get a <u>tremendous</u> amount done? ☐ Yes ☐ No

Did you need less sleep at the same time? ☐ Yes ☐ No

Appetite: ☐ Normal ☐ Up/Down: _____ lbs.

Concentration: ☐ Normal ☐ Poor

(If it seems comfortable and culturally appropriate:) *Libido:* ☐ High ☐ Normal ☐ Low

Mood: ☐ Normal ☐ Other:

_____

Scale of 1-10: Highest:____ Lowest:____

Significant periods of feeling <u>incredibly</u> irritable, agitated? ☐ Yes ☐ No

Ever feel very elated, incredibly powerful or competent, or on top of the world?
□ Yes □ No

> Did you need less sleep at the same time? □ Yes □ No
>
> Have you had this trouble before? □ Yes □ No

History of Treatment: _____ Years _____ Months _____ Days. □ None
> If yes, did it help?

Suicide and Self-injury:

When things get bad, how bad do they get?

Have you ever purposefully hurt yourself such as cutting yourself?
> (if yes, assess most severe and recent actions.)

Have you ever felt <u>so</u> bad that you thought you wanted to die? □ Yes □ No

Have you ever made any type of suicide attempt? □ Yes □ No

> Did you require medical treatment? □ Yes □ No

> Have you felt this way recently? □ Yes □ No
> > If so, how recently?
> > **Assess Risk:**
> > □ Plan?
> > □ Access to means?
> > □ Intent to follow through?

Treatment Plan: If there is a threat to the client's safety, outline treatment plan:_____

Other forms of non-suicidal self-injury to be aware of include the following: cutting, biting, burning, carving, pinching, pulling hair, scratching, banging or hitting self, interfering with wound healing (i.e., picking scabs), rubbing skin against a rough surface, sticking self with needles, swallowing dangerous substances, and more. (Klonsky & Glenn, 2009)

Inquire about past suicide attempts, especially including those that were most recent and most lethal.

Always assess suicide risk with questions about whether they have a plan of potential suicide, access to means to suicide, and intent to suicide. Assess what helps them not act on suicidal urges. It is also important to assess whether the client needs a higher level of care, such as hospitalization.

--------SUMMARIZE the MAIN problem(s) they seem to be struggling with. --------

Family and Social History: *10-20 minutes*

Raised by: □ Mom □ Dad □ Other_____
> > □ Biological □ Adoptive/Foster □ Step- □ Grand-
> □ Mom □ Dad □ Other_____
> > □ Biological □ Adoptive/Foster □ Step- □ Grand-

Are your parents (or caregivers) in good health? □ Yes □ No

Parents'/Caregivers' Relationship: □ Ever married □ Intact □ Divorced □ Blended □ Remarried _____

What is your Mom's / Dad's (or other primary caregiver's) personality like?
        Parent 1 (_____):

        Parent 2 (_____):

How is your relationship with parents: □ Good □ Bad □ Other:

Siblings: □ Yes □ No
        Birth Order:

Is there any sibling you are particularly close to/struggle with?

How is your relationship with siblings: □ Good □ Bad □ Other:

Is there anyone in your family you could go to if you were *really* struggling with something? □ Yes □ No

Is there anyone in your family that you are no longer in contact with? What happened?

Tell me a bit about your closest *friendship*.

Is there a friend you could go to if you are <u>really</u> struggling or upset? □ Yes □ No

How would you describe yourself as a *kid*? Quiet, Loud?

How far did you go in school? _____ grade or year in college.
Did you like school? □ Yes □ No (Friends?)

How did you do with the academic part of school?

How did you get along with teachers?

Where did you feel safe when you were growing up? ⟵

> Assess areas of resilience for the client (e.g., social support and areas and people in their life that felt safe). It may be especially important to find points of resilience for and strengths of those with trauma histories (i.e., what helped them cope?).

Discipline/Trauma: (Be aware of sociocultural norms.)
In your family, how was discipline handled?

Were you spanked, hit, or beaten?
        Did it ever leave any marks or bruises? □ Yes □ No
        Did it ever cause you to have to see a doctor? □ Yes □ No
        Did things ever get worse than that? □ Yes □ No

Did you see family members hit, kick, shove or harm each other?

> If the client did not have enough to eat or were not taken to the doctor when ill, discern if these experiences were due to financial limitations or neglectful caregivers.

Did it ever seem to you that punishments were too strict? □ Yes □ No
As a kid, did you always have enough to eat? □ Yes □ No ⟵
When you were sick, did you get taken to a doctor? □ Yes □ No
        At what age were you left alone without babysitters? _____-years old

As a child, teen, or adult, were you ever approached by someone in a sexual way that made you feel uncomfortable (even if they were the same age, paid, or manipulated into it)? □ Yes □ No_
        About how old were you? _____-years old.
        Can you <u>briefly</u> describe what happened if you are comfortable?

Did you have any major stressors in <u>childhood</u> such as deaths, conflicts, divorces?
□ Yes □ No

Since you've been an <u>adult</u>, has anything traumatic happened to you? (Violence in a relationship, robbery, very serious accidents, natural disasters etc.) □ Yes □ No

How would you describe your race and ethnicity?
If has minoritized racial/ethnic status: Can you share with me a time you were <u>seriously</u> impacted by racism (i.e., experiences where you were concerned about your safety and the event was very upsetting)?

In what ways do you think the [most traumatic event they have told you about] still affects you?

(If trauma history is present, always ask about PTSD symptoms (e.g., hypervigilance, avoidance, flashbacks) & dissociation (e.g., feeling detached from their body, feeling like the world around them is not real, amnesic gaps). If they experience several dissociative symptoms, follow up with a full assessment for dissociative disorders in a later session.)

> If the client is a racial or ethnic minority, it may be clinically relevant to follow up about racial/ethnic trauma. See the UConn Racial/Ethnic Stress and Trauma Survey (Williams et al., 2018) for further semi-structured interview questions regarding racial/ethnic trauma. <u>http:// www.m.mentalhealth disparities.org/docs/ UnRESTS_0716_Eng lish.pdf</u>

------------**BRIEFLY SUMMARIZE the main aspect of what they've told you.** ------------

Life as an Adult: (Listen for symptoms of personality disorders, severity of impairment, and aspects of resiliency.)
Who do you live with now? _____
Have you ever been homeless? □ Yes □ No

Is money a serious stressor for you now? □ Yes □ No

How would you describe your *gender*? _____
    Is it the same as the sex you were assigned at birth? □ Yes □ No
    (If client has minoritized status) Who have you told? How did it go?
    (If client has minoritized status) Can you share with me a time you were <u>seriously</u> impacted by discrimination related to your gender identity (i.e., experiences where you were concerned about your safety and the event was very upsetting)?

> Listen for trauma and stressors related to other minoritized statuses; for example, these may include being transgender, a sexual minority, or other relationship-related minority (e.g., a client identifying as polyamorous).

How do you describe your *sexual orientation*? _____
    (If client has minoritized status) Who have you told? How did it go?
    (If client has minoritized status) Can you share with me a time you were <u>seriously</u> impacted by discrimination related to your sexual orientation

(i.e., experiences where you were concerned about your safety and the event was very upsetting)?

Have you had any significant *romantic relationships*? □ Yes □ No

Have you ever been married? □ Yes □ No _____ years.
Tell me about your marriage(s).

Do you have or have you had any *children*? □ Yes □ No
Age(s) and gender(s):
Describe relationship with them:

Work History:
How are you currently getting your income? (Working? On disability [Medical / Psychiatric]?)

Have you had any jobs in the past? □ Yes □ No
Have you ever been fired? □ Yes □ No (If yes:) what happened?

How well did you get along with coworkers and bosses?

Have you ever been in the *military*? □ Yes □ No
What branch? _____. Active Duty (Combat)? □ Yes □ No
If Active Duty, how did it affect you? (If no longer in the military:) what type of discharge were you given? □ Honorable □ Dishonorable □ Other

Impulsivity and Anger:
How well do you manage anger? □ Good □ Fair □ Bad

Have you ever been so angry that you seriously thought of hurting someone else? □ Yes □ No
Have you ever hurt anyone or tried to?
□ Yes □ No What is the most serious harm you have caused someone?

Inquire about past acts of violence, including those that were most recent and severe.

Always assess violence and homicidal ideation with questions about plan, access to means, and intent to act on violent or homicidal urges. Assess what helps them *not* act on violent urges. Assess whether the client needs a higher level of care, like hospitalization.

Any arrests? □ Yes □ No … For what crime? _____
        Were you convicted? □ Yes □ No … On which crime? What sentence did you get? How much time did you serve? _____

What do you do to cope with [stressor] (e.g., feeling suicidal, very angry, etc.)?

-------------SUMMARIZE what they've told you if a serious issue came up. -------------

Medical:
Major health problems as child? □ Yes □ No

_____
        (If yes:) "How did that impact you?"

Do you have any significant medical problems now? □ Yes □ No

When is the last time you had a general physical examination?

Currently taking any *medications*? □ Yes (List them & dosages.) □ No

> If time is limited at this point in the interview, be directive in especially prompting for psychiatric medications that the client is taking.

        "Do you think your medications help you?" □ Yes □ No Any side-effects?

Substance Use:
How often do you drink alcohol? _____ times per _____
        When you drink, how much at the most? _____ drinks
        How many blackouts? _____
        How many DUI's/DWI's? _____
        Injuries, fights, STIs, relationships problems, legal problems? □ Yes □ No

What drugs have you used? □ _____ □ None (Recreational? Street/prescription?)
        How much and how often?

        Have you ever injected drugs using a needle? □ Yes □ No
        Have you ever taken more of a prescription drug than you were told to? □ Yes □ No
        Are you using any drugs right now? □ Yes □ No _____
        (If they haven't addressed marijuana, ask about smoking or ingesting marijuana.)

Have you ever done something while drunk/high that you wouldn't have done sober (e.g., sex, steal, fights, etc.)?

As a result of drinking or drug use, have you had any problems with school/work, the police, family, health, finances, STIs, unplanned pregnancies, etc. □ Yes □ No

Have you ever wondered about whether you have a drug or alcohol problem?
□ Yes □ No

Does anyone in your family have any emotional problems such as depression, schizophrenia, drug/alcohol problems) □ Yes □ No
(If yes:) Is this a relative you are related to by blood rather than marriage?

(If there is time:)
How much coffee do you drink each day?
Do you smoke or vape? How much?
Do you exercise? How much?
Are you comfortable with your body and weight? If not, are you doing anything to manage your weight?

--------SUMMARIZE anything new/important if they've just told you about it. ---------

Anxiety:
Would you consider yourself a worrier? □ Yes □ No

Phobias:
Is there anything you're *terribly* afraid of? □ Yes □ No _____

Obsessions:
Are there any thoughts that run through your mind *over and over* again? □ Yes □ No

Compulsions:
Is there any kind of (repetitive) behavior that you *have* to do or else you feel very upset?
☐ Yes ☐ No

Panic attacks:
Do you ever feel *completely* panicked like you can't breathe, your heart is racing, you might lose your mind, or die?
☐ Yes ☐ No

Psychosis:
Delusions:
Do you ever have thoughts that some people might think are *really* unusual? ☐ Yes ☐ No

Does it ever seem like people are truly *out to get you*? ☐ Yes ☐ No

> If the client endorses any hallucinations or delusions, assess the range of hallucinations and delusions, including their content and type.

Hallucinations:
Do you ever see things that other people don't *seem* to see? ☐ Yes ☐ No

Do you ever hear voices or other things that others don't *seem* to hear? ☐ Yes ☐ No

Mental Status Exam: (Only if 5+ minutes left)
Where are we? ☐ Correct ☐ Incorrect
Date? ☐ Correct ☐ Incorrect ☐ Close Enough
Count backwards by 3's: ☐ Correct ☐ Incorrect *Concentration*
In general, how's your memory?

3 words repeated (Brown, Eye Dropper, 100 Main Street) *Concentration*
      *Repeat until client gets them all correct. How many tries? _____

Past 3 presidents: ☐ Correct ☐ Incorrect

> Although it is always helpful to conduct a formal mental status exam, much of what is being assessed, such as concentration, can be informally discerned by the clinician throughout the interview.
>
> When conducting the mental status exam and the client gets the answer correct, say "good." If the client gets the answer wrong, say "don't worry, people do it all the time."

In what ways are an apple and an orange alike and different? *Abstract Thought*

What would you do if you smelled smoke in a theater? *Why?* *Judgement*

Ask about the 3 words again. How many right? _____ *Short-term Memory*

Wrap Up:
Is there anything else you think I should know about?

"I'm going to take a couple of minutes to look over my notes to see if there are any further questions."

(Thank the client for coming in and sharing their experiences. Offer empathy and hope about future treatment being able to help them with their concerns.)

REFERENCES

Klonsky, E. D., & Glenn, C. R. (2009). Assessing the functions of non-suicidal self-injury: Psychometric properties of the Inventory of Statements About Self-injury (ISAS). *Journal of Psychopathology and Behavioral Assessment*, *31*(3), 215–219. https://doi.org/10.1007/s10862-008-9107-z

Morrison, J. (2014). *The first interview* (4th ed.). Guilford Press.

Sommers-Flanagan, J., & Sommers-Flanagan, R. (2016). *Clinical interviewing* (6th ed.). Wiley.

Williams, M. T., Metzger, I., Leins, C., & DeLapp, C. (2018). Assessing racial trauma within a DSM-5 framework: The UConn Racial/Ethnic Stress & Trauma Survey. *Practice Innovations*, *3*(4), 242–260. https://doi.org/10.1037/pri0000076

Appendix B

ASSESSMENT MEASURES: PITQ-t AND PITQ-p

HUGO SCHIELKE AND BETHANY L. BRAND

Progress in Treatment Questionnaire—Therapist (PITQ-t)

Circle the number to show what percentage of the time your client has demonstrated the following behaviors, cognitions or experiences in the **last 6 months**.

1. Engages in self-injurious behavior (e.g., cutting, burning) or suicide attempts.

    0%   10   20   30   40   50   60   70   80   90   100%
    (never)   (always)

2. Engages in potentially self-damaging acts such as abusing substances, purging, shoplifting, driving unsafely.

    0%   10   20   30   40   50   60   70   80   90   100%
    (never)   (always)

3. Identity is strongly tied to being a victim of abuse.

    0%   10   20   30   40   50   60   70   80   90   100%
    (never)   (always)

4. Understands that they have a dissociative disorder (DD) and generally acknowledges that this diagnosis is accurate.

    0%   10   20   30   40   50   60   70   80   90   100%
    (never)   (always)

5. Able to maintain a fairly strong treatment alliance, and when there are disruptions to the alliance, able to work productively to repair it.

    0%   10   20   30   40   50   60   70   80   90   100%
    (never)   (always)

6. Knows and uses self-soothing strategies (e.g., any type of calming strategy that is not used explicitly to contain PTSD symptoms or prevent dissociation) when they are needed.

    0%   10   20   30   40   50   60   70   80   90   100%

    (never)   (always)

7. Knows and uses containment strategies (e.g., hypnotic or imagery techniques used to contain intrusive PTSD symptoms) when they are needed.

    0%   10   20   30   40   50   60   70   80   90   100%

    (never)   (always)

8. Knows and uses grounding techniques to prevent self from going numb, zoning out, having amnestic lapses when they are needed (e.g., techniques such as muscle contractions, movement, or touching an object to avoid dissociating).

    0%   10   20   30   40   50   60   70   80   90   100%

    (never)   (always)

9. Keeps oriented in the present (i.e., does NOT get confused about past and present).

    0%   10   20   30   40   50   60   70   80   90   100%

    (never)   (always)

10. Shows good awareness of his/her emotions and feels his/her body sensations.

    0%   10   20   30   40   50   60   70   80   90   100%

    (never)   (always)

11. Shows good affect tolerance (can feel emotions without getting overwhelmed).

    0%   10   20   30   40   50   60   70   80   90   100%

    (never)   (always)

12. Shows good impulse control (e.g., can feel angry or depressed without acting it out).

    0%   10   20   30   40   50   60   70   80   90 100%

    (never)   (always)

13. Is aware that the trauma was not his/her fault.

    0%   10   20   30   40   50   60   70   80   90   100%

    (never)   (always)

14. Manages daily functioning well (e.g., managing hygiene, maintaining a home, paying bills).

0%	10	20	30	40	50	60	70	80	90	100%
(never)										(always)

15. Has continuous awareness of behaviors, that is, the patient does not report time loss or other signs of amnesia (e.g., no behaviors done out of their awareness, no possessions for which they can't recall how they obtained them, etc.).

0%	10	20	30	40	50	60	70	80	90	100%
(never)										(always)

16. Able to deal with stressful situations without dissociating.

0%	10	20	30	40	50	60	70	80	90	100%
(never)										(always)

17. Able to maintain healthy personal and professional relationships with other people.

0%	10	20	30	40	50	60	70	80	90	100%
(never)										(always)

18. Able to experience grief stemming from trauma-related losses.

0%	10	20	30	40	50	60	70	80	90	100%
(never)										(always)

19. Has found ways to make life feel meaningful and rewarding.

0%	10	20	30	40	50	60	70	80	90	100%
(never)										(always)

20. Has a generally positive view of him/herself.

0%	10	20	30	40	50	60	70	80	90	100%
(never)										(always)

21. Has a generally positive view of other people.

0%	10	20	30	40	50	60	70	80	90	100%
(never)										(always)

22. Able to experience sexual intimacy without difficulties such as intense shame, flashbacks or dissociation and with some pleasure.

0%	10	20	30	40	50	60	70	80	90	100%
(never)										(always)

23. Able to tolerate doing trauma focused abreactive work (i.e., able to express intense affect about past trauma, talk in detail about traumatic events, as well as explore the meaning, impact, and conflicts related to trauma).

0%   10   20   30   40   50   60   70   80   90   100%

(never)   (always)

Parts-related questions. The following questions are for persons who have dissociative self-states/"parts." If these items do not apply to your patient, please circle "not applicable." Otherwise, please circle the percentage of time each statement applies to your patient.

24. Has awareness that all dissociative self-states are part of himself/herself and share one body (i.e., does not believe one alter can "kill" another and survive the suicide).

0%   10   20   30   40   50   60   70   80   90   100%

(never or not applicable)   (always)

25. Knows parts and understands their functions (i.e., what purposes they serve, such as helping manage feelings related to trauma).

0%   10   20   30   40   50   60   70   80   90   100%

(never or not applicable)   (always)

26. Shows good internal communication and cooperation among parts.

0%   10   20   30   40   50   60   70   80   90   100%

(never or not applicable)   (always)

27. Has reliable co-consciousness with all parts.

0%   10   20   30   40   50   60   70   80   90   100%

(never or not applicable)   (always)

28. Has integrated at least two parts.

0%   10   20   30   40   50   60   70   80   90   100%

(never or not applicable)   (always)

29. Has integrated all parts and no longer experiences amnesia, voices, passive influence or other signs of identity fragmentation.

0%   10   20   30   40   50   60   70   80   90   100%

(never or not applicable)   (always)

PITQ-t Scoring

To score the PITQ-t, treat the percentages endorsed as points (e.g., 0% = 0 points, 100% = 100 points). *NOTE:* Items 1, 2, and 3 are reverse-scored (i.e., 0 = 100 points, 10 = 90, 20 = 80, 30 = 70, 40 = 60, 50 = 50, 60 = 40, 70 = 30, 80 = 20, 90 = 10, 100 = 0 points).

The procedure for calculating a PITQ-t score is different for patients with and without dissociative self-states.

For patients without dissociative self-states

Add the points corresponding to the percentages endorsed for items 1 through 23 and divide by 23 (i.e., maximum score = 100, minimum score = 0).

For patients with dissociative self-states

Add the points corresponding to the percentages endorsed for items 1 through 29 and then divide the total by 29 (i.e., maximum score = 100, minimum score = 0).

The use of this measure is free of charge. Please note, however, that norms for the PITQ-t have not yet been established. If you use the PITQ-t in research, please share your feedback and findings with BBrand@towson.edu and Hugo. Schielke@gmail.com. Visit https://topddstudy.com/pitq.php

Progress in Treatment Questionnaire—Patient Version (PITQ-p)

Please circle the number that reflects what percentage of time each of the following statements has been true of you in the **last week**.

1. I have been diagnosed with a dissociative disorder and agree that this diagnosis is correct.
   0%   10   20   30   40   50   60   70   80   90   100%
   (never true)   (always true)

2. I collaborate well with my therapist, and when there are problems between us, I talk to my therapist about them so that we can resolve them together.
   0%   10   20   30   40   50   60   70   80   90   100%
   (never true)   (always true)

3. I am compassionate and fair with myself; that is, I respond to myself with as much empathy as I would show someone else in the same situation.
   0%   10   20   30   40   50   60   70   80   90   100%
   (never true)   (always true)

4. I'm aware of the thoughts, feelings, and body sensations that indicate I'm getting anxious or overwhelmed.
   0%   10   20   30   40   50   60   70   80   90   100%
   (never true)   (always true)

5. I use relaxation techniques (such as relaxation exercises, safe place imagery, music) to safely help myself relax and feel better when I begin to get anxious or overwhelmed.
   0%   10   20   30   40   50   60   70   80   90   100%
   (never true)   (always true)

6. I manage intrusive memories and flashbacks using containment strategies (imagery techniques used to contain and manage PTSD symptoms).
   0%   10   20   30   40   50   60   70   80   90   100%
   (never true)   (always true)

7. I use grounding techniques when I need to prevent myself from going numb, zoning out, or losing time. (Examples: focus on my surroundings; pay attention to my five senses; tense and relax my muscles.)
   0%   10   20   30   40   50   60   70   80   90   100%
   (never true)   (always true)

8. If I begin to confuse the past with the present, I notice this and work to see differences between how things are now versus how they were when I was being traumatized.

0%   10   20   30   40   50   60   70   80   90   100%
(never true)   (always true)

9. I am aware of my emotions and body sensations.

0%   10   20   30   40   50   60   70   80   90   100%
(never true)   (always true)

10. I am able to feel my emotions without getting overwhelmed.

0%   10   20   30   40   50   60   70   80   90   100%
(never true)   (always true)

11. I am aware of, able to think about, and can control my impulses. (Example: I can feel angry or depressed without doing something unhealthy.)

0%   10   20   30   40   50   60   70   80   90   100%
(never true)   (always true)

12. I reach out to treatment providers if I have difficulty controlling severe unhealthy impulses despite using recovery-focused coping skills (e.g., grounding, past vs. present, containment).

0%   10   20   30   40   50   60   70   80   90   100%
(never true)   (always true)

13. I know that the traumas that I experienced were not my fault.

0%   10   20   30   40   50   60   70   80   90   100%
(never true)   (always true)

14. I manage everyday life well. (Examples: I regularly eat, bathe, pay bills on time, etc.).

0%   10   20   30   40   50   60   70   80   90   100%
(never true)   (always true)

15. I am able to account for all that I do; that is, I don't "lose time" or find evidence of having done something I do not remember.

0%   10   20   30   40   50   60   70   80   90   100%
(never true)   (always true)

16. I am able to deal with stressful situations without dissociating.

0%   10   20   30   40   50   60   70   80   90   100%
(never true)   (always true)

17. I am able to maintain healthy personal and professional relationships.

0%   10   20   30   40   50   60   70   80   90   100%
(never true)   (always true)

18. I value my physical well-being, and do not do things that hurt my body. (Examples: I don't cut or burn my body or attempt suicide.)

0%   10   20   30   40   50   60   70   80   90   100%
(never true)   (always true)

19. I value my health and do not do things that put me at risk. (Examples: I do not abuse drugs, throw up after eating, drive unsafely, have unsafe sex, etc.)

0%   10   20   30   40   50   60   70   80   90   100%
(never true)   (always true)

20. I am able to experience sadness and grieve the losses related to trauma.

0%   10   20   30   40   50   60   70   80   90   100%
(never true)   (always true)

21. Life feels meaningful and rewarding.

0%   10   20   30   40   50   60   70   80   90   100%
(never true)   (always true)

22. I have a generally positive view of myself.

0%   10   20   30   40   50   60   70   80   90   100%
(never true)   (always true)

23. I have a generally positive view of other people.

0%   10   20   30   40   50   60   70   80   90   100%
(never true)   (always true)

24. My sense of myself includes many important things beyond having been traumatized.

0%   10   20   30   40   50   60   70   80   90   100%
(never true)   (always true)

25. I am able to experience sexual intimacy without intense shame, flashbacks, or dissociation, and with some pleasure.

0%   10   20   30   40   50   60   70   80   90   100%
(never true)   (always true)

26. I can explore the meaning, and impact related to the traumas I experienced; I can feel and express the emotions related to these traumas.

0%   10   20   30   40   50   60   70   80   90   100%
(never true)   (always true)

The following questions are for persons who have dissociated parts/self-states. If these items do not apply to you, please circle "not applicable." Otherwise, please circle the percentage of time the statements apply to you.

27. All parts of myself know that we are part of the same person and that we share one body.
    0%   10   20   30   40   50   60   70   80   90   100%
    (not applicable/never true)   (always true)

28. All parts of myself are oriented to the present (know what day, month, and year it is).
    0%   10   20   30   40   50   60   70   80   90   100%
    (not applicable/never true)   (always true)

29. I pay attention to and am curious about what different parts of myself are feeling.
    0%   10   20   30   40   50   60   70   80   90   100%
    (not applicable/never true)   (always true)

30. I'm aware of which parts of myself are contributing to my actions.
    0%   10   20   30   40   50   60   70   80   90   100%
    (not applicable/never true)   (always true)

31. All parts of myself know and can independently use recovery-focused coping skills (e.g., grounding, past vs. present, containment).
    0%   10   20   30   40   50   60   70   80   90   100%
    (not applicable/never true)   (always true)

32. All parts of myself communicate and cooperate well.
    0%   10   20   30   40   50   60   70   80   90   100%
    (not applicable/never true)   (always true)

PITQ-p Scoring

To score the PITQ-p, treat the percentages endorsed as points (e.g., 0% = 0 points, 100% = 100 points).

The procedure for calculating a PITQ-p score is different for patients with and without dissociative self-states.

For patients without dissociative self-states

Add the points corresponding to the percentages endorsed for items 1 through 26 and divide by 26 (i.e., maximum score = 100, minimum score = 0).

For patients with dissociative self-states

Add the points corresponding to the percentages endorsed for items 1 through 32 and then divide the total by 32 (i.e., maximum score = 100, minimum score = 0).

The use of this measure is free of charge. Please note, however, that norms for the PITQ-p have not yet been established. If you use the PITQ-p in research, please share your feedback and findings with Hugo. Schielke@gmail.com and BBrand@towson.edu. Visit https://topddstudy. com/pitq.php

Appendix C

RESOURCES, TRAINING, AND SUGGESTED READINGS

TRAINING RESOURCES FOR GENERAL TRAUMA-RELATED DISORDERS

- Teachtrauma.com—website with facts about trauma including types of trauma, dissociation, traumatic memory, debates in the trauma field; slideshows for educators; evaluations of textbooks' coverage of trauma; classroom activities to teach about trauma, and additional resources

- International Society for Traumatic Stress Studies: https://ISTSS.org

- International Society for the Study of Trauma and Dissociation: https://ISST-D.org

- American Psychological Association Trauma Division (Division 56): https://apatraumadivision.org/

- The National Child Traumatic Stress Network: https://www.NCTSN.org

- European Society for Trauma & Dissociation: https://www.estd.org/

- Treating Trauma Master Series—National Institute for the Clinical Application of Behavioral Medicine (NICABM): https://www.nicabm.com/program/treating-trauma-master/

- Blue Knot Foundation in Australia: https://www.blueknot.org.au

TRAINING RESOURCES FOR DISSOCIATIVE DISORDERS

- International Society for the Study of Dissociation and Trauma: https://www.ISST-D.org

- European Society for Trauma & Dissociation: https://www.estd.org
- Blue Knot Foundation in Australia: https://www.blueknot.org.au
- Teachtrauma.com—website with facts about trauma including dissociation, dissociative disorders, and traumatic memories; reviews about psychology textbooks including their coverage of dissociation and dissociative disorders

RESOURCES FOR SURVIVORS OF TRAUMA

- Sidran Institute: Traumatic Stress Education and Advocacy: https://www.sidran.org
- Blue Knot Foundation in Australia: https://www.blueknot.org.au
- Male Survivors: Overcoming Sexual Victimization of Boys and Men: https://www.malesurvivor.org
- Site for men who have been sexually abused or assaulted: https://1in6.org/
- Adult Survivors of Child Abuse: https://www.ascasupport.org
- David Baldwin's Trauma Information Pages: https://www.trauma-pages.com/support.php
- Survivors Network of Those Abused by Priests: https://www.snapnetwork.org
- National Sexual Assault Hotline: https://hotline.rainn.org/online
- PTSD Coach Online: https://https://www.ptsd.va.gov/apps/ptsdcoachonline/default.htm

BOOKS AND GUIDELINES ABOUT COMPLEX TRAUMA-RELATED DISORDERS WITH AN EMPHASIS ON DISSOCIATION

Allen, J. G. (2005). *Coping with trauma: Hope through understanding* (2nd ed.). American Psychiatric Publishing.
Allen, J. G. (2013). *Restoring mentalizing in attachment relationships: Treating trauma with plain old therapy*. American Psychiatric Publishing.
Boon, S., & Draijer, N. (1993). *Multiple personality disorder in the Netherlands: A study on reliability and validity of the diagnosis*. Swets & Zeitlinger Publishers.

Boon, S., Steele, K., & van der Hart, O. (2011). *Coping with trauma-related dissociation: Skills training for patients and therapists.* W. W. Norton & Company.

Brenner, I. (2001). *Dissociation of trauma: Theory, phenomenology, and technique.* International Universities Press.

Briere, J. (2004). *Psychological assessment of adult posttraumatic states: Phenomenology, diagnosis, and measurement* (2nd ed.). American Psychological Association.

Briere, J. N., & Scott, C. (2015). *Principles of trauma therapy: A guide to symptoms, evaluation, and treatment* (2nd ed., *DSM-5* update). Sage Publications.

Brown, D. P., & Elliott, D. S. (2016). *Attachment disturbances in adults: Treatment for comprehensive repair.* W. W. Norton & Co.

Brown, L. S. (2008). *Cultural competence in trauma therapy: Beyond the flashback.* American Psychological Association.

Chefetz, R. A. (2015). *Intensive psychotherapy for persistent dissociative processes: The fear of feeling real.* W. W. Norton & Co.

Chu, J. A. (2011). *Rebuilding shattered lives: Treating complex PTSD and dissociative disorders* (2nd ed.). John Wiley & Sons.

Cloitre, M., Courtois, C. A., Charuvastra, A., Carapezza, R., Stolbach, B. C., & Green, B. L. (2011). Treatment of complex PTSD: Results of the ISTSS expert clinician survey on best practices. *Journal of Traumatic Stress, 24*(6), 615–627.

Cloitre, M., Courtois, C. A., Ford, J. D., Green, B. L., Alexander, P., Briere, J., Herman, J. L., Lanius, R., Pearlman, L. A., Stolbach, B., Spinazzola, J., van der Kolk, B., & Van der Hart, O. (2012). *The ISTSS Expert Consensus Treatment Guidelines for Complex PTSD in Adults.* International Society for Traumatic Stress Studies Complex Trauma.

Cook, J. M., & Newman, E. (2017). Training in trauma: New Haven Consensus Conference conclusions on core competencies. In S. N. Gold (Ed.), *APA handbook of trauma psychology: Foundations in knowledge* (Vol. 1, pp. 145–157). American Psychological Association.

Courtois, C. A. (2010). *Healing the incest wound: Adult survivors in therapy* (rev. ed.). W. W. Norton & Co.

Courtois, C. A., & Ford, J. D. (Eds.). (2009). *Treating complex traumatic stress disorders: An evidence-based guide.* Guilford Press.

Courtois, C. A., & Ford, J. D. (2013). *Treatment of complex trauma: A sequenced, relationship-based approach.* Guilford Press.

Courtois, C. A., Ford, J. D., & Cloitre, M. (2009). Best practices in psychotherapy for adults. In C. A. Courtois & J. D. Ford (Eds.), *Treating complex traumatic stress disorders: An evidence-based guide* (pp. 82–103). Guilford Press.

Daitch, C. (2007). *Affect regulation toolbox: Practical and effective hypnotic interventions for the over-reactive client.* W. W. Norton & Co.

Dalenberg, C. J. (2000). *Countertransference and the treatment of trauma.* American Psychological Association.

Davies, J. M., & Frawley, M. G. (1994). *Treating the adult survivor of childhood sexual abuse: A psychoanalytic perspective.* Basic Books.

Dell, P. F., & O'Neil, J. A. (Eds.). (2009). *Dissociation and the dissociative disorders: DSM-5 and beyond.* Routledge.

Dorahy, M. J., Gold, S., & O'Neil, J. (Eds.). (2023). *Dissociation and the dissociative disorders: Past, present, future* (2nd ed.) Routledge Press.

Fisher, J. (2017). *Healing the fragmented selves of trauma survivors: Overcoming internal self-alienation.* Taylor & Francis.

Fisher, J. (2020). *Transforming the living legacy of trauma: A workbook for survivors.* PESI Publishing & Media.

Ford, J. D., & Courtois, C. A. (2020). *Treating complex traumatic stress disorders in adults: Scientific foundations and therapeutic models* (2nd ed.). Guilford Press.

Forner, C. C. (2017). *Dissociation, mindfulness, and creative meditations: Trauma-informed practices to facilitate growth.* Routledge/Taylor & Francis Group.

Frewen, P. A., & Lanius, R. (2015). *Healing the traumatized self: Consciousness, neuroscience, treatment.* W. W. Norton & Co.

Freyd, J. J. (1996). *Betrayal trauma: The logic of forgetting childhood abuse.* Harvard University Press.

Freyd, J. J., & Birrell, P. J. (2013). *Blind to betrayal: Why we fool ourselves we aren't being fooled.* John Wiley & Sons Inc.

Gartner, R. B. (1999). *Betrayed as boys: Psychodynamic treatment of sexually abused men.* Guilford Press.

Gartner, R. B. (2018). *Healing sexually betrayed men and boys: Treatment for sexual abuse, assault, and trauma.* Routledge/Taylor & Francis Group.

Gold, S. N. (2000). *Not trauma alone: Therapy for child abuse survivors in family and social context.* Brunner-Routledge.

Gold, S. N. (2017a). *APA handbook of trauma psychology: Vol. 1. Foundations in knowledge.* American Psychological Association.

Gold, S. N. (2017b). *APA handbook of trauma psychology: Vol. 2. Trauma practice.* American Psychological Association.

Herman, J. L. (1997). *Trauma and recovery: The aftermath of violence—From domestic abuse to political terror.* Basic Books.

Herman, J. L. (2023). *Truth and repair: How trauma survivors envision justice.* Basic Books.

Howell, E. F. (2005). *The dissociative mind.* The Analytic Press/Taylor & Francis Group.

Howell, E. F. (2011). *Understanding and treating dissociative identity disorder: A relational approach.* Routledge/Taylor & Francis Group.

Hunter, M. E. (2004). *Understanding dissociative disorders: A guide for family physicians and healthcare workers.* Crown House Publishing Limited.

International Society for the Study of Trauman and Dissociation. (2011). Guidelines for treating dissociative identity disorder in adults, third revision. *Journal of Trauma and Dissociation, 12*(2), 115–187. https://doi.org/10.1080/15299732.2011.537247

Johnson, S. (2005). *Emotionally focused couple therapy with trauma survivors: Strengthening attachment bonds.* Guilford Press.

Kezelman, C., & Stavropoulos, P. (2019). *Practice guidelines for treatment of complex trauma and trauma informed care and service delivery.* Blue Knot Foundation. Available for purchase at https://blueknot.org.au/product/practice-guidelines-for-clinical-treatment-of-complex-trauma-digital-download/

Kinsler, P. J. (2018). *Complex psychological trauma: The centrality of the relationship.* Routledge.

Kluft, R. P. (Ed.). (1985). *Childhood antecedents of multiple personality.* American Psychiatric Press.

Kluft, R. P. (2013). *Shelter from the storm: Processing the traumatic memories of DID/DDNOS patients with the fractionated abreaction technique (a vademecum for the treatment of DID/DDNOS).* CreateSpace Independent Publishing Platform.

Kluft, R. P., & Fine, C. G. (Eds.). (1993). *Clinical perspectives on multiple personality disorder.* American Psychiatric Press.

Lanius, U. F., Paulsen, S. L., & Corrigan, F. M. (2014). *Neurobiology and treatment of traumatic dissociation: Toward an embodied self.* Springer Publishing Company.

Levine, P. A. (1997). *Waking the tiger: Healing trauma. The innate capacity to transform overwhelming experiences.* North Atlantic Books.

Lewis, L., Kelly, K., & Allen, J. G. (2004). *Restoring hope and trust: An illustrated guide to mastering trauma.* Sidran Press.

Nijenhuis, E. (2015). *The trinity of trauma: Ignorance, fragility, and control.* Vandenhoeck & Ruprecht.

Ogden, P., & Fisher, J. (2015). *Sensorimotor psychotherapy: Interventions for trauma and attachment.* W. W. Norton & Co.

Putnam, F. W. (1989). *Diagnosis and treatment of multiple personality disorder.* Guilford Press.

Putnam, F. W. (1997). *Dissociation in children and adolescents: A developmental perspective.* Guilford Press.

Putnam, F. W. (2016). *The way we are: How states of mind influence our identities, personality, and potential for change.* International Psychoanalytic Books.

Ross, C. A. (1997). *Dissociative identity disorder: Diagnosis, clinical features, and treatment of multiple personality.* John Wiley & Sons.

Rothschild, B. (2000). *The body remembers: The psychophysiology of trauma and trauma treatment.* W. W. Norton & Company.

Rothschild, B. (2017). *The body remembers: Revolutionizing trauma treatment: Vol 2.* W. W. Norton & Co.

Schore, A. N. (2003). *Affect dysregulation and disorders of the self.* W. W. Norton & Company.

Siegel, D. J. (2007). *The mindful brain: Reflection and attunement in the cultivation of well-being.* W. W. Norton & Company.

Siegel, D. J. (2010). *Mindsight: The new science of personal transformation.* Bantam.

Siegel, D. J. (2015). *The developing mind: How relationships and the brain interact to shape who we are.* Guilford Press.

Silberg, J. L. (2013). *The child survivor: Healing developmental trauma and dissociation.* Routledge/Taylor & Francis Group.

Steele, K., Boon, S., & van der Hart, O. (2017). *Treating trauma-related dissociation: A practical, integrative approach.* W. W. Norton & Co.

Steinberg, M. (1994). *Interviewer's guide to the structured clinical interview for* DSM-IV *dissociative disorders (SCID-D)* (rev. ed.). American Psychiatric Press.

Steinberg, M. (1995). *Handbook for the assessment of dissociation: A clinical guide.* American Psychiatric Press.

Steinberg, M. (2000). *The stranger in the mirror: Dissociation—The hidden epidemic* (Vol. 2). Cliff Street/HarperCollins.

Steinberg, M. (2023). *The SCID-D Interview: Dissociation assessment in therapy, forensic, and research.* American Psychiatric Press.

van der Hart, O., Nijenhuis, E. R. S., & Steele, K. (2006). *The haunted self* (Vol. 2). W. W. Norton & Co.

van der Kolk, B. A. (2014). *The body keeps the score: Brain, mind, and body in the healing of trauma*. Viking.

Walker, D., Courtois, C. A., & Aten, J. (Eds.). (2015). *Spirituality oriented psychotherapy for trauma*. American Psychological Association Press.

Watkins, J. G., & Watkins, H. H. (1997). *Ego states: Theory and therapy*. W. W. Norton & Co.

References

Abu-Rayya, H. M., Somer, E., & Knane, H. (2020). Maladaptive daydreaming is associated with intensified psychosocial problems experienced by female survivors of childhood sexual abuse. *Violence Against Women, 26*(8), 825–837. https://doi.org/10.1177/1077801219845532

Abu-Rus, A., Thompson, K. J., Naish, B. L., Brown, C., & Dalenberg, C. (2020). Development of a validity scale for the Dissociative Experiences Scale—Revised: Atypicality, structure, and inconsistency. *Psychological Injury and Law, 13*(2), 167–177. https://doi.org/10.1007/s12207-019-09371-9

Agar, K., Read, J., & Bush, J.-M. (2002). Identification of abuse histories in a community mental health center: The need for policies and training. *Journal of Mental Health, 11*(5), 533–543. https://doi.org/10.1080/09638230020023886

Allen, J. G., & Coyne, L. (1995). Dissociation and vulnerability to psychotic experience: The Dissociative Experiences Scale and the MMPI-2. *Journal of Nervous and Mental Disease, 183*(10), 615–622. https://doi.org/10.1097/00005053-199510000-00001

Allen, J. G., Coyne, L., & Console, D. A. (1996). Dissociation contributes to anxiety and psychoticism on the Brief Symptom Inventory. *Journal of Nervous and Mental Disease, 184*(10), 639–641. https://doi.org/10.1097/00005053-199610000-00010

Allen, J. G., Coyne, L., & Console, D. A. (1997). Dissociative detachment relates to psychotic symptoms and personality decompensation. *Comprehensive Psychiatry, 38*(6), 327–334. https://doi.org/10.1016/S0010-440X(97)90928-7

Allwood, M. A., Ford, J. D., & Levendosky, A. (2021). Introduction to the Special Issue: Disproportionate trauma, stress, and adversities as a pathway to health disparities among disenfranchised groups globally. *Journal of Traumatic Stress, 34*(5), 899–904. https://doi.org/10.1002/jts.22743

Altman, H., Collins, M., & Mundy, P. (1997). Subclinical hallucinations and delusions in nonpsychotic adolescents. *Journal of Child Psychology and Psychiatry, and Allied Disciplines, 38*(4), 413–420. https://doi.org/10.1111/j.1469-7610.1997.tb01526.x

Ambrose, T., Giarratano, K., McCue, M., Brand, B. L., & Dalenberg, C. J. (2023). *Utility of the MMPI-2 in differentiating genuine from feigned dissociative identity disorder* [Manuscript submitted for publication].

American Psychiatric Association. (2013). *Diagnostic and statistical manual of mental disorders* (5th ed.).

American Psychiatric Association. (2022). *Diagnostic and statistical manual of mental disorders* (5th ed., text revision).

American Psychological Association. (2013). Specialty guidelines for forensic psychology. *American Psychologist, 68*(1), 7–19. https://doi.org/10.1037/a0029889

American Psychological Association. (2017). *Ethical principles of psychologists and code of conduct* (2002, Amended June 1, 2010, and January 1, 2017). https://www.apa.org/ethics/code

Anda, R. F., Croft, J. B., Felitti, V. J., Nordenberg, D., Giles, W. H., Williamson, D. F., & Giovino, G. A. (1999). Adverse childhood experiences and smoking during adolescence and adulthood. *JAMA, 282*(17), 1652–1658. https://doi.org/10.1001/jama.282.17.1652

Anderson, R. L., Lyons, J. S., Giles, D. M., Price, J. A., & Estle, G. (2003). Reliability of the Child and Adolescent Needs and Strengths—Mental Health (CANS-MH) scale. *Journal of Child and Family Studies, 12*(3), 279–289. https://doi.org/10.1023/A:1023935726541

Andrews, B., Brewin, C. R., Ochera, J., Morton, J., Bekerian, D. A., Davies, G. M., & Mollon, P. (2000). The timing, triggers and qualities of recovered memories in therapy. *British Journal of Clinical Psychology, 39*(1), 11–26. https://doi.org/10.1348/014466500163077

Anketell, C., Dorahy, M. J., Shannon, M., Elder, R., Hamilton, G., Corry, M., MacSherry, A., Curran, D., & O'Rawe, B. (2010). An exploratory analysis of voice hearing in chronic PTSD: Potential associated mechanisms. *Journal of Trauma & Dissociation, 11*(1), 93–107. https://doi.org/10.1080/15299730903143600

Aponte-Soto, M. R., Vélez-Pastrana, M., Martínez-Taboas, A., & González, R. A. (2014). Psychometric properties of the Cambridge depersonalization scale in Puerto Rico. *Journal of Trauma & Dissociation, 15*(3), 348–363. https://doi.org/10.1080/15299732.2013.856370

Armour, C., Contractor, A. A., Palmieri, P. A., & Elhai, J. D. (2014). Assessing latent level associations between PTSD and dissociative factors: Is depersonalization and derealization related to PTSD factors more so than alternative dissociative factors? *Psychological Injury and Law, 7*(2), 131–142. https://doi.org/10.1007/s12207-014-9196-9

Armstrong, J. (1991). The psychological organization of multiple personality disordered patients as revealed in psychological testing. *The Psychiatric Clinics of North America, 14*(3), 533–546. https://doi.org/10.1016/S0193-953X(18)30288-0

Armstrong, J. G. (1993). *A method for assessing multiple personality disorder through psychological testing.*

Armstrong, J. G. (1994). Reflections on multiple personality disorder as a developmentally complex adaptation. *The Psychoanalytic Study of the Child, 49*(1), 349–364. https://doi.org/10.1080/00797308.1994.11823068

Armstrong, J. G. (1996). Psychological assessment. In J. L. Spira & I. D. Yalom (Eds.), *Treating dissociative identity disorder* (pp. 3–37). Jossey-Bass.

Armstrong, J. G. (2001). The case of Mr. Woods: Psychological contributions to the legal process in defendants with multiple personality/dissociative identity disorder. *Southern California Interdisciplinary Law Journal, 10*(2), 205–224.

Armstrong, J. G. (2002). Deciphering the broken narrative of trauma: Signs of traumatic dissociation on the Rorschach. *Rorschachiana, 25*(1), 11–27. https://doi.org/10.1027/1192-5604.25.1.11

Armstrong, J. G. (2017). Incorporating trauma into an assessment interview. In S. N. Gold (Ed.), *APA handbook of trauma psychology* (Vol. 2, pp. 31–40). American Psychological Association. https://doi.org/10.1037/0000020-002

Armstrong, J. G., & Loewenstein, R. J. (1990). Characteristics of patients with multiple personality and dissociative disorders on psychological testing. *Journal of Nervous and Mental Disease, 178*(7), 448–454. https://doi.org/10.1097/00005053-199007000-00006

Armstrong, J. G., Putnam, F. W., Carlson, E. B., Libero, D. Z., & Smith, S. R. (1997). Development and validation of a measure of adolescent dissociation: The Adolescent Dissociative Experiences Scale. *Journal of Nervous and Mental Disease, 185*(8), 491–497. https://doi.org/10.1097/00005053-199708000-00003

Baars, E. W., van der Hart, O., Nijenhuis, E. R. S., Chu, J. A., Glas, G., & Draijer, N. (2011). Predicting stabilizing treatment outcomes for complex posttraumatic stress disorder and dissociative identity disorder: An expertise-based prognostic model. *Journal of Trauma & Dissociation, 12*(1), 67–87. https://doi.org/10.1080/15299732.2010.514846

Bae, H., Kim, D., & Park, Y. C. (2016). Dissociation predicts treatment response in eye-movement desensitization and reprocessing for posttraumatic stress disorder. *Journal of Trauma & Dissociation, 17*(1), 112–130. https://doi.org/10.1080/15299732.2015.1037039

Bailey, T. D., Boyer, S. M., & Brand, B. L. (2019). Dissociative disorders. In D. L. Segal (Ed.), *Diagnostic interviewing* (pp. 401–424). Springer. https://doi.org/10.1007/978-1-4939-9127-3_16

Bailey, T. D., & Brown, L. S. (2020). Complex trauma: Missed and misdiagnosis in forensic evaluations. *Psychological Injury and Law, 13*(2), 109–123. https://doi.org/10.1007/s12207-020-09383-w

Ballou, M., & Brown, L. S. (Eds.). (2002). *Rethinking mental health and disorder: Feminist perspectives.* Guilford Press.

Barker-Collo, S. L. (2001). Relationship of the Dissociative Experiences Scale to demographics, symptomatology, and coping strategies in a New Zealand student sample. *Journal of Trauma & Dissociation, 2*(3), 79–98. https://doi.org/10.1300/J229v02n03_06

Barth, M. R., Brand, B. L., & Nester, M. S. (2023). Distinguishing clinical and simulated dissociative identity disorder using the Miller Forensic Assessment of Symptoms Test. *Psychological Trauma: Theory, Research, Practice, and Policy.* Advance online publication. https://doi.org/10.1037/tra0001413

Becker-Blease, K., & Freyd, J. J. (2017). Additional questions about the applicability of "false memory" research. *Applied Cognitive Psychology, 31*(1), 34–36. https://doi.org/10.1002/acp.3266

Becker-Blease, K. A., Deater-Deckard, K., Eley, T., Freyd, J. J., Stevenson, J., & Plomin, R. (2004). A genetic analysis of individual differences in dissociative behaviors in childhood and adolescence. *Journal of Child Psychology and Psychiatry, and Allied Disciplines, 45*(3), 522–532. https://doi.org/10.1111/j.1469-7610.2004.00242.x

Bernstein, E. M., & Putnam, F. W. (1986). Development, reliability, and validity of a dissociation scale. *Journal of Nervous and Mental Disease, 174*(12), 727–735. https://doi.org/10.1097/00005053-198612000-00004

Bisson, J. I., Brewin, C. R., Cloitre, M., & Maercker, A. (2020). Diagnosis, assessment, and screening for PTSD and complex PTSD in adults. In D. Forbes, J. I. Bisson, C. M. Monson, & L. Berliner (Eds.), *Effective treatments for PTSD: Practice guidelines from the international society for traumatic stress studies* (3rd ed., pp. 49–68). Guilford Press.

Blevins, C. A., Weathers, F. W., Davis, M. T., Witte, T. K., & Domino, J. L. (2015). The Posttraumatic Stress Disorder Checklist for *DSM-5* (PCL-5): Development and initial psychometric evaluation. *Journal of Traumatic Stress, 28*(6), 489–498. https://doi.org/10.1002/jts.22059

Blevins, C. A., Witte, T. K., & Weathers, F. W. (2013). Factor structure of the Cambridge Depersonalization Scale in trauma-exposed college students. *Journal of Trauma & Dissociation, 14*(3), 288–301. https://doi.org/10.1080/15299732.2012.729555

Bohus, M. J., Landwehrmeyer, G. B., Stiglmayr, C. E., Limberger, M. F., Böhme, R., & Schmahl, C. G. (1999). Naltrexone in the treatment of dissociative symptoms in patients with borderline personality disorder: An open-label trial. *The Journal of Clinical Psychiatry, 60*(9), 598–603. https://doi.org/10.4088/JCP.v60n0906

Bongaerts, H., Voorendonk, E. M., van Minnen, A., & de Jongh, A. (2021). Safety and effectiveness of intensive treatment for complex PTSD delivered via home-based telehealth. *European Journal of Psychotraumatology, 12*(1), 1860346. https://doi.org/10.1080/20008198.2020.1860346

Boon, S., & Draijer, N. (1991). Diagnosing dissociative disorders in The Netherlands: A pilot study with the Structured Clinical Interview for *DSM-III-R* Dissociative Disorders. *The American Journal of Psychiatry, 148*(4), 458–462. https://doi.org/10.1176/ajp.148.4.458

Boon, S., & Draijer, N. (1993a). The differentiation of patients with MPD or DDNOS from patients with a Cluster B personality disorder. *Dissociation*, *6*(2–3), 126–135.

Boon, S., & Draijer, N. (1993b). Multiple personality disorder in The Netherlands: A clinical investigation of 71 patients. *The American Journal of Psychiatry*, *150*(3), 489–494. https://doi.org/10.1176/ajp.150.3.489

Boon, S., & Draijer, N. (1993c). *Multiple personality disorder in the Netherlands: A study on reliability and validity of the diagnosis*. Swets & Zeitlinger Publishers.

Boon, S., Steele, K., & van der Hart, O. (2011). *Coping with trauma-related dissociation: Skills training for patients and therapists*. W. W. Norton & Co.

Bottoms, B. L., Peter-Hagene, L. C., Epstein, M. A., Wiley, T. R. A., Reynolds, C. E., & Rudnicki, A. G. (2016). Abuse characteristics and individual differences related to disclosing childhood sexual, physical, and emotional abuse and witnessed domestic violence. *Journal of Interpersonal Violence*, *31*(7), 1308–1339. https://doi.org/10.1177/0886260514564155

Bourget, D., Gagné, P., & Wood, S. F. (2017). Dissociation: Defining the concept in criminal forensic psychiatry. *The Journal of the American Academy of Psychiatry and the Law*, *45*(2), 147–160.

Bowman, E. S. (2006). Why conversion seizures should be classified as a dissociative disorder. *The Psychiatric Clinics of North America*, *29*(1), 185–211, x. https://doi.org/10.1016/j.psc.2005.10.003

Boyd, J. E., O'Connor, C., Protopopescu, A., Jetly, R., Lanius, R. A., & McKinnon, M. C. (2020). The contributions of emotion regulation difficulties and dissociative symptoms to functional impairment among civilian inpatients with posttraumatic stress symptoms. *Psychological Trauma: Theory, Research, Practice, and Policy*, *12*(7), 739–749. https://doi.org/10.1037/tra0000576

Boyd, J. E., Protopopescu, A., O'Connor, C., Neufeld, R. W. J., Jetly, R., Hood, H. K., Lanius, R. A., & McKinnon, M. C. (2018). Dissociative symptoms mediate the relation between PTSD symptoms and functional impairment in a sample of military members, veterans, and first responders with PTSD. *European Journal of Psychotraumatology*, *9*(1), Article 1463794. https://doi.org/10.1080/20008198.2018.1463794

Bradford, J. M. W., & Smith, S. M. (1979). Amnesia and homicide: The Padola case and a study of thirty cases. *The Bulletin of the American Academy of Psychiatry and the Law*, *7*(3), 219–231.

Brand, B. (2001). Establishing safety with patients with dissociative identity disorder. *Journal of Trauma & Dissociation*, *2*(4), 133–155. https://doi.org/10.1300/J229v02n04_07

Brand, B., & Loewenstein, R. J. (2014). Does phasic trauma treatment make patients with dissociative identity disorder treatment more dissociative? *Journal of Trauma & Dissociation*, *15*(1), 52–65. https://doi.org/10.1080/15299732.2013.828150

Brand, B. L. (2023, April 15). *The Finding Solid Ground program: A promising treatment and training program for trauma-related dissociation*. Keynote talk delivered at the Annual conference of the International Society for the Study of Trauma & Dissociation, Louisville, KY, United States.

Brand, B. L., Armstrong, J. G., & Loewenstein, R. J. (2006). Psychological assessment of patients with dissociative identity disorder. *The Psychiatric Clinics of North America, 29*(1), 145–168, x. https://doi.org/10.1016/j.psc.2005. 10.014

Brand, B. L., Armstrong, J. G., Loewenstein, R. J., & McNary, S. W. (2009). Personality differences on the Rorschach of dissociative identity disorder, borderline personality disorder, and psychotic inpatients. *Psychological Trauma: Theory, Research, Practice, and Policy, 1*(3), 188–205. https://doi.org/10.1037/a0016561

Brand, B. L., Barth, M., Schlumpf, Y. R., Schielke, H., Chalavi, S., Vissia, E. M., Nijenhuis, E. R. S., Jäncke, L., & Reinders, A. A. T. S. (2021). The utility of the Structured Inventory of Malingered Symptomatology for distinguishing individuals with dissociative identity disorder (DID) from DID simulators and healthy controls. *European Journal of Psychotraumatology, 12*(1), 1984048. https://doi.org/10.1080/20008198.2021.1984048

Brand, B. L., & Brown, L. (2023). True drama or true trauma? Forensic trauma assessment and the challenge of detecting malingering. In M. J. Dorahy, S. Gold, & J. O'Neil (Eds.), *Dissociation and the dissociative disorders: Past, present, future* (2nd ed., pp. 673–683). Routledge Press.

Brand, B. L., & Chasson, G. S. (2015). Distinguishing simulated from genuine dissociative identity disorder on the MMPI-2. *Psychological Trauma: Theory, Research, Practice, and Policy, 7*(1), 93–101. https://doi.org/10.1037/a0035181

Brand, B. L., Chasson, G. S., Palermo, C. A., Donato, F. M., Rhodes, K. P., & Voorhees, E. F. (2016). MMPI-2 item endorsements in dissociative identity disorder vs. simulators. *The Journal of the American Academy of Psychiatry and the Law, 44*(1), 63–72.

Brand, B. L., Classen, C. C., Lanius, R. A., Loewenstein, R. J., McNary, S., Pain, C., & Putnam, F. (2009). A naturalistic study of dissociative identity disorder and dissociative disorder not otherwise specified patients treated by community clinicians. *Psychological Trauma: Theory, Research, Practice, and Policy, 1*(2), 153–171. https://doi.org/10.1037/a0016210

Brand, B. L., Classen, C. C., McNary, S. W., & Zaveri, P. (2009). A review of dissociative disorders treatment studies. *Journal of Nervous and Mental Disease, 197*(9), 646–654. https://doi.org/10.1097/NMD.0b013e3181b3afaa

Brand, B. L., Dalenberg, C. J., Frewen, P. A., Loewenstein, R. J., Schielke, H. J., Brams, J. S., & Spiegel, D. (2018). Trauma-related dissociation is no fantasy: Addressing the errors of omission and commission in Merckelbach and Patihis (2018). *Psychological Injury and Law, 11*(4), 377–393. https://doi.org/10.1007/s12207-018-9336-8

Brand, B. L., & Frewen, P. (2017). Dissociation as a trauma-related phenomenon. In S. N. Gold (Ed.), *APA handbook of trauma psychology* (Vol. 1, pp. 215–241). American Psychological Association. https://doi.org/10.1037/0000019-013

Brand, B. L., Frewen, P., Nester, M. S., Dalenberg, C., Loewenstein, R. J., & Spiegel, D. (2021). Challenging myths and bias in Paris (2019). *BJPsych Advances*, *25*(5). https://www.cambridge.org/core/journals/bjpsych-advances/article/dissociative-identity-disorder-validity-and-use-in-the-criminal-justice-system/C1C27EE9731782570E1376A3EDA48CE4#comments

Brand, B. L., Kumar, S. A., & McEwen, L. E. (2019). Coverage of child maltreatment and adult trauma in graduate psychopathology textbooks. *Psychological Trauma: Theory, Research, Practice, and Policy*, *11*(8), 919–926. https://doi.org/10.1037/tra0000454

Brand, B. L., & Lanius, R. A. (2014). Chronic complex dissociative disorders and borderline personality disorder: Disorders of emotion dysregulation? *Borderline Personality Disorder and Emotion Dysregulation*, *1*, 13. https://doi.org/10.1186/2051-6673-1-13

Brand, B. L., Lanius, R., Vermetten, E., Loewenstein, R. J., & Spiegel, D. (2012). Where are we going? An update on assessment, treatment, and neurobiological research in dissociative disorders as we move toward the *DSM-5*. *Journal of Trauma & Dissociation*, *13*(1), 9–31. https://doi.org/10.1080/15299732.2011.620687

Brand, B. L., Loewenstein, R. J., & Lanius, R. (2014). Dissociative identity disorder. In G. Gabbard (Ed.), *Treatments of psychiatric disorders* (5th ed., pp. 439–458). American Psychiatric Publishing.

Brand, B. L., Loewenstein, R. J., & Spiegel, D. (2014). Dispelling myths about dissociative identity disorder treatment: An empirically based approach. *Psychiatry*, *77*(2), 169–189. https://doi.org/10.1521/psyc.2014.77.2.169

Brand, B. L., McNary, S. W., Loewenstein, R. J., Kolos, A. C., & Barr, S. R. (2006). Assessment of genuine and simulated dissociative identity disorder on the structured interview of reported symptoms. *Journal of Trauma & Dissociation*, *7*(1), 63–85. https://doi.org/10.1300/J229v07n01_06

Brand, B. L., McNary, S. W., Myrick, A. C., Classen, C. C., Lanius, R., Loewenstein, R. J., Pain, C., & Putnam, F. W. (2013). A longitudinal naturalistic study of patients with dissociative disorders treated by community clinicians. *Psychological Trauma: Theory, Research, Practice, and Policy*, *5*(4), 301–308. https://doi.org/10.1037/a0027654

Brand, B. L., Myrick, A. C., Loewenstein, R. J., Classen, C. C., Lanius, R., McNary, S. W., Pain, C., & Putnam, F. W. (2012). A survey of practices and recommended treatment interventions among expert therapists treating patients with dissociative identity disorder and dissociative disorder not otherwise specified. *Psychological Trauma: Theory, Research, Practice, and Policy*, *4*(5), 490–500. https://doi.org/10.1037/a0026487

Brand, B. L., & Pasko, D. (2017). *Split* is based on myths about dissociative identity disorder [Review of the film *Split* by M. N. Shyamalan, Dir.]. *PsycCRITIQUES*, *62*(18). https://doi.org/10.1037/a0040801

Brand, B. L., Sar, V., Stavropoulos, P., Krüger, C., Korzekwa, M., Martínez-Taboas, A., & Middleton, W. (2016). Separating fact from fiction: An empirical examination of six myths about dissociative identity disorder. *Harvard Review of Psychiatry*, *24*(4), 257–270. https://doi.org/10.1097/HRP.0000000000000100

Brand, B. L., Schielke, H. J., & Brams, J. S. (2017). Assisting the courts in understanding and connecting with experiences of disconnection: Addressing trauma-related dissociation as a forensic psychologist, Part I. *Psychological Injury and Law*, *10*(4), 283–297. https://doi.org/10.1007/s12207-017-9304-8

Brand, B. L., Schielke, H. J., Brams, J. S., & DiComo, R. A. (2017). Assessing trauma-related dissociation in forensic contexts: Addressing trauma-related dissociation as a forensic psychologist, Part II. *Psychological Injury and Law*, *10*(4), 298–312. https://doi.org/10.1007/s12207-017-9305-7

Brand, B. L., Schielke, H. J., Putnam, K. T., Putnam, F. W., Loewenstein, R. J., Myrick, A., Jepsen, E. K. K., Langeland, W., Steele, K., Classen, C. C., & Lanius, R. A. (2019). An online educational program for individuals with dissociative disorders and their clinicians: 1-year and 2-year follow-up. *Journal of Traumatic Stress*, *32*(1), 156–166. https://doi.org/10.1002/jts.22370

Brand, B. L., Schielke, H. J., Schiavone, F., & Lanius, R. A. (2022). *Finding solid ground: Overcoming obstacles in trauma treatment*. Oxford University Press. https://doi.org/10.1093/med-psych/9780190636081.001.0001

Brand, B. L., Tursich, M., Tzall, D., & Loewenstein, R. J. (2014). Utility of the SIRS-2 in distinguishing genuine from simulated dissociative identity disorder. *Psychological Trauma: Theory, Research, Practice, and Policy*, *6*(4), 308–317. https://doi.org/10.1037/a0036064

Brand, B. L., Vissia, E. M., Chalavi, S., Nijenhuis, E. R. S., Webermann, A. R., Draijer, N., & Reinders, A. A. T. S. (2016). DID is trauma based: Further evidence supporting the trauma model of DID. *Acta Psychiatrica Scandinavica*, *134*(6), 560–563. https://doi.org/10.1111/acps.12653

Brand, B. L., Webermann, A. R., & Frankel, A. S. (2016). Assessment of complex dissociative disorder patients and simulated dissociation in forensic contexts. *International Journal of Law and Psychiatry*, *49*(Part B), 197–204.

Brand, B. L., Webermann, A. R., Snyder, B. L., & Kaliush, P. R. (2019). Detecting clinical and simulated dissociative identity disorder with the Test of Memory Malingering. *Psychological Trauma: Theory, Research, Practice, and Policy*, *11*(5), 513–520. https://doi.org/10.1037/tra0000405

Bremner, J. D., Krystal, J. H., Putnam, F. W., Southwick, S. M., Marmar, C., Charney, D. S., & Mazure, C. M. (1998). Measurement of dissociative states with the Clinician-Administered Dissociative States Scale (CADSS). *Journal of Traumatic Stress*, *11*(1), 125–136. https://doi.org/10.1023/A:1024465317902

Brewin, C. R., & Andrews, B. (2017). Creating memories for false autobiographical events in childhood: A systematic review. *Applied Cognitive Psychology*, *31*(1), 2–23. https://doi.org/10.1002/acp.3220

Brewin, C. R., Dalgleish, T., & Joseph, S. (1996). A dual representation theory of posttraumatic stress disorder. *Psychological Review, 103*(4), 670–686. https://doi.org/10.1037/0033-295X.103.4.670

Briere, J. (1996). *Trauma Symptom Checklist for Children (TSCC): Professional manual*. Psychological Assessment Resources.

Briere, J. (2002). *The Multiscale Dissociation Inventory: Professional manual*. Psychological Assessment Resources.

Briere, J. (2004). *Psychological assessment of adult posttraumatic states: Phenomenology, diagnosis, and measurement* (2nd ed.). American Psychological Association. https://doi.org/10.1037/10809-000

Briere, J. (2011). *Trauma Symptom Inventory–2 (TSI-2): Professional manual*. Psychological Assessment Resources, Inc.

Briere, J. (2019). *Treating risky and compulsive behavior in trauma survivors*. Guilford Press.

Briere, J., Agee, E., & Dietrich, A. (2016). Cumulative trauma and current posttraumatic stress disorder status in general population and inmate samples. *Psychological Trauma: Theory, Research, Practice, and Policy, 8*(4), 439–446. https://doi.org/10.1037/tra0000107

Briere, J., & Armstrong, J. G. (2007). Psychological assessment of posttraumatic dissociation. In E. Vermetten, M. Dorahy, & D. Spiegel (Eds.), *Traumatic dissociation* (pp. 259–274). American Psychiatric Press.

Briere, J., Dietrich, A., & Semple, R. J. (2016). Dissociative complexity: Antecedents and clinical correlates of a new construct. *Psychological Trauma: Theory, Research, Practice, and Policy, 8*(5), 577–584. https://doi.org/10.1037/tra0000126

Briere, J., Johnson, K., Bissada, A., Damon, L., Crouch, J., Gil, E., Hanson, R., & Ernst, V. (2001). The Trauma Symptom Checklist for Young Children (TSCYC): Reliability and association with abuse exposure in a multi-site study. *Child Abuse & Neglect, 25*(8), 1001–1014. https://doi.org/10.1016/S0145-2134(01)00253-8

Briere, J., & Lanktree, C. B. (1995). *The Trauma Symptom Checklist for Children (TSCC): Preliminary psychometric characteristics* [Unpublished manuscript]. Department of Psychiatry, University of Southern California School of Medicine.

Briere, J., & Runtz, M. (2015). Dissociation in individuals denying trauma exposure: Findings from two samples. *Journal of Nervous and Mental Disease, 203*(6), 439–442. https://doi.org/10.1097/NMD.0000000000000303

Briere, J., Runtz, M., Eadie, E. M., Bigras, N., & Godbout, N. (2019). The Disorganized Response Scale: Construct validity of a potential self-report measure of disorganized attachment. *Psychological Trauma: Theory, Research, Practice, and Policy, 11*(5), 486–494. https://doi.org/10.1037/tra0000396

Briere, J., Runtz, M., Rassart, C. A., Rodd, K., & Godbout, N. (2020). Sexual assault trauma: Does prior childhood maltreatment increase the risk and exacerbate the outcome? *Child Abuse & Neglect, 103*, Article 104421. https://doi.org/10.1016/j.chiabu.2020.104421

Briere, J., & Scott, C. (2012). *Principles of trauma therapy.* Sage Publications.

Briere, J., & Scott, C. (2015). Complex trauma in adolescents and adults: Effects and treatment. *The Psychiatric Clinics of North America, 38*(3), 515–527. https://doi.org/10.1016/j.psc.2015.05.004

Briere, J., Scott, C., & Weathers, F. (2005). Peritraumatic and persistent dissociation in the presumed etiology of PTSD. *The American Journal of Psychiatry, 162*(12), 2295–2301. https://doi.org/10.1176/appi.ajp.162.12.2295

Briere, J., & Spinazzola, J. (2009). Assessment of the sequelae of complex trauma: Evidence-based measures. In C. A. Courtois & J. D. Ford (Eds.), *Treating complex traumatic stress disorders: An evidence-based guide* (pp. 104–123). Guilford Press.

Briere, J., Weathers, F. W., & Runtz, M. (2005). Is dissociation a multidimensional construct? Data from the Multiscale Dissociation Inventory. *Journal of Traumatic Stress, 18*(3), 221–231. https://doi.org/10.1002/jts.20024

Brooks, R., Bryant, R. A., Silove, D., Creamer, M., O'Donnell, M., McFarlane, A. C., & Marmar, C. R. (2009). The latent structure of the Peritraumatic Dissociative Experiences Questionnaire. *Journal of Traumatic Stress, 22*(2), 153–157. https://doi.org/10.1002/jts.20414

Brown, D. P., & Elliott, D. S. (2016). *Attachment disturbances in adults: Treatment for comprehensive repair.* W. W. Norton & Co.

Brown, D. W., Anda, R. F., Edwards, V. J., Felitti, V. J., Dube, S. R., & Giles, W. H. (2007). Adverse childhood experiences and childhood autobiographical memory disturbance. *Child Abuse & Neglect, 31*(9), 961–969. https://doi.org/10.1016/j.chiabu.2007.02.011

Brown, L. (2023). *Decolonizing trauma healing: Towards a humble, culturally responsive trauma practice* [Manuscript in preparation]. American Psychological Association.

Brown, L. S. (2009). True drama or true trauma? Forensic trauma assessment and the challenge of detecting malingering. In P. F. Dell & J. A. O'Neil (Eds.), *Dissociation and the dissociative disorders: DSM-V and beyond* (pp. 585–595). Routledge/Taylor & Francis Group.

Bryant, R. (2022). Acute stress disorder in adults: Epidemiology, pathogenesis, clinical manifestations, course, and diagnosis. *Up-to-Date.* https://www.uptodate.com/contents/acute-stress-disorder-in-adults-epidemiology-pathogenesis-clinical-manifestations-course-and-diagnosis?search=acute%20stress%20disorder&source=search_result&selectedTitle=1~43&usage_type=default&display_rank=1

Bryant, R. A. (2007). Does dissociation further our understanding of PTSD? *Journal of Anxiety Disorders, 21*(2), 183–191. https://doi.org/10.1016/j.janxdis.2006.09.012

Bury, A. S., & Bagby, R. M. (2002). The detection of feigned uncoached and coached posttraumatic stress disorder with the MMPI-2 in a sample of workplace accident victims. *Psychological Assessment, 14*(4), 472–484. https://doi.org/10.1037/1040-3590.14.4.472

Bush, S. S., Connell, M., & Denney, R. L. (2020). *Ethical practice in forensic psychology: A guide for mental health professionals* (2nd ed.). American Psychological Association.

Butcher, J. N., Graham, J. R., Ben-Porath, Y. S., Tellegen, A., & Dahlstrom, W. G. (2001). *Manual for the administration and scoring of the MMPI-2*. Minnesota University Press.

Butler, L. D., Duran, R. E., Jasiukaitis, P., Koopman, C., & Spiegel, D. (1996). Hypnotizability and traumatic experience: A diathesis-stress model of dissociative symptomatology. *The American Journal of Psychiatry, 153*(7, Suppl.), 42–63. https://doi.org/10.1176/ajp.153.7.42

Byun, S., Brumariu, L. E., & Lyons-Ruth, K. (2016). Disorganized attachment in young adulthood as a partial mediator of relations between severity of childhood abuse and dissociation. *Journal of Trauma & Dissociation, 17*(4), 460–479. https://doi.org/10.1080/15299732.2016.1141149

Calati, R., Bensassi, I., & Courtet, P. (2017). The link between dissociation and both suicide attempts and non-suicidal self-injury: Meta-analyses. *Psychiatry Research, 251*, 103–114. https://doi.org/10.1016/j.psychres.2017.01.035

Caldwell, A. B. (2001). What do the MMPI scales fundamentally measure? Some hypotheses. *Journal of Personality Assessment, 76*(1), 1–17. https://doi.org/10.1207/S15327752JPA7601_1

Cardeña, E., & Carlson, E. (2011). Acute stress disorder revisited. *Annual Review of Clinical Psychology, 7*(1), 245–267. https://doi.org/10.1146/annurev-clinpsy-032210-104502

Carlson, E. A. (1998). A prospective longitudinal study of attachment disorganization/disorientation. *Child Development, 69*(4), 1107–1128. https://doi.org/10.1111/j.1467-8624.1998.tb06163.x

Carlson, E. B., Dalenberg, C. J., & McDade-Montez, E. (2012). Dissociation in posttraumatic stress disorder Part I: Definitions and review of research. *Psychological Trauma: Theory, Research, Practice, and Policy, 4*(5), 479–489. https://doi.org/10.1037/a0027748

Carlson, E. B., Newman, E., Daniels, J. W., Armstrong, J. G., Roth, D., & Loewenstein, R. J. (2003). Distress in response to and perceived usefulness of trauma research interviews. *Journal of Trauma & Dissociation, 4*(2), 131–142. https://doi.org/10.1300/J229v04n02_08

Carlson, E. B., & Putnam, F. W. (1993). An update on the Dissociative Experiences Scale. *Dissociation, 6*, 16–27.

Carlson, E. B., Putnam, F. W., Ross, C. A., Torem, M., Coons, P., Dill, D. L., Loewenstein, R. J., & Braun, B. G. (1993). Validity of the Dissociative Experiences Scale in screening for multiple personality disorder: A multicenter study. *The American Journal of Psychiatry, 150*(7), 1030–1036. https://doi.org/10.1176/ajp.150.7.1030

Carlson, E. B., Smith, S. R., & Dalenberg, C. J. (2013). Can sudden, severe emotional loss be a traumatic stressor? *Journal of Trauma & Dissociation, 14*(5), 519–528. https://doi.org/10.1080/15299732.2013.773475

Carlson, E. B., Smith, S. R., Palmieri, P. A., Dalenberg, C., Ruzek, J. I., Kimerling, R., Burling, T. A., & Spain, D. A. (2011). Development and validation of a brief self-report measure of trauma exposure: The Trauma History Screen. *Psychological Assessment, 23*(2), 463–477. https://doi.org/10.1037/a0022294

Carlson, E. B., Waelde, L. C., Palmieri, P. A., Macia, K. S., Smith, S. R., & McDade-Montez, E. (2018). Development and validation of the Dissociative Symptoms Scale. *Assessment, 25*(1), 84–98. https://doi.org/10.1177/1073191116645904

Carrion, V. G., & Steiner, H. (2000). Trauma and dissociation in delinquent adolescents. *Journal of the American Academy of Child & Adolescent Psychiatry, 39*(3), 353–359. https://doi.org/10.1097/00004583-200003000-00018

Cassiers, L. L. M., Sabbe, B. G. C., Schmaal, L., Veltman, D. J., Penninx, B. W. J. H., & Van Den Eede, F. (2018). Structural and functional brain abnormalities associated with exposure to different childhood trauma subtypes: A systematic review of neuroimaging findings. *Frontiers in Psychiatry, 9*, 329. https://doi.org/10.3389/fpsyt.2018.00329

Cavicchioli, M., Scalabrini, A., Northoff, G., Mucci, C., Ogliari, A., & Maffei, C. (2021). Dissociation and emotion regulation strategies: A meta-analytic review. *Journal of Psychiatric Research, 143*, 370–387. https://doi.org/10.1016/j.jpsychires.2021.09.011

Černis, E., Chan, C., & Cooper, M. (2019). What is the relationship between dissociation and self-harming behaviour in adolescents? *Clinical Psychology & Psychotherapy, 26*(3), 328–338. https://doi.org/10.1002/cpp.2354

Cernovsky, Z. Z., & Diamond, D. M. (2020). High risk of false classification of injured people as malingerers by the Structured Inventory of Malingered Symptomatology (SIMS): A review. *Archives of Psychiatry and Behavioral Sciences, 3*(2), 30–38.

Cernovsky, Z., Mendonca, J., Oyewumi, L. K., Ferrari, J. R., Sidhu, G., & Campbell, R. (2019). Content validity of the Psychosis subscale of the Structured Inventory of Malingered Symptomatology (SIMS). *International Journal of Psychology and Cognitive Science, 5*(3), 121–127.

Chefetz, R. A. (1997a). Abreaction: Baby or bathwater? *Dissociation, 10*(4), 203–213.

Chefetz, R. A. (1997b). Special case transferences and countertransferences in the treatment of dissociative disorders. *Dissociation, 10*(4), 255–264.

Chefetz, R. A. (2015). *Intensive psychotherapy for persistent dissociative processes: The fear of feeling real.* W. W. Norton & Co.

Chessell, Z. J., Brady, F., Akbar, S., Stevens, A., & Young, K. (2019). A protocol for managing dissociative symptoms in refugee populations. *Cognitive Behaviour Therapist, 12*, 1–16.

Chiu, C.-D., Meg Tseng, M.-C., Chien, Y.-L., Liao, S.-C., Liu, C.-M., Yeh, Y.-Y., Hwu, H.-G., & Ross, C. A. (2017). Dissociative disorders in acute psychiatric inpatients in Taiwan. *Psychiatry Research, 250*, 285–290. https://doi.org/10.1016/j.psychres.2017.01.082

Chlebowski, S. M., & Gregory, R. J. (2012). Three cases of dissociative identity disorder and co-occurring borderline personality disorder treated with dynamic deconstructive psychotherapy. *American Journal of Psychotherapy*, *66*(2), 165–180. https://doi.org/10.1176/appi.psychotherapy.2012.66.2.165

Christensen, E. M. (2022). The online community: DID and plurality. *European Journal of Trauma & Dissociation*, *6*(2), Article 100257. https://doi.org/10.1016/j.ejtd.2021.100257

Chu, J. A. (1988). Ten traps for therapists in the treatment of trauma survivors. *Dissociation*, *1*(4), 24–32.

Cintron, G., Salloum, A., Blair-Andrews, Z., & Storch, E. A. (2018). Parents' descriptions of young children's dissociative reactions after trauma. *Journal of Trauma & Dissociation*, *19*(5), 500–513. https://doi.org/10.1080/15299732.2017.1387886

Cloitre, M., Courtois, C. A., Charuvastra, A., Carapezza, R., Stolbach, B. C., & Green, B. L. (2011). Treatment of complex PTSD: Results of the ISTSS expert clinician survey on best practices. *Journal of Traumatic Stress*, *24*(6), 615–627. https://doi.org/10.1002/jts.20697

Cloitre, M., Courtois, C. A., Ford, J. D., Green, B. L., Alexander, P., Briere, J., Herman, J. L., Lanius, R. A., Stolbach, B., Spinazzola, J., Van der Kolk, B. A., & Van der Hart, O. (2012). *The ISTSS expert consensus treatment guidelines for complex PTSD in adults*. https://istss.org/ISTSS_Main/media/Documents/ComplexPTSD.pdf

Cloitre, M., Petkova, E., Wang, J., & Lu Lassell, F. (2012). An examination of the influence of a sequential treatment on the course and impact of dissociation among women with PTSD related to childhood abuse. *Depression and Anxiety*, *29*(8), 709–717. https://doi.org/10.1002/da.21920

Cloitre, M., Shevlin, M., Brewin, C. R., Bisson, J. I., Roberts, N. P., Maercker, A., Karatzias, T., & Hyland, P. (2018). The International Trauma Questionnaire: Development of a self-report measure of *ICD-11* PTSD and complex PTSD. *Acta Psychiatrica Scandinavica*, *138*(6), 536–546. https://doi.org/10.1111/acps.12956

Cloitre, M., Stovall-McClough, K. C., Nooner, K., Zorbas, P., Cherry, S., Jackson, C. L., Gan, W., & Petkova, E. (2010). Treatment for PTSD related to childhood abuse: A randomized controlled trial. *The American Journal of Psychiatry*, *167*(8), 915–924. https://doi.org/10.1176/appi.ajp.2010.09081247

Coe, M. T., Dalenberg, C. J., Aransky, K. M., & Reto, C. S. (1995). Adult attachment style, reported childhood violence history and types of dissociative experiences. *Dissociation*, *8*(3), 142–154.

Cook, J. M., Rehman, O., Bufka, L., Dinnen, S., & Courtois, C. (2011). Responses of a sample of practicing psychologists to questions about clinical work with trauma and interest in specialized training. *Psychological Trauma: Theory, Research, Practice, and Policy*, *3*(3), 253–257. https://doi.org/10.1037/a0025048

Coons, P. M., & Milstein, V. (1994). Factitious or malingered multiple personality disorder: Eleven cases. *Dissociation, 7*(2), 81–85.

Corrigan, F. M., & Christie-Sands, J. (2020). An innate brainstem self-other system involving orienting, affective responding, and polyvalent relational seeking: Some clinical implications for a "Deep Brain Reorienting" trauma psychotherapy approach. *Medical Hypotheses, 136*, Article 109502. https://doi.org/10.1016/j.mehy.2019.109502

Courtois, C. A., & Brown, L. S. (2019). Guideline orthodoxy and resulting limitations of the American Psychological Association's clinical practice guideline for the treatment of PTSD in adults [*APA Clinical Practice Guideline for PTSD: Coordinated Special Issue With Psychotherapy and Practice Innovations*]. *Psychotherapy: Theory, Research, & Practice, 56*(3), 329–339. https://doi.org/10.1037/pst0000239

Courtois, C. A., & Ford, J. D. (Eds.). (2009). *Treating complex traumatic stress disorders: An evidence-based guide*. Guilford Press.

Courtois, C. A., & Ford, J. D. (2013). *Treatment of complex trauma: A sequenced, relationship-based approach*. Guilford Press.

Coy, D. M., Madere, J. A., & Dell, P. F. (2020). *An interpretive manual for the Multidimensional Inventory of Dissociation (MID)*. https://www.mid-assessment.com/

Craske, M. G., Kircanski, K., Zelikowsky, M., Mystkowski, J., Chowdhury, N., & Baker, A. (2008). Optimizing inhibitory learning during exposure therapy. *Behaviour Research and Therapy, 46*(1), 5–27. https://doi.org/10.1016/j.brat.2007.10.003

Cromer, L. D., Freyd, J. J., Binder, A. K., DePrince, A. P., & Becker-Blease, K. (2006). What's the risk in asking? Participant reaction to trauma history questions compared with reaction to other personal questions. *Ethics & Behavior, 16*(4), 347–362. https://doi.org/10.1207/s15327019eb1604_5

Cronin, E., Brand, B. L., & Mattanah, J. F. (2014). The impact of the therapeutic alliance on treatment outcome in patients with dissociative disorders. *European Journal of Psychotraumatology, 5*(1), Article 22676. https://doi.org/10.3402/ejpt.v5.22676

Dalenberg, C. (2006). Recovered memory and the Daubert criteria: Recovered memory as professionally tested, peer reviewed, and accepted in the relevant scientific community. *Trauma, Violence & Abuse, 7*(4), 274–310. https://doi.org/10.1177/1524838006294572

Dalenberg, C., & Carlson, E. B. (2010). *DES-B modified for DSM-5*. https://www.psychiatry.org/File%20Library/Psychiatrists/Practice/DSM/APA_DSM5_Severity-of-Dissociative-Symptoms-Adult.pdf

Dalenberg, C. J. (1996). Accuracy, timing, and circumstances of disclosure in therapy of recovered and continuous memories of abuse. *The Journal of Psychiatry & Law, 24*(2), 229–276. https://doi.org/10.1177/009318539602400206

Dalenberg, C. J. (2000). *Countertransference and the treatment of trauma*. American Psychological Association. https://doi.org/10.1037/10380-000

Dalenberg, C. J. (2004). Maintaining the safe and effective therapeutic relationship in the context of distrust and anger: Countertransference and complex trauma. *Psychotherapy: Theory, Research, & Practice, 41*(4), 438–447. https://doi.org/10.1037/0033-3204.41.4.438

Dalenberg, C. J., Brand, B. L., Gleaves, D. H., Dorahy, M. J., Loewenstein, R. J., Cardeña, E., Frewen, P. A., Carlson, E. B., & Spiegel, D. (2012). Evaluation of the evidence for the trauma and fantasy models of dissociation. *Psychological Bulletin, 138*(3), 550–588. https://doi.org/10.1037/a0027447

Dalenberg, C. J., Brand, B. L., Loewenstein, R. J., Frewen, P. A., & Spiegel, D. (2020). Inviting scientific discourse on traumatic dissociation: Progress made and obstacles to further resolution. *Psychological Injury and Law, 13*(2), 135–154. https://doi.org/10.1007/s12207-020-09376-9

Dalenberg, C. J., & Briere, J. (2017). Psychometric assessment of trauma. In S. N. Gold (Ed.), *APA handbook of trauma psychology* (Vol. 2, pp. 41–63). American Psychological Association. https://doi.org/10.1037/0000020-003

Dalenberg, C. J., & Carlson, E. (2010). *Brief Dissociative Experiences Scale (DES-B)—Modified*. https://www.psychiatry.org/File%20Library/Psychiatrists/Practice/DSM/APA_DSM5_Severity-of-Dissociative-Symptoms-Adult.pdf

Dalenberg, C. J., Coe, M. T., Reto, C. S., Aransky, K. M., Duvenage, C., & Weber, R. (1994, January). *The development of a measure of dissociation for use on general psychiatric and nonpsychiatric populations*. Presented at the Eighth Annual Conference on Responding to Child Maltreatment, San Diego, CA, United States.

Dalenberg, C. J., & Palesh, O. G. (2010). Scientific progress and methodological issues in the study of recovered and false memories of trauma. In R. A. Lanius, E. Vermetten, & C. Pain (Eds.), *The hidden epidemic: The impact of early life trauma on health and disease* (pp. 225–233). Cambridge University Press. https://doi.org/10.1017/CBO9780511777042.026

Dalenberg, C. J., & Paulson, K. (2009). The case for the study of "normal" dissociation processes. In P. F. Dell & J. A. O'Neil (Eds.), *Dissociation and the dissociative disorders:* DSM-V *and beyond* (pp. 145–154). Routledge/Taylor & Francis Group.

Dalenberg, C. J., Straus, E., & Ardill, M. (2017). Forensic psychology in the context of trauma. In S. N. Gold (Ed.), *APA handbook of trauma psychology* (Vol. 2, pp. 543–563). American Psychological Association. https://doi.org/10.1037/0000020-026

Dalenberg, C. J., Straus, E., & Carlson, E. B. (2017). Defining trauma. In S. N. Gold (Ed.), *APA handbook of trauma psychology* (Vol. 1, pp. 15–33). American Psychological Association. https://doi.org/10.1037/0000019-002

D'Andrea, W., & Pole, N. (2012). A naturalistic study of the relation of psychotherapy process to changes in symptoms, information processing, and physiological activity in complex trauma. *Psychological Trauma: Theory, Research, Practice, and Policy, 4*(4), 438–446. https://doi.org/10.1037/a0025067

Daubert v. Merrell Dow Pharmaceuticals, 61 U.S.L.W. 4805 (1993).

DeCou, C. R., Cole, T. T., Lynch, S. M., Wong, M. M., & Matthews, K. C. (2017). Assault-related shame mediates the association between negative social reactions to disclosure of sexual assault and psychological distress. *Psychological Trauma: Theory, Research, Practice, and Policy, 9*(2), 166–172. https://doi.org/10.1037/tra0000186

De Jongh, A., Resick, P. A., Zoellner, L. A., van Minnen, A., Lee, C. W., Monson, C. M., Foa, E. B., Wheeler, K., Broeke, E. T., Feeny, N., Rauch, S. A. M., Chard, K. M., Mueser, K. T., Sloan, D. M., van der Gaag, M., Rothbaum, B. O., Neuner, F., de Roos, C., Hehenkamp, L. M. J., . . . Bicanic, I. A. E. (2016). Critical analysis of the current treatment guidelines for complex PTSD in adults. *Depression and Anxiety, 33*(5), 359–369. https://doi.org/10.1002/da.22469

Dell, P. F. (1998). Axis II pathology in outpatients with dissociative identity disorder. *Journal of Nervous and Mental Disease, 186*(6), 352–356. https://doi.org/10.1097/00005053-199806000-00005

Dell, P. F. (2002). Dissociative phenomenology of dissociative identity disorder. *The Journal of Nervous and Mental Disease, 190*(1), 10–15.

Dell, P. F. (2006a). The Multidimensional Inventory of Dissociation (MID): A comprehensive measure of pathological dissociation. *Journal of Trauma & Dissociation, 7*(2), 77–106. https://doi.org/10.1300/J229v07n02_06

Dell, P. F. (2006b). A new model of dissociative identity disorder. *The Psychiatric Clinics of North America, 29*(1), 1–26, vii. https://doi.org/10.1016/j.psc.2005.10.013

Dell, P. F. (2009). The phenomena of pathological dissociation. In P. F. Dell & J. A. O'Neil (Eds.), *Dissociation and the dissociative disorders: DSM-V and beyond* (pp. 225–237). Routledge/Taylor & Francis Group.

Dell, P. F. (2011, April). *How to use the Multidimensional Inventory of Dissociation (MID)*. Presented at International Society for the Study of Trauma and Dissociation 29th Annual International Conference, Montreal, Canada.

Dell, P. F. (2017). Is high hypnotizability a necessary diathesis for pathological dissociation? *Journal of Trauma & Dissociation, 18*(1), 58–87.

Dell, P. F., & Lawson, D. (2009). An empirical delineation of the domain of pathological dissociation. In P. F. Dell & J. A. O'Neil (Eds.), *Dissociation and the dissociative disorders: DSM-V and beyond* (pp. 667–692). Routledge/Taylor & Francis Group.

Demakis, G. J., & Elhai, J. D. (2011). Neuropsychological and psychological aspects of malingered posttraumatic stress disorder. *Psychological Injury and Law, 4*(1), 24–31. https://doi.org/10.1007/s12207-011-9099-y

Dietz, T. J., Davis, D., & Pennings, J. (2012). Evaluating animal-assisted therapy in group treatment for child sexual abuse. *Journal of Child Sexual Abuse, 21*(6), 665–683. https://doi.org/10.1080/10538712.2012.726700

Dorahy, M. J., Gorgas, J., Seager, L., & Middleton, W. (2017). Engendered responses to, and interventions for, shame in dissociative disorders: A survey and experimental investigation. *Journal of Nervous and Mental Disease, 205*(11), 886–892. https://doi.org/10.1097/NMD.0000000000000740

Dorahy, M. J., Lewis, C. A., & Mulholland, C. (2005). The detection of dissociative identity disorder by Northern Irish clinical psychologists and psychiatrists: A clinical vignettes study. *Journal of Trauma & Dissociation, 6*(4), 39–50. https://doi.org/10.1300/J229v06n04_03

Dorahy, M. J., Shannon, C., Seagar, L., Corr, M., Stewart, K., Hanna, D., Mulholland, C., & Middleton, W. (2009). Auditory hallucinations in dissociative identity disorder and schizophrenia with and without a childhood trauma history: Similarities and differences. *Journal of Nervous and Mental Disease, 197*(12), 892–898. https://doi.org/10.1097/NMD.0b013e3181c299ea

Dorrepaal, E., Thomaes, K., Smit, J. H., Hoogendoorn, A., Veltman, D. J., van Balkom, A. J. L. M., & Draijer, N. (2012). Clinical phenomenology of childhood abuse-related complex PTSD in a population of female patients: Patterns of personality disturbance. *Journal of Trauma & Dissociation, 13*(3), 271–290. https://doi.org/10.1080/15299732.2011.641496

Douglas, A. N. (2009). Racial and ethnic differences in dissociation: An examination of the dissociative experiences scale in a nonclinical population. *Journal of Trauma & Dissociation, 10*(1), 24–37. https://doi.org/10.1080/15299730802488452

Draijer, N., & Boon, S. (1993). The validation of the Dissociative Experiences Scale against the criterion of the SCID-D, using receiver operating characteristics (ROC) analysis. *Dissociation, 6*(1), 28–37.

Draijer, N., & Boon, S. (1999). The imitation of dissociative identity disorder: Patients at risk, therapists at risk. *The Journal of Psychiatry & Law, 27*(3–4), 423–458. https://doi.org/10.1177/009318539902700304

Dunn, G. E., Dunn, C. E., Ryan, J. J., & Van Fleet, J. N. (1998). Cultural differences on three measures of dissociation in a substance abuse population. *Journal of Clinical Psychology, 54*(8), 1109–1116. https://doi.org/10.1002/(SICI)1097-4679(199812)54:8<1109::AID-JCLP10>3.0.CO;2-3

Dutra, L., Bureau, J. F., Holmes, B., Lyubchik, A., & Lyons-Ruth, K. (2009). Quality of early care and childhood trauma: A prospective study of developmental pathways to dissociation. *Journal of Nervous and Mental Disease, 197*(6), 383–390. https://doi.org/10.1097/NMD.0b013e3181a653b7

Eadie, E., & Briere, J. (2023). *Psychological assessment of adult posttraumatic states: Phenomenology, diagnosis, and measurement* (3rd ed.) [Manuscript in preparation]. American Psychological Association.

Ehlers, A., & Clark, D. M. (2000). A cognitive model of posttraumatic stress disorder. *Behaviour Research and Therapy, 38*(4), 319–345. https://doi.org/10.1016/S0005-7967(99)00123-0

Eidhof, M. B., Ter Heide, F. J. J., van Der Aa, N., Schreckenbach, M., Schmidt, U., Brand, B. L., Lanius, R. A., Loewenstein, R. J., Spiegel, D., & Vermetten, E. (2019). The dissociative subtype of PTSD interview (DSP-I): Development and psychometric properties. *Journal of Trauma & Dissociation, 20*(5), 564–581. https://doi.org/10.1080/15299732.2019.1597806

Elhai, J. D., Gold, S. N., Mateus, L. F., & Astaphan, T. A. (2001). Scale 8 elevations on the MMPI-2 among women survivors of childhood sexual abuse: Evaluating posttraumatic stress, depression, and dissociation as predictors. *Journal of Family Violence, 16*(1), 47–57. https://doi.org/10.1023/A:1026576425986

Elhai, J. D., Gold, S. N., Sellers, A. H., & Dorfman, W. I. (2001). The detection of malingered posttraumatic stress disorder with MMPI-2 fake bad indices. *Assessment, 8*(2), 221–236. https://doi.org/10.1177/107319110100800210

Elhai, J. D., Naifeh, J. A., Zucker, I. S., Gold, S. N., Deitsch, S. E., & Frueh, B. C. (2004). Discriminating malingered from genuine civilian posttraumatic stress disorder: A validation of three MMPI-2 Infrequency scales (F, Fp, and Fptsd). *Assessment, 11*(2), 139–144. https://doi.org/10.1177/1073191104264965

Ellason, J. W., & Ross, C. A. (1997). Two-year follow-up of inpatients with dissociative identity disorder. *The American Journal of Psychiatry, 154*(6), 832–839. https://doi.org/10.1176/ajp.154.6.832

Ellason, J. W., Ross, C. A., & Fuchs, D. L. (1996). Lifetime Axis I and II comorbidity and childhood trauma history in dissociative identity disorder. *Psychiatry: Interpersonal and Biological Processes, 59*(3), 255–266.

Ellickson-Larew, S., Escarfulleri, S., & Wolf, E. J. (2020). The dissociative subtype of posttraumatic stress disorder: Forensic considerations and recent controversies. *Psychological Injury and Law, 13*(2), 178–186. https://doi.org/10.1007/s12207-020-09381-y

Ellickson-Larew, S., Stasik-O'Brien, S. M., Stanton, K., & Watson, D. (2020). Dissociation as a multidimensional transdiagnostic symptom. *Psychology of Consciousness, 7*(2), 126–150. https://doi.org/10.1037/cns0000218

Engelberg, J. C., & Brand, B. L. (2012). The effect of depression on self-harm and treatment outcome in patients with severe dissociative disorders. *Psi Chi Journal of Psychological Research, 17*(3), 115–124. https://doi.org/10.24839/2164-8204.JN17.3.115

Espirito-Santo, H., & Pio-Abreu, J. L. (2009). Psychiatric symptoms and dissociation in conversion, somatization and dissociative disorders. *The Australian and New Zealand Journal of Psychiatry, 43*(3), 270–276. https://doi.org/10.1080/00048670802653307

Evans, F. B., Brand, B. L., & Kaser-Boyd, N. (2023). Differentiating bipolar spectrum and psychological trauma spectrum disorders. In J. H. Kleiger & I. B. Weiner (Eds.), *Psychological assessment of bipolar spectrum disorders* (pp. 233–252). American Psychological Association.

Evans, F. B., & Finn, S. E. (2017). Training and consultation in psychological assessment with professional psychologists: Suggestions for enhancing the profession and individual practices. *Journal of Personality Assessment, 99*(2), 175–185. https://doi.org/10.1080/00223891.2016.1187156

Evans, R. W., & Whitlow, C. T. (2022). Acute mild traumatic brain injury (concussion) in adults. *Up-to-Date.* https://www.medilib.ir/uptodate/show/4828

Evers-Szostak, M., & Sanders, S. (1992). The children's perceptual alteration scale (CPAS): A measure of children's dissociation. *Dissociation, 5*(2), 91–97.

Exner, J. E., Jr. (2003). *The Rorschach: A comprehensive system* (4th ed.). John Wiley & Sons Inc.

Exner, J. E., Jr., & Erdberg, P. (2005). *The Rorschach: A comprehensive system* (3rd ed.). John Wiley & Sons.

Felitti, V. J., & Anda, R. F. (2010). The relationship of adverse childhood experiences to adult medical disease, psychiatric disorders and sexual behavior. In R. A. Lanius, E. Vermetten, & C. Pain (Eds.), *The hidden epidemic: The impact of early life trauma on health and disease* (pp. 77–87). Cambridge University Press. https://doi.org/10.1017/CBO9780511777042.010

Felitti, V. J., Anda, R. F., Nordenberg, D., Williamson, D. F., Spitz, A. M., Edwards, V., Koss, M. P., & Marks, J. S. (1998). Relationship of childhood abuse and household dysfunction to many of the leading causes of death in adults: The Adverse Childhood Experiences (ACE) Study. *American Journal of Preventive Medicine, 14*(4), 245–258. https://doi.org/10.1016/S0749-3797(98)00017-8

Ferentz, L. (2012). *Treating self-destructive behaviors in trauma survivors: A clinician's guide*. Routledge. https://doi.org/10.4324/9780203833414

Ferrante, E., Marino, A., Guglielmucci, F., & Schimmenti, A. (2022). The mediating role of dissociation and shame in the relationship between emotional trauma and maladaptive daydreaming. *Psychology of Consciousness, 9*(1), 27–39. https://doi.org/10.1037/cns0000253

Finn, S. E. (2015). *In our clients' shoes: Theory and techniques of therapeutic assessment*. Routledge.

Finn, S. E., & Tonsager, M. E. (1997). Information-gathering and therapeutic models of assessment: Complementary paradigms. *Psychological Assessment, 9*(4), 374–385. https://doi.org/10.1037/1040-3590.9.4.374

Fischer, C. T. (1985). *Individualizing psychological assessment*. Brooks/Cole Publishing Company.

Foa, E. B., Molnar, C., & Cashman, L. (1995). Change in rape narratives during exposure therapy for posttraumatic stress disorder. *Journal of Traumatic Stress, 8*(4), 675–690. https://doi.org/10.1002/jts.2490080409

Foltz, R., Kaeley, A., Kupchan, J., Mills, A., Murray, K., Pope, A., Rahman, H., & Rubright, C. (2023). Trauma-informed care? Identifying training deficits in accredited doctoral programs. *Psychological Trauma: Theory, Research, Practice, and Policy*. Advance online publication. https://doi.org/10.1037/tra0001461

Fonagy, P., Gergely, G., Jurist, E. L., & Target, M. (2002). *Affect regulation, mentalization, and the development of the self*. Other Press.

Foote, B. (2022). Dissociative identity disorder: Epidemiology, pathogenesis, clinical manifestations, course, assessment, and diagnosis. *UpToDate*. https://www.uptodate.com/contents/dissociative-identity-disorder-epidemiology-pathogenesis-clinical-manifestations-course-assessment-and-diagnosis

Foote, B., & Park, J. (2008). Dissociative identity disorder and schizophrenia: Differential diagnosis and theoretical issues. *Current Psychiatry Reports, 10*(3), 217–222.

Foote, B., Smolin, Y., Kaplan, M., Legatt, M. E., & Lipschitz, D. (2006). Prevalence of dissociative disorders in psychiatric outpatients. *The American Journal of Psychiatry, 163*(4), 623–629. https://doi.org/10.1176/ajp.2006.163.4.623

Foote, B., Smolin, Y., Neft, D. I., & Lipschitz, D. (2008). Dissociative disorders and suicidality in psychiatric outpatients. *Journal of Nervous and Mental Disease, 196*(1), 29–36. https://doi.org/10.1097/NMD.0b013e31815fa4e7

Ford, J. D. (2021). Why we need a developmentally appropriate trauma diagnosis for children: A 10-year update on developmental trauma disorder. *Journal of Child & Adolescent Trauma, 16*(4), 403–418. https://doi.org/10.1007/s40653-021-00415-4

Ford, J. D., & Courtois, C. A. (2013). *Treating complex traumatic stress disorders in children and adolescents: Scientific foundations and therapeutic models*. Guilford Press.

Ford, J. D., & Courtois, C. A. (2020a). Defining and understanding complex trauma and complex traumatic stress disorders. In J. D. Ford & C. A. Courtois (Eds.), *Treating complex traumatic stress disorders in adults: Scientific foundations and therapeutic models* (2nd ed., pp. 3–34). Guilford Press.

Ford, J. D., & Courtois, C. A. (2020b). *Treating complex traumatic stress disorders in adults: Scientific foundations and therapeutic models* (2nd ed.). Guilford Press.

Ford, J. D., & Gómez, J. M. (2015). The relationship of psychological trauma, and dissociative and posttraumatic stress disorders to non-suicidal self-injury and suicidality: A review. *Journal of Trauma & Dissociation, 16*(3), 232–271. https://doi.org/10.1080/15299732.2015.989563

Frankel, A. S. (2009). Dissociation and dissociative disorders: Clinical and forensic assessment with adults. In P. F. Dell & J. A. O'Neil (Eds.), *Dissociation and the dissociative disorders: DSM-V and beyond* (pp. 571–583). Routledge/Taylor & Francis Group.

Frankel, A. S., & Dalenberg, C. (2006). The forensic evaluation of dissociation and persons diagnosed with dissociative identity disorder: Searching for convergence. *The Psychiatric Clinics of North America, 29*(1), 169–184, x. https://doi.org/10.1016/j.psc.2005.10.002

Frewen, P. A., Brown, M. F. D., & Lanius, R. A. (2017). Trauma-related altered states of consciousness (TRASC) in an online community sample: Further support for the 4-D model of trauma-related dissociation. *Psychology of Consciousness, 4*(1), 92–114. https://doi.org/10.1037/cns0000091

Frewen, P. A., & Lanius, R. A. (2015). *Healing the traumatized self: Consciousness, neuroscience, treatment*. W. W. Norton & Co.

Freyd, J. J. (1996). *Betrayal trauma: The logic of forgetting childhood abuse*. Harvard University Press.

Friedl, M. C., Draijer, N., & de Jonge, P. (2000). Prevalence of dissociative disorders in psychiatric in-patients: The impact of study characteristics. *Acta Psychiatrica Scandinavica, 102*(6), 423–428. https://doi.org/10.1034/j.1600-0447.2000.102006423.x

Frost, J., Silberg, J. L., & McIntee, J. (1996, November). *Imaginary friends in normal and traumatized children.* Presented at the 13th International Conference of the International Society for the Study of Dissociation, San Francisco, CA, United States.

Fung, H. W., Chien, W. T., Chan, C., & Ross, C. A. (2022). A cross-cultural investigation of the association between betrayal trauma and dissociative features. *Journal of Interpersonal Violence, 38*(1–2), NP1630–NP1653. https://doi.org/10.1177/08862605221090568

Gast, U., Rodenwald, F., Dehner-Rau, C., Kowalewsky, E., Engl, V., Reddemann, L., & Emrich, H. M. (2003, April). *Validation of the German version of the Multidimensional Inventory of Dissociation (MID-d).* Presented at the Annual Meeting of the International Society for the Study of Dissociation, Chicago, IL, United States.

Gee, T., Allen, K., & Powell, R. A. (2003). Questioning premorbid dissociative symptomatology in dissociative identity disorder: Comment on Gleaves, Hernandez and Warner (1999). *Professional Psychology, Research and Practice, 34*(1), 114–116. https://doi.org/10.1037/0735-7028.34.1.114

Geng, F., Lu, H., Zhang, Y., Zhan, N., Zhang, L., & Liu, M. (2022). Dissociative depression and its related clinical and psychological characteristics among Chinese prisoners: A latent class analysis. *Current Psychology.* Advance online publication. https://doi.org/10.1007/s12144-022-02751-6

George, C., Kaplan, N., & Main, M. (1996). *Adult Attachment Interview protocol* (3rd ed.). University of California at Berkeley.

Giesbrecht, T., Lynn, S. J., Lilienfeld, S. O., & Merckelbach, H. (2008). Cognitive processes in dissociation: An analysis of core theoretical assumptions. *Psychological Bulletin, 134*(5), 617–647. https://doi.org/10.1037/0033-2909.134.5.617

Giesbrecht, T., Lynn, S. J., Lilienfeld, S. O., & Merckelbach, H. (2010). Cognitive processes, trauma, and dissociation—Misconceptions and misrepresentations: Reply to Bremner (2010). *Psychological Bulletin, 136*(1), 7–11. https://doi.org/10.1037/a0018068

Gilbert, A. M. (2004). Psychometric properties of the Trauma Symptom Checklist for Young Children (TSCYC). *Dissertation Abstracts International: Section B: The Sciences and Engineering, 65*(1-B), 478.

Ginzburg, K., Koopman, C., Butler, L. D., Palesh, O., Kraemer, H. C., Classen, C. C., & Spiegel, D. (2006). Evidence for a dissociative subtype of post-traumatic stress disorder among help-seeking childhood sexual abuse survivors. *Journal of Trauma and Dissociation, 7*(2), 7–27.

Gleaves, D. H. (2007). What are students learning about trauma, memory, and dissociation? *Journal of Trauma & Dissociation, 8*(4), 1–5. https://doi.org/10.1300/J229v08n04_01

Gleaves, D. H., & Eberenz, K. P. (1995). Correlates of dissociative symptoms among women with eating disorders. *Journal of Psychiatric Research, 29*(5), 417–426.

Goffinet, S. J. L., & Beine, A. (2018). Prevalence of dissociative symptoms in adolescent psychiatric inpatients. *European Journal of Trauma & Dissociation, 2*(1), 39–45. https://doi.org/10.1016/j.ejtd.2017.10.008

Gold, S. N. (Ed.). (2017). *APA handbook of trauma psychology: Trauma practice* (Vol. 2). American Psychological Association. https://doi.org/10.1037/0000020-000

Golier, J. A., Yehuda, R., Bierer, L. M., Mitropoulou, V., New, A. S., Schmeidler, J., Silverman, J. M., & Siever, L. J. (2003). The relationship of borderline personality disorder to posttraumatic stress disorder and traumatic events. *The American Journal of Psychiatry, 160*(11), 2018–2024. https://doi.org/10.1176/appi.ajp.160.11.2018

González-Vázquez, A. I., Del Río-Casanova, L., Seijo-Ameneiros, N., Cabaleiro-Fernández, P., Seoane-Pillado, T., Justo-Alonso, A., & Santed-Germán, M. A. (2017). Validity and reliability of the Spanish version of the Somatoform Dissociation Questionnaire (SDQ-20). *Psicothema, 29*(2), 275–280.

Goodman-Brown, T. B., Edelstein, R. S., Goodman, G. S., Jones, D. P. H., & Gordon, D. S. (2003). Why children tell: A model of children's disclosure of sexual abuse. *Child Abuse & Neglect, 27*(5), 525–540. https://doi.org/10.1016/S0145-2134(03)00037-1

Granqvist, P., Sroufe, L. A., Dozier, M., Hesse, E., Steele, M., van Ijzendoorn, M., Solomon, J., Schuengel, C., Fearon, P., Bakermans-Kranenburg, M., Steele, H., Cassidy, J., Carlson, E., Madigan, S., Jacobvitz, D., Foster, S., Behrens, K., Rifkin-Graboi, A., Gribneau, N., . . . Duschinsky, R. (2017). Disorganized attachment in infancy: A review of the phenomenon and its implications for clinicians and policy-makers. *Attachment & Human Development, 19*(6), 534–558. https://doi.org/10.1080/14616734.2017.1354040

Green, J. G., McLaughlin, K. A., Berglund, P. A., Gruber, M. J., Sampson, N. A., Zaslavsky, A. M., & Kessler, R. C. (2010). Childhood adversities and adult psychiatric disorders in the national comorbidity survey replication I: Associations with first onset of *DSM-IV* disorders. *Archives of General Psychiatry, 67*(2), 113–123. https://doi.org/10.1001/archgenpsychiatry.2009.186

Greenberg, S. A., & Shuman, D. W. (1997). Irreconcilable conflict between therapeutic and forensic roles. *Professional Psychology, Research and Practice, 28*(1), 50–57. https://doi.org/10.1037/0735-7028.28.1.50

Greenberg, S. A., & Shuman, D. W. (2007). When worlds collide: Therapeutic and forensic roles. *Professional Psychology, Research and Practice, 38*(2), 129–132. https://doi.org/10.1037/0735-7028.38.2.129

Hagenaars, M. A., van Minnen, A., & Hoogduin, K. A. (2010). The impact of dissociation and depression on the efficacy of prolonged exposure treatment for PTSD. *Behaviour Research and Therapy, 48*(1), 19–27. https://doi.org/10.1016/j.brat.2009.09.001

Halligan, S. L., Michael, T., Clark, D. M., & Ehlers, A. (2003). Posttraumatic stress disorder following assault: The role of cognitive processing, trauma memory, and appraisals. *Journal of Consulting and Clinical Psychology, 71*(3), 419–431. https://doi.org/10.1037/0022-006X.71.3.419

Halvorsen, J. O., Stenmark, H., Neuner, F., & Nordahl, H. M. (2014). Does dissociation moderate treatment outcomes of narrative exposure therapy for PTSD? A secondary analysis from a randomized controlled clinical trial. *Behaviour Research and Therapy, 57*, 21–28. https://doi.org/10.1016/j.brat.2014.03.010

Hammond, D. C. (1990). *Handbook of hypnotic suggestions and metaphors.* W. W. Norton & Co.

Hansen, N. B., Lambert, M. J., & Forman, E. M. (2002). The psychotherapy dose–response effect and its implications for treatment delivery services. *Clinical Psychology: Science and Practice, 9*(3), 329–343. https://doi.org/10.1093/clipsy.9.3.329

Harricharan, S., McKinnon, M. C., & Lanius, R. A. (2021). How processing of sensory information from the internal and external worlds shape the perception and engagement with the world in the aftermath of trauma: Implications for PTSD. *Frontiers in Neuroscience, 15*, Article 625490. https://doi.org/10.3389/fnins.2021.625490

Harvey, A. G., & Bryant, R. A. (1999). A qualitative investigation of the organization of traumatic memories. *British Journal of Clinical Psychology, 38*(4), 401–405. https://doi.org/10.1348/014466599162999

Hébert, M., Langevin, R., Guidi, E., Bernard-Bonnin, A. C., & Allard-Dansereau, C. (2017). Sleep problems and dissociation in preschool victims of sexual abuse. *Journal of Trauma & Dissociation, 18*(4), 507–521. https://doi.org/10.1080/15299732.2016.1240739

Hediger, K., Wagner, J., Künzi, P., Haefeli, A., Theis, F., Grob, C., Pauli, E., & Gerger, H. (2021). Effectiveness of animal-assisted interventions for children and adults with post-traumatic stress disorder symptoms: A systematic review and meta-analysis. *European Journal of Psychotraumatology, 12*(1), Article 1879713. https://doi.org/10.1080/20008198.2021.1879713

Heilbrun, K., Grisso, T., & Goldstein, A. (2009). *Foundations of forensic mental health assessment.* Oxford University Press.

Heilbrun, K., Phillips, S., & Thornewill, A. (2016). Professional standards' citations in law and the behavioral sciences: Implications for policy and practice. *Professional Psychology, Research and Practice, 47*(4), 287–294. https://doi.org/10.1037/pro0000080

Henning, J. A., Brand, B., & Courtois, C. A. (2022). Graduate training and certification in trauma treatment for clinical practitioners. *Training and Education in Professional Psychology, 16*(4), 362–375.

Hepworth, I., & McGowan, L. (2013). Do mental health professionals enquire about childhood sexual abuse during routine mental health assessment in acute mental health settings? A substantive literature review. *Journal of Psychiatric and Mental Health Nursing, 20*(6), 473–483. https://doi.org/10.1111/j.1365-2850.2012.01939.x

Herman, J. L. (1992a). Complex PTSD: A syndrome in survivors of prolonged and repeated trauma. *Journal of Traumatic Stress, 5*(3), 377–391. https://doi.org/10.1002/jts.2490050305

Herman, J. L. (1992b). *Trauma and recovery.* Basic Books.

Herman, J. L. (2020). Foreword. In J. D. Ford & C. A. Courtois (Eds.), *Treating complex traumatic stress disorders in adults: Scientific foundations and therapeutic models* (2nd ed., pp. xi–xvii). Guilford Press.

Herman, J. L. (2023). *Truth and repair: How trauma survivors envision justice.* Basic Books.

Herzog, S., Fogle, B. M., Harpaz-Rotem, I., Tsai, J., & Pietrzak, R. H. (2020). Dissociative symptoms in a nationally representative sample of trauma-exposed U.S. Military veterans: Prevalence, comorbidities, and suicidality. *Journal of Affective Disorders, 272,* 138–145. https://doi.org/10.1016/j.jad.2020.03.177

Hoeboer, C. M., De Kleine, R. A., Molendijk, M. L., Schoorl, M., Oprel, D. A. C., Mouthaan, J., Van der Does, W., & Van Minnen, A. (2020). Impact of dissociation on the effectiveness of psychotherapy for post-traumatic stress disorder: Meta-analysis. *BJPsych Open, 6*(3), e53. https://doi.org/10.1192/bjo.2020.30

Holgersen, K. H., Klöckner, C. A., Boe, H. J., Weisaeth, L., & Holen, A. (2011). Disaster survivors in their third decade: Trajectories of initial stress responses and long-term course of mental health. *Journal of Traumatic Stress, 24*(3), 334–341. https://doi.org/10.1002/jts.20636

Holmes, E. A., Brown, R. J., Mansell, W., Fearon, R. P., Hunter, E. C. M., Frasquilho, F., & Oakley, D. A. (2005). Are there two qualitatively distinct forms of dissociation? A review and some clinical implications. *Clinical Psychology Review, 25*(1), 1–23. https://doi.org/10.1016/j.cpr.2004.08.006

Hornstein, N. L. (1996). Complexities of psychiatric differential diagnosis in children with dissociative symptoms and disorders. In J. L. Silberg (Ed.), *The dissociative child: Diagnosis, treatment, and management* (2nd ed., pp. 27–45). The Sidran Press.

Hoyos, C., Mancini, V., Furlong, Y., Medford, N., Critchley, H., & Chen, W. (2019). The role of dissociation and abuse among adolescents who self-harm. *The Australian and New Zealand Journal of Psychiatry, 53*(10), 989–999. https://doi.org/10.1177/0004867419851869

Hunter, E. C. M., Baker, D., Phillips, M. L., Sierra, M., & David, A. S. (2005). Cognitive-behaviour therapy for depersonalisation disorder: An open study. *Behaviour Research and Therapy, 43*(9), 1121–1130. https://doi.org/10.1016/j.brat.2004.08.003

International Society for the Study of Trauma and Dissociation. (2011). Guidelines for treating dissociative identity disorder in adults, third revision: Summary version. *Journal of Trauma & Dissociation, 12*(2), 188–212. https://doi.org/10.1080/15299732.2011.537248

James, B. (1994). *Handbook for treatment of attachment-trauma problems in children.* Lexington Books.

Janet, P. (1907). *The major symptoms of hysteria*. The Macmillan Company. https://doi.org/10.1037/10008-000

Jang, K. L., Paris, J., Zweig-Frank, H., & Livesley, W. J. (1998). Twin study of dissociative experience. *Journal of Nervous and Mental Disease, 186*(6), 345–351. https://doi.org/10.1097/00005053-199806000-00004

Jaycox, L. H., Foa, E. B., & Morral, A. R. (1998). Influence of emotional engagement and habituation on exposure therapy for PTSD. *Journal of Consulting and Clinical Psychology, 66*(1), 185–192. https://doi.org/10.1037/0022-006X.66.1.185

Jepsen, E. K. K., Langeland, W., & Heir, T. (2013). Impact of dissociation and interpersonal functioning on inpatient treatment for early sexually abused adults. *European Journal of Psychotraumatology, 4*(1), Article 22825. https://doi.org/10.3402/ejpt.v4i0.22825

Jepsen, E. K. K., Langeland, W., Sexton, H., & Heir, T. (2014). Inpatient treatment for early sexually abused adults: A naturalistic 12-month follow-up study. *Psychological Trauma: Theory, Research, Practice, and Policy, 6*(2), 142–151. https://doi.org/10.1037/a0031646

The John Praed Foundation. (n.d.). *TCOM tools*. https://praedfoundation.org/tcom/tcom-tools/the-child-and-adolecsent-needs-and-strengths-cans/

Johnson, J. G., Cohen, P., Kasen, S., & Brook, J. S. (2006). Dissociative disorders among adults in the community, impaired functioning, and Axis I and II comorbidity. *Journal of Psychiatric Research, 40*(2), 131–140. https://doi.org/10.1016/j.jpsychires.2005.03.003

Jones, C., Harvey, A. G., & Brewin, C. R. (2005). Traumatic brain injury, dissociation, and posttraumatic stress disorder in road traffic accident survivors. *Journal of Traumatic Stress, 18*(3), 181–191. https://doi.org/10.1002/jts.20031

Kamaradova, D., Prasko, J., Cerna, M., Grambal, A., Jelenova, D., Latalova, K., & Sigmundova, Z. (2013). 835—Prediction of outcome in complex treatment program for pharmacoresistant panic disorder patients [Abstract]. *European Psychiatry, 28*, 1. https://doi.org/10.1016/S0924-9338(13)76009-7

Kaser-Boyd, N., & Evans, F. B. (2008). Rorschach assessment of psychological trauma. In C. B. Gacono & F. B. Evans (Eds.), *The handbook of forensic Rorschach assessment* (pp. 255–277). Routledge/Taylor & Francis Group.

Kassin, S. M., Dror, I. E., & Kukucka, J. (2013). The forensic confirmation bias: Problems, perspectives, and proposed solutions. *Journal of Applied Research in Memory and Cognition, 2*(1), 42–52. https://doi.org/10.1016/j.jarmac.2013.01.001

Kate, M.-A., Jamieson, G., Dorahy, M. J., & Middleton, W. (2021). Measuring dissociative symptoms and experiences in an Australian college sample using a short version of the multidimensional inventory of dissociation. *Journal of Trauma & Dissociation, 22*(3), 265–287.

Kaysen, D. L., Bedard-Gilligan, M. A., & Saxon, A. J. (2019). Use of prolonged exposure and sertraline in the treatment of posttraumatic stress disorder for veterans.

JAMA Psychiatry, 76(2), 109–110. https://doi.org/10.1001/jamapsychiatry.2018.3410

Kearney, B. E., Corrigan, F. M., Frewen, P. A., Nevill, S., Harricharan, S., Andrews, K., Jetly, R., McKinnon, M. C., & Lanius, R. A. (2023). A randomized controlled trial of Deep Brain Reorienting: A neuroscientifically guided treatment for post-traumatic stress disorder. *European Journal of Psychotraumatology, 14*(2), 2240691. https://doi.org/10.1080/20008066.2023.2240691

Kearney, B. E., & Lanius, R. A. (2022). The brain–body disconnect: A somatic sensory basis for trauma-related disorders. *Frontiers in Neuroscience, 16,* Article 1015749. https://doi.org/10.3389/fnins.2022.1015749

Kessler, R. C., McLaughlin, K. A., Green, J. G., Gruber, M. J., Sampson, N. A., Zaslavsky, A. M., Aguilar-Gaxiola, S., Alhamzawi, A. O., Alonso, J., Angermeyer, M., Benjet, C., Bromet, E., Chatterji, S., de Girolamo, G., Demyttenaere, K., Fayyad, J., Florescu, S., Gal, G., Gureje, O., . . . Williams, D. R. (2010). Childhood adversities and adult psychopathology in the WHO World Mental Health Surveys. *The British Journal of Psychiatry, 197*(5), 378–385. https://doi.org/10.1192/bjp.bp.110.080499

Kessler, R. C., Warner, C. H., Ivany, C., Petukhova, M. V., Rose, S., Bromet, E. J., Brown, M., III, Cai, T., Colpe, L. J., Cox, K. L., Fullerton, C. S., Gilman, S. E., Gruber, M. J., Heeringa, S. G., Lewandowski-Romps, L., Li, J., Millikan-Bell, A. M., Naifeh, J. A., Nock, M. K., . . . the Army STARRS Collaborators. (2015). Predicting suicides after psychiatric hospitalization in US Army soldiers: The Army Study to Assess Risk and Resilience in Servicemembers (Army STARRS). *JAMA Psychiatry, 72*(1), 49–57. https://doi.org/10.1001/jamapsychiatry.2014.1754

Kezelman, C., & Stavropoulos, P. (2012). *Practice guidelines for treatment of complex trauma and trauma informed care and service delivery.* Blue Knot Foundation.

Kezelman, C., & Stavropoulos, P. (2019). *Practice guidelines for clinical treatment of complex trauma* (2nd ed.). Blue Knot Foundation.

Khantzian, E. J. (1985). The self-medication hypothesis of addictive disorders: Focus on heroin and cocaine dependence. *The American Journal of Psychiatry, 142*(11), 1259–1264. https://doi.org/10.1176/ajp.142.11.1259

King, C. D., Hill, S. B., Wolff, J. D., Bigony, C. E., Winternitz, S., Ressler, K. J., Kaufman, M. L., & Lebois, L. A. M. (2020). Childhood maltreatment type and severity predict depersonalization and derealization in treatment-seeking women with posttraumatic stress disorder. *Psychiatry Research, 292,* Article 113301. https://doi.org/10.1016/j.psychres.2020.113301

Kinsler, P. J. (2018). *Complex psychological trauma: The centrality of the relationship.* Routledge.

Kisiel, C. L., & Lyons, J. S. (2001). Dissociation as a mediator of psychopathology among sexually abused children and adolescents. *The American Journal of Psychiatry, 158*(7), 1034–1039. https://doi.org/10.1176/appi.ajp.158.7.1034

Kisiel, C. L., Torgersen, E., & McClelland, G. (2020). Understanding dissociation in relation to child trauma, mental health needs, and intensity of services in child welfare: A possible missing link. *Journal of Family Trauma,*

Child Custody & Child Development, 17(3), 189–218. https://doi.org/10.1080/26904586.2020.1816867

Kissee, J. L., Isaacson, L. J., & Miller-Perrin, C. (2014). An analysis of child maltreatment content in introductory psychology textbooks. *Journal of Aggression, Maltreatment & Trauma, 23*(3), 215–228. https://doi.org/10.1080/10926771.2014.878891

Kleindienst, N., Limberger, M. F., Ebner-Priemer, U. W., Keibel-Mauchnik, J., Dyer, A., Berger, M., Schmahl, C., & Bohus, M. (2011). Dissociation predicts poor response to dialectial behavioral therapy in female patients with borderline personality disorder. *Journal of Personality Disorders, 25*(4), 432–447. https://doi.org/10.1521/pedi.2011.25.4.432

Kleindienst, N., Priebe, K., Görg, N., Dyer, A., Steil, R., Lyssenko, L., Winter, D., Schmahl, C., & Bohus, M. (2016). State dissociation moderates response to dialectical behavior therapy for posttraumatic stress disorder in women with and without borderline personality disorder. *European Journal of Psychotraumatology, 7*(1), 30375. https://doi.org/10.3402/ejpt.v7.30375

Klotz Flitter, J. M., Elhai, J. D., & Gold, S. N. (2003). MMPI-2 *F* scale elevations in adult victims of child sexual abuse. *Journal of Traumatic Stress, 16*(3), 269–274. https://doi.org/10.1023/A:1023700208696

Kluemper, N. S., & Dalenberg, C. (2014). Is the dissociative adult suggestible? A test of the trauma and fantasy models of dissociation. *Journal of Trauma & Dissociation, 15*(4), 457–476. https://doi.org/10.1080/15299732.2014.880772

Kluft, R. P. (1982). Varieties of hypnotic interventions in the treatment of multiple personality. *The American Journal of Clinical Hypnosis, 24*(4), 230–240. https://doi.org/10.1080/00029157.1982.10403310

Kluft, R. P. (1984). Multiple personality in childhood. *The Psychiatric Clinics of North America, 7*(1), 121–134. https://doi.org/10.1016/S0193-953X(18)30785-8

Kluft, R. P. (1985). The natural history of multiple personality disorder. In R. P. Kluft (Ed.), *Childhood antecedents of multiple personality* (pp. 197–238). American Psychiatric Press.

Kluft, R. P. (1987a). First-rank symptoms as a diagnostic clue to multiple personality disorder. *The American Journal of Psychiatry, 144*(3), 293–298. https://doi.org/10.1176/ajp.144.3.293

Kluft, R. P. (1987b). The simulation and dissimulation of multiple personality disorder. *The American Journal of Clinical Hypnosis, 30*(2), 104–118. https://doi.org/10.1080/00029157.1987.10404170

Kluft, R. P. (1989). Playing for time: Temporizing techniques in the treatment of multiple personality disorder. *The American Journal of Clinical Hypnosis, 32*(2), 90–98. https://doi.org/10.1080/00029157.1989.10402806

Kluft, R. P. (1991). Clinical presentations of multiple personality disorder. *The Psychiatric Clinics of North America, 14*(3), 605–629. https://doi.org/10.1016/S0193-953X(18)30291-0

Kluft, R. P. (1992). Paradigm exhaustion and paradigm shift: Thinking through the therapeutic impasse. *Psychiatric Annals, 22*(10), 502–508. https://doi.org/10.3928/0048-5713-19921001-06

Kluft, R. P. (1993a). Basic principles in conducing the psychotherapy of multiple personality disorder. In R. P. Kluft & C. G. Fine (Eds.), *Clinical perspectives on multiple personality disorder* (pp. 19–50). American Psychiatric Press.

Kluft, R. P. (1993b). The initial stages of psychotherapy in the treatment of multiple personality disorder patients. *Dissociation, 6*(2–3), 145–161.

Kluft, R. P. (1994a). Clinical observations on the use of the CSDS Dimensions of Therapeutic Movement Instrument (DTMI). *Dissociation, 7*(4), 272–283.

Kluft, R. P. (1994b). Countertransference in the treatment of multiple personality disorder. In J. P. Wilson & J. D. Lindy (Eds.), *Countertransference in the treatment of PTSD* (pp. 122–150). Guilford Press.

Kluft, R. P. (1994c). Treatment trajectories in multiple personality disorder. *Dissociation, 7*, 63–76.

Kluft, R. P. (1997). On the treatment of traumatic memories of DID patients: Always? Never? Sometimes? Now? Later? *Dissociation, 10*(2), 80–90.

Kluft, R. P. (2007). Applications of innate affect theory to the understanding and treatment of dissociative identity disorder. In E. Vermetten, M. Dorahy, D. Spiegel, E. Vermetten, M. Dorahy, & D. Spiegel (Eds.), *Traumatic dissociation: Neurobiology and treatment* (pp. 301–316). American Psychiatric Publishing.

Kluft, R. P. (2013). *Shelter from the storm: Processing the traumatic memories of DID/DDNOS patients with the fractionated abreaction technique (a vademecum for the treatment of DID/DDNOS)*. CreateSpace Independent Publishing Platform.

Korgaonkar, M. S., Breukelaar, I. A., Felmingham, K., Williams, L. M., & Bryant, R. A. (2023). Association of neural connectome with early experiences of abuse in adults. *JAMA Network Open, 6*(1), Article e2253082. https://doi.org/10.1001/jamanetworkopen.2022.53082

Korzekwa, M. I., Dell, P. F., Links, P. S., Thabane, L., & Fougere, P. (2009). Dissociation in borderline personality disorder: A detailed look. *Journal of Trauma & Dissociation, 10*(3), 346–367. https://doi.org/10.1080/15299730902956838

Kritchevsky, M., Chang, J., & Squire, L. R. (2004). Functional amnesia: Clinical description and neuropsychological profile of 10 cases. *Learning & Memory, 11*(2), 213–226. https://doi.org/10.1101/lm.71404

Krüger, C. (2020). Culture, trauma and dissociation: A broadening perspective for our field. *Journal of Trauma & Dissociation, 21*(1), 1–13. https://doi.org/10.1080/15299732.2020.1675134

Krüger, C., & Fletcher, L. (2017). Predicting a dissociative disorder from type of childhood maltreatment and abuser–abused relational tie. *Journal of Trauma & Dissociation, 18*(3), 356–372. https://doi.org/10.1080/15299732.2017.1295420

Krüger, C., & Mace, C. J. (2002). Psychometric validation of the State Scale of Dissociation (SSD). *Psychology and Psychotherapy: Theory, Research and Practice, 75*(Pt. 1), 33–51. https://doi.org/10.1348/147608302169535

Kumar, S. A., Brand, B. L., & Courtois, C. A. (2022). The need for trauma training: Clinicians' reactions to training on complex trauma. *Psychological Trauma:*

Theory, Research, Practice, and Policy, 14(8), 1387–1394. https://doi.org/10.1037/tra0000515

Kundakçi, T., Şar, V., Kiziltan, E., Yargiç, I. L., & Tutkun, H. (2014). Reliability and validity of the Turkish version of the Structured Clinical Interview for *DSM-IV* Dissociative Disorders (SCID-D): A preliminary study. *Journal of Trauma & Dissociation, 15*(1), 24–34. https://doi.org/10.1080/15299732.2013.821434

Kutateladze, B. L., Andiloro, N. R., Johnson, B. D., & Spohn, C. C. (2014). Cumulative disadvantage: Examining racial and ethnic disparity in prosecution and sentencing. *Criminology, 52*(3), 514–551. https://doi.org/10.1111/1745-9125.12047

Lab, D. D., Feigenbaum, J. D., & De Silva, P. (2000). Mental health professionals' attitudes and practices towards male childhood sexual abuse. *Child Abuse & Neglect, 24*(3), 391–409. https://doi.org/10.1016/S0145-2134(99)00152-0

Laddis, A., & Dell, P. F. (2012). Dissociation and psychosis in dissociative identity disorder and schizophrenia. *Journal of Trauma & Dissociation, 13*(4), 397–413. https://doi.org/10.1080/15299732.2012.664967

Lahtinen, H.-M., Laitila, A., Korkman, J., & Ellonen, N. (2018). Children's disclosures of sexual abuse in a population-based sample. *Child Abuse & Neglect, 76*, 84–94. https://doi.org/10.1016/j.chiabu.2017.10.011

Lahtinen, H.-M., Laitila, A., Korkman, J., Ellonen, N., & Honkalampi, K. (2022). Children's disclosures of physical abuse in a population-based sample. *Journal of Interpersonal Violence, 37*(5–6), 2011–2036. https://doi.org/10.1177/0886260520934443

Langeland, W., Jepsen, E. K. K., Brand, B. L., Kleven, L., Loewenstein, R. J., Putnam, F. W., Schielke, H. J., Myrick, A., Lanius, R. A., & Heir, T. (2020). The economic burden of dissociative disorders: A qualitative systematic review of empirical studies. *Psychological Trauma: Theory, Research, Practice, and Policy, 12*(7), 730–738. https://doi.org/10.1037/tra0000556

Lanius, R. A., Boyd, J. E., McKinnon, M. C., Nicholson, A. A., Frewen, P., Vermetten, E., Jetly, R., & Spiegel, D. (2018). A review of the neurobiological basis of trauma-related dissociation and its relation to cannabinoid- and opioid-mediated stress response: A transdiagnostic, translational approach. *Current Psychiatry Reports, 20*(12), 118. https://doi.org/10.1007/s11920-018-0983-y

Lanius, R. A., Brand, B., Vermetten, E., Frewen, P. A., & Spiegel, D. (2012). The dissociative subtype of posttraumatic stress disorder: Rationale, clinical and neurobiological evidence, and implications. *Depression and Anxiety, 29*(8), 701–708. https://doi.org/10.1002/da.21889

Lanius, R. A., Terpou, B. A., & McKinnon, M. C. (2020). The sense of self in the aftermath of trauma: Lessons from the default mode network in post-traumatic stress disorder. *European Journal of Psychotraumatology, 11*(1), Article 1807703. https://doi.org/10.1080/20008198.2020.1807703

Lanius, R. A., Vermetten, E., Loewenstein, R. J., Brand, B., Schmahl, C., Bremner, J. D., & Spiegel, D. (2010). Emotion modulation in PTSD: Clinical and neurobiological evidence for a dissociative subtype. *The American Journal of Psychiatry, 167*(6), 640–647. https://doi.org/10.1176/appi.ajp.2009. 09081168

Lanius, R. A., Wolf, E. J., Miller, M. W., Frewen, P. A., Vermetten, E., Brand, B. L., & Spiegel, D. (2014). The dissociative subtype of PTSD. In M. J. Friedman, T. M. Keane, & P. A. Resick (Eds.), *Handbook of PTSD: Science and practice* (2nd ed., pp. 234–250). Guilford Press.

Lanius, U. F., Paulsen, S. L., & Corrigan, F. M. (Eds.). (2014). *Neurobiology and treatment of traumatic dissociation: Toward an embodied self.* Springer Publishing Company. https://doi.org/10.1891/9780826106322

Leavitt, F. (1997). False attribution of suggestibility to explain recovered memory of childhood sexual abuse following extended amnesia. *Child Abuse & Neglect, 21*(3), 265–272. https://doi.org/10.1016/S0145-2134(96)00171-8

Leavitt, F. (1999). Dissociative experiences scale taxon and measurement of dissociative pathology: Does the taxon add to an understanding of dissociation and its associated pathologies? *Journal of Clinical Psychology in Medical Settings, 6*(4), 427–440. https://doi.org/10.1023/A:1026275916184

Leavitt, F. (2001). MMPI profile characteristics of women with varying levels of normal dissociation. *Journal of Clinical Psychology, 57*(12), 1469–1477. https://doi.org/10.1002/jclp.1110

Lebois, L. A. M., Kumar, P., Palermo, C. A., Lambros, A. M., O'Connor, L., Wolff, J. D., Baker, J. T., Gruber, S. A., Lewis-Schroeder, N., Ressler, K. J., Robinson, M. A., Winternitz, S., Nickerson, L. D., & Kaufman, M. L. (2022). Deconstructing dissociation: A triple network model of trauma-related dissociation and its subtypes. *Neuropsychopharmacology, 47*(13), 2261–2270. https://doi.org/10.1038/s41386-022-01468-1

Lebois, L. A. M., Li, M., Baker, J. T., Wolff, J. D., Wang, D., Lambros, A. M., Grinspoon, E., Winternitz, S., Ren, J., Gönenç, A., Gruber, S. A., Ressler, K. J., Liu, H., & Kaufman, M. L. (2021). Large-scale functional brain network architecture changes associated with trauma-related dissociation. *The American Journal of Psychiatry, 178*(2), 165–173. https://doi.org/10.1176/appi.ajp.2020. 19060647

Lebois, L. A. M., Palermo, C. A., Scheuer, L. S., Lebois, E. P., Winternitz, S. R., Germine, L., & Kaufman, M. L. (2020). Higher integration scores are associated with facial emotion perception differences in dissociative identity disorder. *Journal of Psychiatric Research, 123*, 164–170. https://doi.org/10.1016/j.jpsychires.2020.02.007

Lebois, L. A. M., Wolff, J. D., Hill, S. B., Bigony, C. E., Winternitz, S., Ressler, K. J., & Kaufman, M. L. (2019). Preliminary evidence of a missing self bias in face perception for individuals with dissociative identity disorder. *Journal of Trauma & Dissociation, 20*(2), 140–164. https://doi.org/10.1080/15299732. 2018.1547807

Leonard, D., Brann, S., & Tiller, J. (2005). Dissociative disorders: Pathways to diagnosis, clinician attitudes and their impact. *The Australian and New*

Zealand Journal of Psychiatry, *39*(10), 940–946. https://doi.org/10.1080/ j.1440-1614.2005.01700.x

Lewis, D. O., Pincus, J. H., Bard, B., Richardson, E., Prichep, L. S., Feldman, M., & Yeager, C. (1988). Neuropsychiatric, psychoeducational, and family characteristics of 14 juveniles condemned to death in the United States. *The American Journal of Psychiatry*, *145*(5), 584–589. https://doi.org/10.1176/ ajp.145.5.584

Lewis, D. O., Pincus, J. H., Feldman, M., Jackson, L., & Bard, B. (1986). Psychiatric, neurological, and psychoeducational characteristics of 15 death row inmates in the United States. *The American Journal of Psychiatry*, *143*(7), 838–845. https://doi.org/10.1176/ajp.143.7.838

Lewis, D. O., Yeager, C. A., Blake, P., Bard, B., & Strenziok, M. (2004). Ethics questions raised by the neuropsychiatric, neuropsychological, educational, developmental, and family characteristics of 18 juveniles awaiting execution in Texas. *The Journal of the American Academy of Psychiatry and the Law*, *32*(4), 408–429.

Lewis, D. O., Yeager, C. A., Swica, Y., Pincus, J. H., & Lewis, M. (1997). Objective documentation of child abuse and dissociation in 12 murderers with dissociative identity disorder. *The American Journal of Psychiatry*, *154*(12), 1703–1710. https://doi.org/10.1176/ajp.154.12.1703

Lewis, M., & Rudolph, K. D. (Eds.). (2014). *Handbook of developmental psychopathology* (3rd ed.). Springer. https://doi.org/10.1007/978-1-4614-9608-3

Lewis-Fernández, R., Martínez-Taboas, A., Şar, V., Patel, S., & Boatin, A. (2007). The cross-cultural assessment of dissociation. In J. P. Wilson & C. S.-K. Tang (Eds.), *Cross-cultural assessment of psychological trauma and PTSD* (pp. 279–317). Springer Science + Business Media. https://doi.org/10.1007/978-0-387- 70990-1_12

Lilienfeld, S. O. (2007). Psychological treatments that cause harm. *Perspectives on Psychological Science*, *2*(1), 53–70. https://doi.org/10.1111/j.1745-6916. 2007.00029.x

Liotti, G. (1992). Disorganized/disoriented attachment in the etiology of the dissociative disorders. *Dissociation: Progress in the Dissociative Disorders*, *5*(4), 196–204.

Liotti, G. (2006). A model of dissociation based on attachment theory and research. *Journal of Trauma & Dissociation*, *7*(4), 55–73. https://doi.org/ 10.1300/J229v07n04_04

Lloyd, C. S., Lanius, R. A., Brown, M. F., Neufeld, R. J., Frewen, P. A., & McKinnon, M. C. (2019). Assessing post-traumatic tonic immobility responses: The Scale for Tonic Immobility Ocurring Post-trauma. *Chronic Stress*, *3*, 2470547018822492. https://doi.org/10.1177/2470547018822492

Lloyd, M. (2016). Reducing the cost of dissociative identity disorder: Measuring the effectiveness of specialized treatment by frequency of contacts with mental health services. *Journal of Trauma & Dissociation*, *17*(3), 362–370. https://doi.org/10.1080/15299732.2015.1108947

Loewenstein, R. J. (Ed.). (1991a). Multiple personality disorder. *Psychiatric Clinics of North America, 14*(3). W. B. Saunders.

Loewenstein, R. J. (1991b). An office mental status examination for complex chronic dissociative symptoms and multiple personality disorder. *The Psychiatric Clinics of North America, 14*(3), 567–604. https://doi.org/10.1016/S0193-953X(18)30290-9

Loewenstein, R. J. (1993). Posttraumatic and dissociative aspects of transference and countertransference in the treatment of multiple personality disorder. In R. P. Kluft & C. G. Fine (Eds.), *Clinical perspectives on multiple personality disorder* (pp. 51–85). American Psychiatric Press.

Loewenstein, R. J. (2005). Psychopharmacologic treatments for dissociative identity disorder. *Psychiatric Annals, 35*(8), 666–673. https://doi.org/10.3928/00485713-20050801-08

Loewenstein, R. J. (2006). DID 101: A hands-on clinical guide to the stabilization phase of dissociative identity disorder treatment. *The Psychiatric Clinics of North America, 29*(1), 305–332, xii. https://doi.org/10.1016/j.psc.2005.10.005

Loewenstein, R. J. (2016, October). *Rational and irrational psychopharmacology for complex trauma and dissociative disorders.* Annual Conference of the International Society for the Study of Trauma and Dissociation, Louisville, KY, United States.

Loewenstein, R. J. (2018). Dissociation debates: Everything you know is wrong. *Dialogues in Clinical Neuroscience, 20*(3), 229–242. https://doi.org/10.31887/DCNS.2018.20.3/rloewenstein

Loewenstein, R. J. (2020). Firebug! Dissociative identity disorder? Malingering? Or . . .? An intensive case study of an arsonist. *Psychological Injury and Law, 13*(2), 187–224. https://doi.org/10.1007/s12207-020-09377-8

Loewenstein, R. J. (2022). Conceptual foundations for long-term psychotherapy of dissociative identity. In M. Dorahy, S. Gold, & J. A. O'Neill (Eds.), *Dissociation and the dissociative disorders: Past, present, future* (2nd ed., pp. 770–789). Routledge.

Loewenstein, R. J., Frewen, P. A., & Lewis-Fernández, R. (2017). Dissociative disorders. In B. J. Sadock, V. A. Sadock, & P. Ruiz (Eds.), *Kaplan & Sadock's comprehensive textbook of psychiatry* (10th ed., Vol. 1, pp. 1866–1952). Wolters Kluwer/Lippincott Williams & Wilkens.

Loewenstein, R. J., Hamilton, J., Alagna, S., Reid, N., & deVries, M. (1987). Experiential sampling in the study of multiple personality disorder. *The American Journal of Psychiatry, 144*(1), 19–24. https://doi.org/10.1176/ajp.144.1.19

Loewenstein, R. J., Lewis-Fernandez, R., & Frewen, P. (in press). Dissociative disorders. In B. J. Sadock, V. A. Sadock, & P. Ruiz (Eds.), *Kaplan & Sadock's comprehensive textbook of psychiatry* (11th ed.). Wolters Kluwer/Lippincott.

Loewenstein, R. J., & Putnam, F. W. (1990). The clinical phenomenology of males with multiple personality disorder: A report of 21 cases. *Dissociation, 3*(3), 135–143.

Loewenstein, R. J., & Putnam, F. W. (2023). Discrete behavioral states theory. In M. Dorahy, S. Gold, & J. A. O'Neill (Eds.), *Dissociation and the dissociative disorders: Past, present, future* (2nd ed., pp. 281–296). Routledge.

Loewenstein, R. J., Vermetten, E., Wilson, K., & Bremner, J. D. (2002, November 11). *Suggestibility in dissociative identity disorder: Relationship to factitious and "iatrogenic" DID*. 19th International Fall Conference of the ISSTD: The Complexities of Dissociation: Trauma, Adaptation and Creativity, Baltimore, MD, United States.

Longden, E., Branitsky, A., Moskowitz, A., Berry, K., Bucci, S., & Varese, F. (2020). The relationship between dissociation and symptoms of psychosis: A meta-analysis. *Schizophrenia Bulletin, 46*(5), 1104–1113. https://doi.org/10.1093/schbul/sbaa037

Longden, E., Madill, A., & Waterman, M. G. (2012). Dissociation, trauma, and the role of lived experience: Toward a new conceptualization of voice hearing. *Psychological Bulletin, 138*(1), 28–76. https://doi.org/10.1037/a0025995

Lui, P. P., & Quezada, L. (2019). Associations between microaggression and adjustment outcomes: A meta-analytic and narrative review. *Psychological Bulletin, 145*(1), 45–78. https://doi.org/10.1037/bul0000172

Luxenberg, T., Spinazzola, J., & van der Kolk, B. (2001). Complex trauma and disorders of extreme stress (DESNOS) diagnosis, part one: Assessment. *Directions in Psychiatry, 21*(26), 373–393.

Lynn, S. J., Lilienfeld, S. O., Merckelbach, H., Giesbrecht, T., McNally, R. J., Loftus, E. F., Bruck, M., Garry, M., & Malaktaris, A. (2014). The trauma model of dissociation: Inconvenient truths and stubborn fictions. Comment on Dalenberg et al. (2012). *Psychological Bulletin, 140*(3), 896–910. https://doi.org/10.1037/a0035570

Lynn, S. J., Lilienfeld, S. O., Merckelbach, H., Giesbrecht, T., & van der Kloet, D. (2012). Dissociation and dissociative disorders: Challenging conventional wisdom. *Current Directions in Psychological Science, 21*(1), 48–53. https://doi.org/10.1177/0963721411429457

Lyons, J. S., & Fernando, A. D. (2021). *Child and Adolescent Needs and Strengths: Standard CANS comprehensive 3.0, 2021 reference guide*. The Praed Foundation.

Lyons, J. S., Gawron, T., & Kisiel, C. L. (2005). *Child and Adolescent Needs and Strengths: Comprehensive assessment for Illinois Department of Children and Family Services manual*. The Praed Foundation.

Lyons, J. S., Weiner, D. A., & Lyons, M. B. (2004). Measurement as communication in outcomes management: The Child and Adolescent Needs and Strengths (CANS). In M. E. Maruish (Ed.), *The use of psychological testing for treatment planning and outcomes assessment: Instruments for children and adolescents* (3rd ed., Vol. 2, pp. 461–476). Lawrence Erlbaum Associates Publishers.

Lyons-Ruth, K. (2008). Contributions of the mother–infant relationship to dissociative, borderline, and conduct symptoms in young adulthood. *Infant Mental Health Journal, 29*(3), 203–218. https://doi.org/10.1002/imhj.20173

Lyons-Ruth, K., Dutra, L., Schuder, M. R., & Bianchi, I. (2006). From infant attachment disorganization to adult dissociation: Relational adaptations or traumatic experiences? *The Psychiatric Clinics of North America, 29*(1), 63–86, viii. https://doi.org/10.1016/j.psc.2005.10.011

Lyssenko, L., Schmahl, C., Bockhacker, L., Vonderlin, R., Bohus, M., & Kleindienst, N. (2018). Dissociation in psychiatric disorders: A meta-analysis of studies using the Dissociative Experiences Scale. *The American Journal of Psychiatry, 175*(1), 37–46. https://doi.org/10.1176/appi.ajp.2017.17010025

Maaranen, P., Tanskanen, A., Hintikka, J., Honkalampi, K., Haatainen, K., Koivumaa-Honkanen, H., & Viinamäki, H. (2008). The course of dissociation in the general population: A 3-year follow-up study. *Comprehensive Psychiatry, 49*(3), 269–274. https://doi.org/10.1016/j.comppsych.2007.04.010

Maaranen, P., Tanskanen, A., Honkalampi, K., Haatainen, K., Hintikka, J., & Viinamäki, H. (2005). Factors associated with pathological dissociation in the general population. *The Australian and New Zealand Journal of Psychiatry, 39*(5), 387–394. https://doi.org/10.1080/j.1440-1614.2005.01586.x

Macia, K. S., Carlson, E. B., Palmieri, P. A., Smith, S. R., Anglin, D. M., Ghosh Ippen, C., Lieberman, A. F., Wong, E. C., Schell, T. L., & Waelde, L. C. (2022). Development of a brief version of the Dissociative Symptoms Scale and the reliability and validity of DSS-B Scores in diverse clinical and community samples. *Assessment*. Advance online publication. https://doi.org/10.1177/10731911221133317

Malmo, C., & Laidlaw, T. S. (2010). Symptoms of trauma and traumatic memory retrieval in adult survivors of childhood sexual abuse. *Journal of Trauma & Dissociation, 11*(1), 22–43. https://doi.org/10.1080/15299730903318467

Mansfield, A. J., Kaufman, J. S., Marshall, S. W., Gaynes, B. N., Morrissey, J. P., & Engel, C. C. (2010). Deployment and the use of mental health services among U.S. Army wives. *The New England Journal of Medicine, 362*(2), 101–109. https://doi.org/10.1056/NEJMoa0900177

Mantovani, A., Simeon, D., Urban, N., Bulow, P., Allart, A., & Lisanby, S. (2011). Temporoparietal junction stimulation in the treatment of depersonalization disorder. *Psychiatry Research, 186*(1), 138–140. https://doi.org/10.1016/j.psychres.2010.08.022

Marmar, C. R., Weiss, D. S., & Metzler, T. J. (1997). The Peritraumatic Dissociative Experiences Questionnaire. In J. P. Wilson & T. M. Keane (Eds.), *Assessing psychological trauma and PTSD* (pp. 412–428). Guilford Press.

Martínez-Taboas, A., Shrout, P. E., Canino, G., Chavez, L. M., Ramírez, R., Bravo, M., Bauermeister, J. J., & Ribera, J. C. (2004). The psychometric properties of a shortened version of the Spanish Adolescent Dissociative Experiences Scale. *Journal of Trauma & Dissociation, 5*(4), 33–54. https://doi.org/10.1300/J229v05n04_03

Mayou, R. A., Ehlers, A., & Bryant, B. (2002). Posttraumatic stress disorder after motor vehicle accidents: 3-year follow-up of a prospective longitudinal study. *Behaviour Research and Therapy, 40*(6), 665–675. https://doi.org/10.1016/S0005-7967(01)00069-9

McElroy, L. P. (1992). Early indicators of pathological dissociation in sexually abused children. *Child Abuse & Neglect, 16*(6), 833–846. https://doi.org/10.1016/0145-2134(92)90085-6

McFarlane, A. (2010). Synopsis. In R. Lanius, E. Vermetten, & C. Pain (Eds.), *The impact of early life trauma on health and disease: The hidden epidemic* (pp. 43–47). Cambridge University Press. https://doi.org/10.1017/CBO9780511777042.006

McHugh, P. R., & Putnam, F. W. (1995). Resolved: Multiple personality disorder is an individually and socially created artifact. *Journal of the American Academy of Child & Adolescent Psychiatry, 34*(7), 957–962. https://doi.org/10.1097/00004583-199507000-00020

McKinnon, M. C., Boyd, J. E., Frewen, P. A., Lanius, U. F., Jetly, R., Richardson, J. D., & Lanius, R. A. (2016). A review of the relation between dissociation, memory, executive functioning and social cognition in military members and civilians with neuropsychiatric conditions. *Neuropsychologia, 90*, 210–234. https://doi.org/10.1016/j.neuropsychologia.2016.07.017

Mendelsohn, M., Herman, J. L., Schatzow, E., Coco, M., Kallivayalil, D., & Levitan, J. (2011). *The trauma recovery group: A guide for practitioners.* Guilford Press.

Mendez, N., Martinez-Taboas, A., & Pedrosa, O. (2000). Experiences, beliefs and attitudes of Puerto Rican psychologists toward dissociative identity disorder. *Ciencias de la Conducta, 15*, 69–84.

Merckelbach, H., Boskovic, I., Pesy, D., Dalsklev, M., & Lynn, S. J. (2017). Symptom overreporting and dissociative experiences: A qualitative review. *Consciousness and Cognition: An International Journal, 49*, 132–144. https://doi.org/10.1016/j.concog.2017.01.007

Merckelbach, H., Giesbrecht, T., van Heugten-van der Kloet, D., de Jong, J., Meyer, T., & Rietman, K. (2015). The overlap between dissociative symptoms and symptom over-reporting. *European Journal of Psychiatry, 29*(3), 165–172. https://doi.org/10.4321/S0213-61632015000300001

Merckelbach, H., Horselenberg, R., & Muris, P. (2001). The Creative Experiences Questionnaire (CEQ): A brief self-report measure of fantasy proneness. *Personality and Individual Differences, 31*(6), 987–995. https://doi.org/10.1016/S0191-8869(00)00201-4

Merckelbach, H., & Patihis, L. (2018). Why "trauma-related dissociation" is a misnomer in courts: A critical analysis of Brand et al. (2017a, b). *Psychological Injury and Law, 11*(4), 370–376. https://doi.org/10.1007/s12207-018-9328-8

Meyer, G. J., Viglione, D. J., & Mihura, J. L. (2017). Psychometric foundations of the Rorschach Performance Assessment System (R-PAS). In R. E. Erard & F. B. Evans (Eds.), *The Rorschach in multimethod forensic assessment: Conceptual foundations and practical applications* (pp. 23–91). Routledge/Taylor & Francis Group.

Michelson, L., June, K., Vives, A., Testa, S., & Marchione, N. (1998). The role of trauma and dissociation in cognitive-behavioral psychotherapy outcome and maintenance for panic disorder with agoraphobia. *Behaviour Research and Therapy, 36*(11), 1011–1050. https://doi.org/10.1016/S0005-7967(98) 00073-4

Miller, H. A. (2001). *M-FAST Miller Forensic Assessment of Symptoms Test professional manual.* Psychological Assessment Resources.

Miller, T. J., McGlashan, T. H., Rosen, J. L., Cadenhead, K., Cannon, T., Ventura, J., McFarlane, W., Perkins, D. O., Pearlson, G. D., & Woods, S. W. (2003). Prodromal assessment with the structured interview for prodromal syndromes and the scale of prodromal symptoms: Predictive validity, interrater reliability, and training to reliability. *Schizophrenia Bulletin, 29*(4), 703–715. https://doi.org/10.1093/oxfordjournals.schbul.a007040

Millon, T. (1997). *The Millon inventories: Clinical and personality assessment.* Guilford Press.

Monnier, J., Elhai, J. D., Frueh, B. C., Sauvageot, J. A., & Magruder, K. M. (2002). Replication and expansion of findings related to racial differences in veterans with combat-related PTSD. *Depression and Anxiety, 16*(2), 64–70. https://doi.org/10.1002/da.10060

Morales, T. I., & Viglione, D. J. (2022). Using quantitative and qualitative Rorschach data within a multi-method, forensic assessment of dissociative posttraumatic stress disorder. *Psychological Injury and Law.* Advance online publication. https://doi.org/10.1007/s12207-022-09453-1

Morey, L. C. (1991). *Personality Assessment Inventory: Professional Manual.* Psychological Assessment Resources.

Moskowitz, A. K. (2004). Dissociative pathways to homicide: Clinical and forensic implications. *Journal of Trauma & Dissociation, 5*(3), 5–32. https://doi.org/10.1300/J229v05n03_02

Moskowitz, A., & Corstens, D. (2007). Auditory hallucinations: Psychotic symptom or dissociative experience? *Journal of Psychological Trauma, 6*(2–3), 35–63. https://doi.org/10.1300/J513v06n02_04

Mueller, C., Moergeli, H., Assaloni, H., Schneider, R., & Rufer, M. (2007). Dissociative disorders among chronic and severely impaired psychiatric outpatients. *Psychopathology, 40*(6), 470–471. https://doi.org/10.1159/000108129

Mueller-Pfeiffer, C., Rufibach, K., Perron, N., Wyss, D., Kuenzler, C., Prezewowsky, C., Pitman, R. K., & Rufer, M. (2012). Global functioning and disability in dissociative disorders. *Psychiatry Research, 200*(2–3), 475–481. https://doi.org/10.1016/j.psychres.2012.04.028

Mueller-Pfeiffer, C., Rufibach, K., Wyss, D., Perron, N., Pitman, R. K., & Rufer, M. (2013). Screening for dissociative disorders in psychiatric out- and day care-patients. *Journal of Psychopathology and Behavioral Assessment, 35*(4), 592–602. https://doi.org/10.1007/s10862-013-9367-0

Mulder, R. T., Beautrais, A. L., Joyce, P. R., & Fergusson, D. M. (1998). Relationship between dissociation, childhood sexual abuse, childhood physical abuse, and mental illness in a general population sample. *The American Journal of*

Psychiatry, 155(6), 806–811. https://ajp.psychiatryonline.org/cgi/content/abstract/155/6/806

Murray, H. A. (1943). *Thematic Apperception Test: Manual.* Harvard University Press.

Murray, J., Ehlers, A., & Mayou, R. A. (2002). Dissociation and post-traumatic stress disorder: Two prospective studies of road traffic accident survivors. *The British Journal of Psychiatry, 180*(4), 363–368. https://doi.org/10.1192/bjp.180.4.363

Mychailyszyn, M. P., Brand, B. L., Webermann, A. R., Şar, V., & Draijer, N. (2021). Differentiating dissociative from non-dissociative disorders: A meta-analysis of the Structured Clinical Interview for *DSM* Dissociative Disorders (SCID-D). *Journal of Trauma & Dissociation, 22*(1), 19–34.

Myrick, A. C., Brand, B. L., McNary, S. W., Classen, C. C., Lanius, R., Loewenstein, R. J., Pain, C., & Putnam, F. W. (2012). An exploration of young adults' progress in treatment for dissociative disorder. *Journal of Trauma & Dissociation, 13*(5), 582–595. https://doi.org/10.1080/15299732.2012.694841

Myrick, A. C., Brand, B. L., & Putnam, F. W. (2013). For better or worse: The role of revictimization and stress in the course of treatment for dissociative disorders. *Journal of Trauma & Dissociation, 14*(4), 375–389. https://doi.org/10.1080/15299732.2012.736931

Myrick, A. C., Webermann, A. R., Langeland, W., Putnam, F. W., & Brand, B. L. (2017). Treatment of dissociative disorders and reported changes in inpatient and outpatient cost estimates. *European Journal of Psychotraumatology, 8*(1), 1375829. https://doi.org/10.1080/20008198.2017.1375829

Myrick, A. C., Webermann, A. R., Loewenstein, R. J., Lanius, R., Putnam, F. W., & Brand, B. L. (2017). Six-year follow-up of the treatment of patients with dissociative disorders study. *European Journal of Psychotraumatology, 8*(1), 1344080. https://doi.org/10.1080/20008198.2017.1344080

Nadal, K. L. (2018). *Microaggressions and traumatic stress: Theory, research, and clinical treatment.* American Psychological Association. https://doi.org/10.1037/0000073-000

Narang, D. S., & Contreras, J. M. (2005). The relationships of dissociation and affective family environment with the intergenerational cycle of child abuse. *Child Abuse & Neglect, 29*(6), 683–699. https://doi.org/10.1016/j.chiabu.2004.11.003

Neal, T. M. S., Lienert, P., Denne, E., & Singh, J. P. (2022). A general model of cognitive bias in human judgment and systematic review specific to forensic mental health. *Law and Human Behavior, 46*(2), 99–120. https://doi.org/10.1037/lhb0000482

Nemeroff, C. B., Heim, C. M., Thase, M. E., Klein, D. N., Rush, A. J., Schatzberg, A. F., Ninan, P. T., McCullough, J. P., Jr., Weiss, P. M., Dunner, D. L., Rothbaum, B. O., Kornstein, S., Keitner, G., & Keller, M. B. (2003). Differential responses to psychotherapy versus pharmacotherapy in patients with chronic forms of major depression and childhood trauma. *Proceedings of the National Academy of Sciences of the United States of America, 100*(24), 14293–14296. https://doi.org/10.1073/pnas.2336126100

Nester, M. S., Boi, C., Brand, B. L., & Schielke, H. J. (2022). The reasons dissociative disorder patients self-injure. *European Journal of Psychotraumatology, 13*(1), 2026738. https://doi.org/10.1080/20008198.2022.2026738

Nester, M. S., Brand, B. L., Schielke, H. J., & Kumar, S. (2022). An examination of the relations between emotion dysregulation, dissociation, and self-injury among dissociative disorder patients. *European Journal of Psychotraumatology, 13*(1), Article 2031592. https://doi.org/10.1080/20008198.2022.2031592

Nester, M. S., Hawkins, S. L., & Brand, B. L. (2022). Barriers to accessing and continuing mental health treatment among individuals with dissociative symptoms. *European Journal of Psychotraumatology, 13*(1), Article 2031594. https://doi.org/10.1080/20008198.2022.2031594

Nester, M. S., Pierorazio, N. A., Shandler, G., & Brand, B. L. (2023). Characteristics, methods, and functions of non-suicidal self-injury among highly dissociative individuals. *Journal of Trauma & Dissociation, 24*(3), 333–347. https://doi.org/10.1080/15299732.2023.2181475

Nester, M. S., Schielke, H. J., Brand, B. L., & Loewenstein, R. J. (2021). Dissociative identity disorder: Diagnostic accuracy and *DSM-5* criteria change implications. *Journal of Trauma & Dissociation*, 1–13. Advance online publication. https://pubmed.ncbi.nlm.nih.gov/34661505/

Newman, E., Briere, J., & Kirlic, N. (2012). Clinical assessment as a form of listening and intervention. In R. A. McMackin, E. Newman, J. M. Fogler, & T. M. Keane (Eds.), *Trauma therapy in context: The science and craft of evidence-based practice* (pp. 51–71). American Psychological Association. https://doi.org/10.1037/13746-003

Newman, E., Walker, E. A., & Gefland, A. (1999). Assessing the ethical costs and benefits of trauma-focused research. *General Hospital Psychiatry, 21*(3), 187–196. https://doi.org/10.1016/S0163-8343(99)00011-0

Nijenhuis, E. R. S., Spinhoven, P., Van Dyck, R., Van der Hart, O., & Vanderlinden, J. (1996). The development and psychometric characteristics of the Somatoform Dissociation Questionnaire (SDQ-20). *Journal of Nervous and Mental Disease, 184*(11), 688–694. https://doi.org/10.1097/00005053-199611000-00006

Nijenhuis, E. R. S., Spinhoven, P., van Dyck, R., van der Hart, O., & Vanderlinden, J. (1997). The development of the Somatoform Dissociation Questionnaire (SDQ-5) as a screening instrument for dissociative disorders. *Acta Psychiatrica Scandinavica, 96*(5), 311–318. https://doi.org/10.1111/j.1600-0447.1997.tb09922.x

Nijenhuis, E. R. S., Spinhoven, P., van Dyck, R., van der Hart, O., & Vanderlinden, J. (1998). Psychometric characteristics of the somatoform dissociation questionnaire: A replication study. *Psychotherapy and Psychosomatics, 67*(1), 17–23. https://doi.org/10.1159/000012254

Nijenhuis, E. R. S., van der Hart, O., & Steele, K. (2002). The emerging psychobiology of trauma-related dissociation and dissociative disorders. In H. D'Haenen, J. A. den Boer, & P. Willner (Eds.), *Biological psychiatry* (pp. 1079–1098). John Wiley & Sons.

Nijenhuis, E. R. S., Vanderlinden, J., & Spinhoven, P. (1998). Animal defensive reactions as a model for trauma-induced dissociative reactions. *Journal of Traumatic Stress, 11*(2), 243–260. https://doi.org/10.1023/A:1024447003022

Nilsson, D., Lejonclou, A., Svedin, C. G., Jonsson, M., & Holmqvist, R. (2015). Somatoform dissociation among Swedish adolescents and young adults: The psychometric properties of the Swedish versions of the SDQ-20 and SDQ-5. *Nordic Journal of Psychiatry, 69*(2), 152–160. https://doi.org/10.3109/080 39488.2014.949851

Nilsson, D., & Svedin, C. G. (2006). Dissociation among Swedish adolescents and the connection to trauma: An evaluation of the Swedish version of Adolescent Dissociative Experience Scale. *Journal of Nervous and Mental Disease, 194*(9), 684–689. https://doi.org/10.1097/01.nmd.0000235774.08690.dc

Noll, J. G., Trickett, P. K., Harris, W. W., & Putnam, F. W. (2009). The cumulative burden borne by offspring whose mothers were sexually abused as children: Descriptive results from a multigenerational study. *Journal of Interpersonal Violence, 24*(3), 424–449. https://doi.org/10.1177/0886260508317194

Ogawa, J. R., Sroufe, L. A., Weinfield, N. S., Carlson, E. A., & Egeland, B. (1997). Development and the fragmented self: Longitudinal study of dissociative symptomatology in a nonclinical sample. *Development and Psychopathology, 9*(4), 855–879. https://doi.org/10.1017/S0954579497001478

Ogden, P., Minton, K., & Pain, C. (2006). *Trauma and the body: A sensorimotor approach to psychotherapy*. W. W. Norton & Co.

Ortiz, R., Gilgoff, R., & Burke Harris, N. (2022). Adverse childhood experiences, toxic stress, and trauma-informed neurology. *JAMA Neurology, 79*(6), 539–540. https://doi.org/10.1001/jamaneurol.2022.0769

Ozer, E. J., Best, S. R., Lipsey, T. L., & Weiss, D. S. (2003). Predictors of posttraumatic stress disorder and symptoms in adults: A meta-analysis. *Psychological Bulletin, 129*(1), 52–73. https://doi.org/10.1037/0033-2909.129.1.52

Ozer, E. J., Best, S. R., Lipsey, T. L., & Weiss, D. S. (2008). Predictors of posttraumatic stress disorder and symptoms in adults: A meta-analysis. *Psychological Trauma: Theory, Research, Practice, and Policy, S*(1), 3–36. https://doi.org/10.1037/1942-9681.S.1.3

Palermo, C. A., & Brand, B. L. (2019). Can the Trauma Symptom Inventory–2 distinguish coached simulators from dissociative disorder patients? *Psychological Trauma: Theory, Research, Practice, and Policy, 11*(5), 477–485. https://doi.org/10.1037/tra0000382

Paris, J. (2019). Dissociative identity disorder: Validity and use in the criminal justice system. *BJPsych Advances, 25*(5), 287–293. https://doi.org/10.1192/bja.2019.12

Patel, H., O'Connor, C., Andrews, K., Amlung, M., Lanius, R., & McKinnon, M. C. (2022). Dissociative symptomatology mediates the relation between posttraumatic stress disorder severity and alcohol-related problems. *Alcoholism, Clinical and Experimental Research, 46*(2), 289–299. https://doi.org/10.1111/acer.14764

Patihis, L., & Lynn, S. J. (2017). Psychometric comparison of Dissociative Experiences Scales II and C: A weak trauma–dissociation link. *Applied Cognitive Psychology, 31*(4), 392–403. https://doi.org/10.1002/acp.3337

Peltonen, K., Kangaslampi, S., Saranpää, J., Qouta, S., & Punamäki, R.-L. (2017). Peritraumatic dissociation predicts posttraumatic stress disorder symptoms via dysfunctional trauma-related memory among war-affected children. *European Journal of Psychotraumatology, 8*(Suppl. 3), Article 1375828. https://doi.org/10.1080/20008198.2017.1375828

People v. Henderson, Teresa Marie [CR168054] (Superior Court of Napa—Criminal 2015).

Perniciaro, L. A. (2014). *The influence of skepticism and clinical experience on the detection of dissociative identity disorder by mental health clinicians* [Doctoral dissertation, Massachusetts School of Professional Psychology]. ProQuest Dissertations and Theses Global. https://www.proquest.com/openview/02d0968fb8a5c77fdb74779c2b200341/1?pq-origsite=gscholar&cbl=18750

Perry, B. D., Pollard, R. A., Blakley, T. L., Baker, W. L., & Vigilante, D. (1995). Childhood trauma, the neurobiology of adaptation, and "use-dependent" development of the brain: How "states" become "traits." *Infant Mental Health Journal, 16*(4), 271–291. https://doi.org/10.1002/1097-0355(199524)16:4<271::AID-IMHJ2280160404>3.0.CO;2-B

Pica, M., Beere, D., Lovinger, S., & Dush, D. (2001). The responses of dissociative patients on the thematic apperception test. *Journal of Clinical Psychology, 57*(7), 847–864. https://doi.org/10.1002/jclp.1054

Piedfort-Marin, O., Tarquinio, C., Steinberg, M., Azarmsa, S., Cuttelod, T., Piot, M., Wisler, D., Zimmermann, E., & Nater, J. (2022). Reliability and validity study of the French-language version of the SCID-D semi-structured clinical interview for diagnosing *DSM-5* and *ICD-11* dissociative disorders. *Annales Médico-Psychologiques, Revue Psychiatrique, 180*(6, Suppl.), S1–S9. https://doi.org/10.1016/j.amp.2020.12.012

Pietkiewicz, I. J., Helka, A. M., & Tomalski, R. (2019). Validity and reliability of the Polish online and pen-and-paper versions of the Somatoform Dissociation Questionnaires (SDQ-20 and PSDQ-5). *European Journal of Trauma & Dissociation, 3*(1), 23–31. https://doi.org/10.1016/j.ejtd.2018.05.002

Pilton, M., Varese, F., Berry, K., & Bucci, S. (2015). The relationship between dissociation and voices: A systematic literature review and meta-analysis. *Clinical Psychology Review, 40*, 138–155. https://doi.org/10.1016/j.cpr.2015.06.004

Porter, C., Palmier-Claus, J., Branitsky, A., Mansell, W., Warwick, H., & Varese, F. (2020). Childhood adversity and borderline personality disorder: A meta-analysis. *Acta Psychiatrica Scandinavica, 141*(1), 6–20. https://doi.org/10.1111/acps.13118

Powell, R. A., & Gee, T. L. (1999). The effects of hypnosis on dissociative identity disorder: A reexamination of the evidence. *Canadian Journal of Psychiatry*, *44*(9), 914–916. https://doi.org/10.1177/070674379904400908

Powers, A., Cross, D., Fani, N., & Bradley, B. (2015). PTSD, emotion dysregulation, and dissociative symptoms in a highly traumatized sample. *Journal of Psychiatric Research*, *61*, 174–179. https://doi.org/10.1016/j.jpsychires.2014.12.011

Price, M., Kearns, M., Houry, D., & Rothbaum, B. O. (2014). Emergency department predictors of posttraumatic stress reduction for trauma-exposed individuals with and without an early intervention. *Journal of Consulting and Clinical Psychology*, *82*(2), 336–341. https://doi.org/10.1037/a0035537

Putnam, F. W. (1984). The psychophysiologic investigation of multiple personality disorder. A review. *The Psychiatric Clinics of North America*, *7*(1), 31–39. https://doi.org/10.1016/S0193-953X(18)30778-0

Putnam, F. W. (1992). Discussion: Are alter personalities fragments or figments? *Psychoanalytic Inquiry*, *12*(1), 95–111. https://doi.org/10.1080/07351699209533884

Putnam, F. W. (1994). The switch process in multiple personality disorder and other state-change disorders. In R. M. Klein & B. K. Doane (Eds.), *Psychological concepts and dissociative disorders* (pp. 283–304). Lawrence Erlbaum Associates.

Putnam, F. W. (1997). *Dissociation in children and adolescents: A developmental perspective*. Guilford Press.

Putnam, F. W. (2016). *The way we are: How states of mind influence our identities, personality, and potential for change*. International Psychoanalytic Books.

Putnam, F. W., Amaya-Jackson, L., Putnam, K. T., & Briggs, E. C. (2020). Synergistic adversities and behavioral problems in traumatized children and adolescents. *Child Abuse & Neglect*, *106*, Article 104492. https://doi.org/10.1016/j.chiabu.2020.104492

Putnam, F. W., Guroff, J. J., Silberman, E. K., Barban, L., & Post, R. M. (1986). The clinical phenomenology of multiple personality disorder: Review of 100 recent cases. *The Journal of Clinical Psychiatry*, *47*(6), 285–293.

Putnam, F. W., Helmers, K., & Trickett, P. K. (1993). Development, reliability, and validity of a child dissociation scale. *Child Abuse & Neglect*, *17*(6), 731–741. https://doi.org/10.1016/S0145-2134(08)80004-X

Putnam, F. W., Hornstein, N. L., & Peterson, G. (1996). Clinical phenomenology of child and adolescent dissociative disorders: Gender and age effects. *Child and Adolescent Psychiatric Clinics of North America*, *5*(2), 351–360. https://doi.org/10.1016/S1056-4993(18)30370-5

Putnam, F. W., & Peterson, G. (1994). Further validation of the Child Dissociative Checklist. *Dissociation*, *7*(4), 204–211.

Putnam, K. T., Harris, W. W., & Putnam, F. W. (2013). Synergistic childhood adversities and complex adult psychopathology. *Journal of Traumatic Stress*, *26*(4), 435–442. https://doi.org/10.1002/jts.21833

Quimby, L. G., Andrei, A., & Putnam, F. W., Jr. (1993). The deinstitutionalization of patients with chronic multiple personality disorder. In R. P. Kluft & C. G. Fine (Eds.), *Clinical perspectives on multiple personality disorder* (pp. 201–225). American Psychiatric Association.

Ratnamohan, L., MacKinnon, L., Lim, M., Webster, R., Waters, K., Kozlowska, K., Silberg, J., Greenwald, R., & Ribeiro, M. (2018). Ambushed by memories of trauma: Memory-processing interventions in an adolescent boy with nocturnal dissociative episodes. *Harvard Review of Psychiatry*, *26*(4), 228–236. https://doi.org/10.1097/HRP.0000000000000195

Rauch, S. A. M., Kim, H. M., Powell, C., Tuerk, P. W., Simon, N. M., Acierno, R., Allard, C. B., Norman, S. B., Venners, M. R., Rothbaum, B. O., Stein, M. B., Porter, K., Martis, B., King, A. P., Liberzon, I., Phan, K. L., & Hoge, C. W. (2019). Efficacy of prolonged exposure therapy, sertraline hydrochloride, and their combination among combat veterans with posttraumatic stress disorder: A randomized clinical trial. *JAMA Psychiatry*, *76*(2), 117–126. https://doi.org/10.1001/jamapsychiatry.2018.3412

Reinders, A. A. (2008). Cross-examining dissociative identity disorder: Neuroimaging and etiology on trial. *Neurocase*, *14*(1), 44–53. https://doi.org/10.1080/13554790801992768

Reinders, A. A., Nijenhuis, E. R. S., Paans, A. M. J., Korf, J., Willemsen, A. T. M., & den Boer, J. A. (2003). One brain, two selves. *NeuroImage*, *20*(4), 2119–2125. https://doi.org/10.1016/j.neuroimage.2003.08.021

Reinders, A. A., Nijenhuis, E. R. S., Quak, J., Korf, J., Haaksma, J., Paans, A. M. J., Willemsen, A. T. M., & den Boer, J. A. (2006). Psychobiological characteristics of dissociative identity disorder: A symptom provocation study. *Biological Psychiatry*, *60*(7), 730–740. https://doi.org/10.1016/j.biopsych.2005.12.019

Reinders, A. A., Willemsen, A. T. M., den Boer, J. A., Vos, H. P. J., Veltman, D. J., & Loewenstein, R. J. (2014). Opposite brain emotion-regulation patterns in identity states of dissociative identity disorder: A PET study and neurobiological model. *Psychiatry Research: Neuroimaging*, *223*(3), 236–243. https://doi.org/10.1016/j.pscychresns.2014.05.005

Reinders, A. A. T. S., Willemsen, A. T. M., Vos, H. P. J., den Boer, J. A., & Nijenhuis, E. R. S. (2012). Fact or factitious? A psychobiological study of authentic and simulated dissociative identity states [erratum at *PLOS ONE*. 2012;7(7): doi/10.1371/annotation/4f2000ce-ff9e-48e8-8de0-893b67efa3a4].*PLOS ONE*, *7*(6), e39279. https://doi.org/10.1371/journal.pone.0039279

Repetti, R. L., Taylor, S. E., & Seeman, T. E. (2002). Risky families: Family social environments and the mental and physical health of offspring. *Psychological Bulletin*, *128*(2), 330–366. https://doi.org/10.1037/0033-2909.128.2.330

Rettew, D. (2022, March 17). *The TikTok-inspired surge of dissociative identity disorder.* https://www.psychologytoday.com/au/blog/abcs-child-psychiatry/202203/the-tiktok-inspired-surge-dissociative-identity-disorder

Riley, K. C. (1988). Measurement of dissociation. *Journal of Nervous and Mental Disease,176*(7),449–450.https://doi.org/10.1097/00005053-198807000-00008

Riley, R. L., & Mead, J. (1988). The development of symptoms of multiple personality disorder in a child of three. *Dissociation, 1*(3), 41–46.

Rivera v. Bado, July Term 2014, No. 1548.

Roberts, A. L., Gilman, S. E., Breslau, J., Breslau, N., & Koenen, K. C. (2011). Race/ethnic differences in exposure to traumatic events, development of post-traumatic stress disorder, and treatment-seeking for post-traumatic stress disorder in the United States. *Psychological Medicine, 41*(1), 71–83. https://doi.org/10.1017/S0033291710000401

Rocchio, L. M. (2020). Ethical and professional considerations in the forensic assessment of complex trauma and dissociation. *Psychological Injury and Law, 13*(2), 124–134. https://doi.org/10.1007/s12207-020-09384-9

Rodewald, F., Gast, U., & Emrich, H. M. (2006). Screening auf Komplexe Dissoziative Störungen mit dem Fragebogen für dissoziative Symptome (FDS) [Screening for major dissociative disorders with the FDS, the German version of the Dissociative Experience Scale]. *Psychotherapie, Psychosomatik, Medizinische Psychologie, 56*(6), 249–258. https://doi.org/10.1055/s-2006-932590

Rogers, R., Bagby, R. M., & Dickens, S. E. (1992). *Structured Interview of Reported Symptoms: Professional manual.* Psychological Assessment Resources.

Rogers, R., & Bender, S. D. (2018). *Clinical assessment of malingering and deception* (4th ed.). Guilford Press.

Rogers, R., Payne, J. W., Correa, A. A., Gillard, N. D., & Ross, C. A. (2009). A study of the SIRS with severely traumatized patients. *Journal of Personality Assessment, 91*(5), 429–438. https://doi.org/10.1080/00223890903087745

Rogers, R., Sewell, K. W., & Gillard, N. D. (2010). *Structured Interview of Reported Symptoms—2 (SIRS-2) and professional manual.* Psychological Assessment Resources.

Rogers, R., Sewell, K. W., Martin, M. A., & Vitacco, M. J. (2003). Detection of feigned mental disorders: A meta-analysis of the MMPI-2 and malingering. *Assessment, 10*(2), 160–177. https://doi.org/10.1177/1073191103010002007

Root, M. (1992). Reconstructing the impact of trauma on personality. In L. S. Brown & M. Ballou (Eds.), *Personality and psychopathology: Feminist reappraisals* (pp. 229–265). Guilford Press.

Ross, C. A. (2007). Borderline personality disorder and dissociation. *Journal of Trauma & Dissociation, 8*(1), 71–80. https://doi.org/10.1300/J229v08n01_05

Ross, C. A. (2011). Possession experiences in dissociative identity disorder: A preliminary study. *Journal of Trauma & Dissociation, 12*(4), 393–400. https://doi.org/10.1080/15299732.2011.573762

Ross, C. A., & Browning, E. (2017). The self-report Dissociative Disorders Interview Schedule: A preliminary report. *Journal of Trauma & Dissociation, 18*(1), 31–37. https://doi.org/10.1080/15299732.2016.1172538

Ross, C. A., Duffy, C., & Ellason, J. W. (2002). Prevalence, reliability and validity of dissociative disorders in an inpatient setting. *Journal of Trauma & Dissociation, 3*(1), 7–17. https://doi.org/10.1300/J229v03n01_02

Ross, C. A., Ferrell, L., & Schroeder, E. (2014). Co-occurrence of dissociative identity disorder and borderline personality disorder. *Journal of Trauma & Dissociation, 15*(1), 79–90. https://doi.org/10.1080/15299732.2013.834861

Ross, C. A., Heber, S., Norton, G. R., Anderson, D., Anderson, G., & Barchet, P. (1989). The Dissociative Disorders Interview Schedule: A structured interview. *Dissociation, 2*(3), 169–189.

Ross, C. A., Joshi, S., & Currie, R. (1990). Dissociative experiences in the general population. *The American Journal of Psychiatry, 147*(11), 1547–1552. https://doi.org/10.1176/ajp.147.11.1547

Ross, C. A., Ridgway, J., & George, N. (2020). Maladaptive daydreaming, dissociation, and the dissociative disorders. *Psychiatric Research and Clinical Practice, 2*(2), 53–61. https://doi.org/10.1176/appi.prcp.20190050

Rossiter, A., Byrne, F., Wota, A. P., Nisar, Z., Ofuafor, T., Murray, I., Byrne, C., & Hallahan, B. (2015). Childhood trauma levels in individuals attending adult mental health services: An evaluation of clinical records and structured measurement of childhood trauma. *Child Abuse & Neglect, 44*, 36–45. https://doi.org/10.1016/j.chiabu.2015.01.001

Roydeva, M. I., & Reinders, A. A. T. S. (2021). Biomarkers of pathological dissociation: A systematic review. *Neuroscience and Biobehavioral Reviews, 123*, 120–202. https://doi.org/10.1016/j.neubiorev.2020.11.019

Rufer, M., Held, D., Cremer, J., Fricke, S., Moritz, S., Peter, H., & Hand, I. (2006). Dissociation as a predictor of cognitive behavior therapy outcome in patients with obsessive-compulsive disorder. *Psychotherapy and Psychosomatics, 75*(1), 40–46. https://doi.org/10.1159/000089225

Ruths, S., Silberg, J. L., Dell, P. F., & Jenkins, C. (2002, April). *Adolescent DID: An elucidation of symptomatology and validation of the MID*. Presented at the 19th meeting of the International Society for the Study of Dissociation, Baltimore, MD, United States.

Saakvitne, K. W. (2017). Relational theory: The cornerstone of integrative trauma practice. In S. N. Gold (Ed.), *APA handbook of trauma psychology* (Vol. 2, pp. 117–142). American Psychological Association. https://doi.org/10.1037/0000020-006

Sack, M., Sachsse, U., Overkamp, B., & Dulz, B. (2013). Traumafolgestörungen bei Patienten mit Borderline-Persönlichkeitsstörung: Ergebnisse einer Multicenterstudie [Trauma-related disorders in patients with borderline personality disorders. Results of a multicenter study]. *Der Nervenarzt, 84*(5), 608–614. https://doi.org/10.1007/s00115-012-3489-6

Saks, E. (1995). The criminal responsibility of people with multiple personality disorder. *Psychiatric Quarterly, 66*(2), 119–131. https://doi.org/10.1007/BF02238859

Saks, E. R. (1994). Does multiple personality disorder exist? The beliefs, the data, and the law. *International Journal of Law and Psychiatry, 17*(1), 43–78. https://doi.org/10.1016/0160-2527(94)90037-X

Saks, E. R. (1997). *Jekyll on trial: Multiple personality and criminal law*. New York University.

Salinger, T. (2015, November 19). Indiana girl, 12, killed stepmother because creepy clown character "Laughing Jack" told her to do it. *New York Daily News*. https://www.nydailynews.com/news/crime/indiana-girl-12-killed-stepmom-laughing-jack-article-1.2440821

Sanders, S. (1986). The Perceptual Alteration Scale: A scale measuring dissociation. *The American Journal of Clinical Hypnosis, 29*(2), 95–102. https://doi.org/10.1080/00029157.1986.10402691

Şar, V., Akyüz, G., & Doğan, O. (2007). Prevalence of dissociative disorders among women in the general population. *Psychiatry Research, 149*(1–3), 169–176. https://doi.org/10.1016/j.psychres.2006.01.005

Şar, V., Akyüz, G., Kugu, N., Öztürk, E., & Ertem-Vehid, H. (2006). Axis I dissociative disorder comorbidity in borderline personality disorder and reports of childhood trauma. *The Journal of Clinical Psychiatry, 67*(10), 1583–1590. https://doi.org/10.4088/JCP.v67n1014

Şar, V., Alioğlu, F., & Akyüz, G. (2014). Experiences of possession and paranormal phenomena among women in the general population: Are they related to traumatic stress and dissociation? *Journal of Trauma & Dissociation, 15*(3), 303–318. https://doi.org/10.1080/15299732.2013.849321

Şar, V., Alioğlu, F., Akyüz, G., & Karabulut, S. (2014). Dissociative amnesia in dissociative disorders and borderline personality disorder: Self-rating assessment in a college population. *Journal of Trauma & Dissociation, 15*(4), 477–493. https://doi.org/10.1080/15299732.2014.902415

Şar, V., Dorahy, M. J., & Krüger, C. (2017). Revisiting the etiological aspects of dissociative identity disorder: A biopsychosocial perspective. *Psychology Research and Behavior Management, 10*, 137–146. https://doi.org/10.2147/PRBM.S113743

Şar, V., Koyuncu, A., Öztürk, E., Yargic, L. I., Kundakçi, T., Yazici, A., Kuskonmaz, E., & Aksüt, D. (2007). Dissociative disorders in the psychiatric emergency ward. *General Hospital Psychiatry, 29*(1), 45–50. https://doi.org/10.1016/j.genhosppsych.2006.10.009

Şar, V., Kundakçi, T., Kiziltan, E., Bakim, B., & Bozkurt, O. (2001). Differentiating dissociative disorders from other diagnostic groups through somatoform dissociation in Turkey. *Journal of Trauma & Dissociation, 1*(4), 67–80. https://doi.org/10.1300/J229v01n04_04

Şar, V., Önder, C., Kilincaslan, A., Zoroglu, S. S., & Alyanak, B. (2014). Dissociative identity disorder among adolescents: Prevalence in a university psychiatric outpatient unit. *Journal of Trauma & Dissociation, 15*(4), 402–419. https://doi.org/10.1080/15299732.2013.864748

Şar, V., Tutkun, H., Alyanak, B., Bakim, B., & Baral, I. (2000). Frequency of dissociative disorders among psychiatric outpatients in Turkey. *Comprehensive Psychiatry, 41*(3), 216–222. https://doi.org/10.1016/s0010-440x(00)90050-6

Saxe, G. N., Chinman, G., Berkowitz, R., Hall, K., Lieberg, G., Schwartz, J., & van der Kolk, B. A. (1994). Somatization in patients with dissociative disorders. *The*

American Journal of Psychiatry, 151(9), 1329–1334. https://doi.org/10.1176/ajp.151.9.1329

Schalinski, I., Schauer, M., & Elbert, T. (2015). The Shutdown Dissociation Scale (Shut-D). *European Journal of Psychotraumatology, 6.* https://doi.org/10.3402/ejpt.v6.25652

Schauer, M., & Elbert, T. (2010). Dissociation following traumatic stress: Etiology and treatment. *Zeitschrift für Psychologie, 218*(2), 109–127.

Schiavone, F. L., McKinnon, M. C., & Lanius, R. A. (2018). Psychotic-like symptoms and the temporal lobe in trauma-related disorders: Diagnosis, treatment, and assessment of potential malingering. *Chronic Stress, 2,* 2470547018797046. https://doi.org/10.1177/2470547018797046

Schielke, H., Brand, B., & Marsic, A. (2017). Assessing therapeutic change in patients with severe dissociative disorders: The progress in treatment questionnaire, therapist and patient measures. *European Journal of Psychotraumatology, 8*(1), Article 1380471. https://doi.org/10.1080/20008198.2017.1380471

Schielke, H. J., Brand, B. L., & Lanius, R. A. (2022). *The Finding Solid Ground program workbook: Overcoming obstacles in trauma recovery.* Oxford University Press. https://doi.org/10.1093/med-psych/9780197629031.001.0001

Schlumpf, Y. R., Nijenhuis, E. R. S., Klein, C., Jäncke, L., & Bachmann, S. (2019). Functional reorganization of neural networks involved in emotion regulation following trauma therapy for complex trauma disorders. *NeuroImage: Clinical, 23,* 101807. https://doi.org/10.1016/j.nicl.2019.101807

Schlumpf, Y. R., Reinders, A. A. T. S., Nijenhuis, E. R. S., Luechinger, R., van Osch, M. J. P., & Jäncke, L. (2014). Dissociative part-dependent resting-state activity in dissociative identity disorder: A controlled FMRI perfusion study. *PLOS ONE, 9*(6), e98795. https://doi.org/10.1371/journal.pone.0098795

Schmahl, C., Kleindienst, N., Limberger, M., Ludäscher, P., Mauchnik, J., Deibler, P., Brünen, S., Hiemke, C., Lieb, K., Herpertz, S., Reicherzer, M., Berger, M., & Bohus, M. (2012). Evaluation of naltrexone for dissociative symptoms in borderline personality disorder. *International Clinical Psychopharmacology, 27*(1), 61–68. https://doi.org/10.1097/YIC.0b013e32834d0e50

Schnyder, U., Bryant, R. A., Ehlers, A., Foa, E. B., Hasan, A., Mwiti, G., Kristensen, C. H., Neuner, F., Oe, M., & Yule, W. (2016). Culture-sensitive psychotraumatology. *European Journal of Psychotraumatology, 7*(1), Article 31179. https://doi.org/10.3402/ejpt.v7.31179

Schweizer, J. (2013). Racial disparity in capital punishment and its impact on family members of capital defendants. *Journal of Evidence-Based Social Work, 10*(2), 91–99. https://doi.org/10.1080/15433714.2011.581549

Sedlak, A. J., Mettenbug, J., Basena, M., Petta, I., McPherson, K., Greene, A., & Li, S. (2010). *Fourth National Incidence Study of Child Abuse and Neglect (NIS-4): Report to Congress.* https://www.acf.hhs.gov/opre/report/fourth-national-incidence-study-child-abuse-and-neglect-nis-4-report-congress

Sege, R. D. (2021). Reasons for HOPE. *Pediatrics, 147*(5), e2020013987. Advance online publication. https://doi.org/10.1542/peds.2020-013987

Shapiro, D. L., Schumacher, L., Davis, J., & Caezza, J. (2013, August). *Mitigating psychological factors in capital cases* [Poster presentation]. 121st Annual Convention of the American Psychological Association, Honolulu, HI, United States.

Shinn, A. K., Wolff, J. D., Hwang, M., Lebois, L. A. M., Robinson, M. A., Winternitz, S. R., Öngür, D., Ressler, K. J., & Kaufman, M. L. (2020). Assessing voice hearing in trauma spectrum disorders: A comparison of two measures and a review of the literature. *Frontiers in Psychiatry, 10*, 1011. https://doi.org/10.3389/fpsyt.2019.01011

Shipherd, J. C., Maguen, S., Skidmore, W. C., & Abramovitz, S. M. (2011). Potentially traumatic events in a transgender sample: Frequency and associated symptoms. *Traumatology, 17*(2), 56–67. https://doi.org/10.1177/1534765610395614

Shirar, L. (1996). *Dissociative children: Bridging the inner and outer worlds.* W. W. Norton & Co.

Siegel, D. J. (1999). *The developing mind.* Guilford Press.

Sierra, M., Baker, D., Medford, N., & David, A. S. (2005). Unpacking the depersonalization syndrome: An exploratory factor analysis on the Cambridge Depersonalization Scale. *Psychological Medicine, 35*(10), 1523–1532. https://doi.org/10.1017/S0033291705005325

Sierra, M., & Berrios, G. E. (2000). The Cambridge Depersonalization Scale: A new instrument for the measurement of depersonalization. *Psychiatry Research, 93*(2), 153–164. https://doi.org/10.1016/S0165-1781(00)00100-1

Sierra, M., Medford, N., Wyatt, G., & David, A. S. (2012). Depersonalization disorder and anxiety: A special relationship? *Psychiatry Research, 197*(1–2), 123–127. https://doi.org/10.1016/j.psychres.2011.12.017

Silberg, J. L. (1998). Dissociative symptomatology in children and adolescents as displayed on psychological testing. *Journal of Personality Assessment, 71*(3), 421–439. https://doi.org/10.1207/s15327752jpa7103_10

Silberg, J. L. (2001). A presidents' perspective: The human face of the diagnostic controversy. *Journal of Trauma & Dissociation, 2*(1), 1–5. https://doi.org/10.1300/J229v02n01_01

Silberg, J. L. (2013). *The child survivor: Healing developmental trauma and dissociation.* Routledge/Taylor & Francis Group.

Silberg, J. L. (2022). *The child survivor: Healing developmental trauma and dissociation* (2nd ed.). Routledge/Taylor & Francis Group.

Silberg, J. L., Stipic, D., & Tagizadeh, F. (1997). Dissociative disorders in children and adolescents. In J. Noshpitz (Ed.), *The handbook of child and adolescent psychiatry* (pp. 329–355). John Wiley & Sons.

Silberman, E. K., Putnam, F. W., Weingartner, H., Braun, B. G., & Post, R. M. (1985). Dissociative states in multiple personality disorder: A quantitative study. *Psychiatry Research, 15*(4), 253–260. https://doi.org/10.1016/0165-1781(85)90062-9

Simeon, D. (2004). Depersonalisation disorder: A contemporary overview. *CNS Drugs, 18*(6), 343–354. https://doi.org/10.2165/00023210-200418060-00002

Simeon, D. (2009). Depersonalization disorder. In P. F. Dell & J. A. O'Neil (Eds.), *Dissociation and dissociative disorders: DSM-V and beyond* (pp. 441–442). Routledge.

Simeon, D., & Abugel, J. (2006). *Feeling unreal: Depersonalization disorder and the loss of the self.* Oxford University Press.

Simeon, D., Guralnik, O., & Schmeidler, J. (2001). Development of a depersonalization severity scale. *Journal of Traumatic Stress, 14*(2), 341–349. https://doi.org/10.1023/A:1011169019614

Simeon, D., Guralnik, O., Schmeidler, J., Sirof, B., & Knutelska, M. (2001). The role of childhood interpersonal trauma in depersonalization disorder. *The American Journal of Psychiatry, 158*(7), 1027–1033. https://doi.org/10.1176/appi.ajp.158.7.1027

Simeon, D., & Knutelska, M. (2005). An open trial of naltrexone in the treatment of depersonalization disorder. *Journal of Clinical Psychopharmacology, 25*(3), 267–270. https://doi.org/10.1097/01.jcp.0000162803.61700.4f

Simeon, D., Kozin, D. S., Segal, K., Lerch, B., Dujour, R., & Giesbrecht, T. (2008). De-constructing depersonalization: Further evidence for symptom clusters. *Psychiatry Research, 157*(1–3), 303–306. https://doi.org/10.1016/j.psychres.2007.07.007

Simeon, D., & Putnam, F. (2022). Pathological Dissociation in the National Comorbidity Survey Replication (NCS-R): Prevalence, morbidity, comorbidity, and childhood maltreatment. *Journal of Trauma & Dissociation, 23*(5), 490–503. https://doi.org/10.1080/15299732.2022.2064580

Sinason, V., & Marks, R. P. (2021). *Treating children with dissociative disorders: Attachment trauma, theory and practice.* Routledge. https://doi.org/10.4324/9781003246541

Smith, G. P., & Burger, G. K. (1997). Detection of malingering: Validation of the Structured Inventory of Malingered Symptomatology (SIMS). *The Journal of the American Academy of Psychiatry and the Law, 25*(2), 183–189.

Soffer-Dudek, N., & Somer, E. (2023). Maladaptive daydreaming is a dissociative disorder: Supporting evidence and theory. In M. J. Dorahy, S. Gold, & J. O'Neil (Eds.), *Dissociation and the dissociative disorders: Past, present, future* (2nd ed., pp. 449–563). Routledge Press.

Somer, E., Abu-Rayya, H. M., & Brenner, R. (2021). Childhood trauma and maladaptive daydreaming: Fantasy functions and themes in a multi-country sample. *Journal of Trauma & Dissociation, 22*(3), 288–303. https://doi.org/10.1080/15299732.2020.1809599

Somer, E., Amos-Williams, T., & Stein, D. J. (2013). Evidence-based treatment for depersonalisation-derealisation disorder (DPRD). *BMC Psychology, 1*(1), 20. https://doi.org/10.1186/2050-7283-1-20

Somer, E., Cardeña, E., Catelan, R. F., & Soffer-Dudek, N. (2021). Reality shifting: Psychological features of an emergent online daydreaming culture. *Current Psychology.* Advance online publication. https://doi.org/10.1007/s12144-021-02439-3

Somer, E., & Dell, P. F. (2005). Development of the Hebrew-Multidimensional Inventory of Dissociation (H-MID): A valid and reliable measure of pathological dissociation. *Journal of Trauma & Dissociation, 6*(1), 31–53. https://doi.org/10.1300/J229v06n01_03

Somer, E., Lehrfeld, J., Bigelsen, J., & Jopp, D. S. (2016). Development and validation of the Maladaptive Daydreaming Scale (MDS). *Consciousness and Cognition, 39*, 77–91. https://doi.org/10.1016/j.concog.2015.12.001

Somer, E., Somer, L., & Jopp, D. S. (2016). Childhood antecedents and maintaining factors in maladaptive daydreaming. *Journal of Nervous and Mental Disease, 204*(6), 471–478. https://doi.org/10.1097/NMD.0000000000000507

Speckens, A. E., Ehlers, A., Hackmann, A., & Clark, D. M. (2006). Changes in intrusive memories associated with imaginal reliving in posttraumatic stress disorder. *Journal of Anxiety Disorders, 20*(3), 328–341. https://doi.org/10.1016/j.janxdis.2005.02.004

Spiegel, D. (1984). Multiple personality as a post-traumatic stress disorder. *Psychiatric Clinics of North America, 7*, 101–110.

Spiegel, D., Loewenstein, R. J., Lewis-Fernández, R., Şar, V., Simeon, D., Vermetten, E., Cardeña, E., Brown, R. J., & Dell, P. F. (2011). Dissociative disorders in DSM-5. *Depression and Anxiety, 28*(12), E17–E45 [correction in *Depression and Anxiety, 29*(8), 747]. https://doi.org/10.1002/da.20923

Spiegel, H. (1972). An eye-roll test for hypnotizability. *American Journal of Clinical Hypnosis, 15*, 25–28. https://doi.org/10.1080/00029157.1972.10402206

Spitzer, C., Barnow, S., Freyberger, H. J., & Grabe, H. J. (2007). Dissociation predicts symptom-related treatment outcome in short-term inpatient psychotherapy. *The Australian and New Zealand Journal of Psychiatry, 41*(8), 682–687. https://doi.org/10.1080/00048670701449146

Stadnik, R. D., Brand, B., & Savoca, A. (2013). Personality Assessment Inventory profile and predictors of elevations among dissociative disorder patients. *Journal of Trauma & Dissociation, 14*(5), 546–561. https://doi.org/10.1080/15299732.2013.792310

Staniloiu, A., & Markowitsch, H. J. (2014). Dissociative amnesia. *The Lancet Psychiatry, 1*(3), 226–241. https://doi.org/10.1016/S2215-0366(14)70279-2

Staniloiu, A., Markowitsch, H. J., & Kordon, A. (2018). Psychological causes of autobiographical amnesia: A study of 28 cases. *Neuropsychologia, 110*, 134–147. https://doi.org/10.1016/j.neuropsychologia.2017.10.017

Steele, K., Boon, S., & van der Hart, O. (2017). *Treating trauma-related dissociation: A practical, integrative approach*. W. W. Norton & Co.

Steele, K., van der Hart, O., & Nijenhuis, E. R. S. (2005). Phase-oriented treatment of structural dissociation in complex traumatization: Overcoming trauma-related phobias. *Journal of Trauma & Dissociation, 6*(3), 11–53. https://doi.org/10.1300/J229v06n03_02

Stein, D. J., Koenen, K. C., Friedman, M. J., Hill, E., McLaughlin, K. A., Petukhova, M., Ruscio, A. M., Shahly, V., Spiegel, D., Borges, G., Bunting, B., Caldas-de-Almeida, J. M., de Girolamo, G., Demyttenaere, K., Florescu, S., Haro, J. M., Karam, E. G.,

Kovess-Masfety, V., Lee, S., . . . Kessler, R. C. (2013). Dissociation in posttraumatic stress disorder: Evidence from the world mental health surveys. *Biological Psychiatry, 73*(4), 302–312. https://doi.org/10.1016/j.biopsych.2012.08.022

Steinberg, M. (1994a). *Interviewer's guide to the structured clinical interview for* DSM-IV *dissociative disorders (SCID-D)* (rev. ed.). American Psychiatric Association.

Steinberg, M. (1994b). *The Structured Clinical Interview for* DSM-IV *Dissociative Disorders—Revised (SCID-D-R)*. American Psychiatric Association.

Steinberg, M. (1996). Diagnosis and assessment of dissociation in children and adolescents. *Child and Adolescent Psychiatric Clinics of North America, 5*(2), 333–350.

Steinberg, M. (2000). Advances in the clinical assessment of dissociation: The SCID-D-R. *Bulletin of the Menninger Clinic, 64*(2), 146–163.

Steinberg, M. (2023). *The SCID-D Interview: Dissociation assessment in therapy, forensics, and research*. American Psychiatric Association Press.

Steinberg, M., Rounsaville, B., & Cicchetti, D. (1991). Detection of dissociative disorders in psychiatric patients by a screening instrument and a structured diagnostic interview. *The American Journal of Psychiatry, 148*(8), 1050–1054. https://doi.org/10.1176/ajp.148.8.1050

Steinberg, M., Rounsaville, B., & Cicchetti, D. V. (1990). The Structured Clinical Interview for *DSM-III-R* Dissociative Disorders: Preliminary report on a new diagnostic instrument. *The American Journal of Psychiatry, 147*(1), 76–82. https://doi.org/10.1176/ajp.147.1.76

Steinberg, M., & Steinberg, A. (1995). Using the SCID-D to assess dissociative identity disorder in adolescents: Three case studies. *Bulletin of the Menninger Clinic, 59*(2), 221–231.

Steuwe, C., Lanius, R. A., & Frewen, P. A. (2012). Evidence for a dissociative subtype of PTSD by latent profile and confirmatory factor analyses in a civilian sample. *Depression and Anxiety, 29*(8), 689–700. https://doi.org/10.1002/da.21944

Stiglmayr, C., Schimke, P., Wagner, T., Braakmann, D., Schweiger, U., Sipos, V., Fydrich, T., Schmahl, C., Ebner-Priemer, U., Kleindienst, N., Bischkopf, J., Auckenthaler, A., & Kienast, T. (2010). Development and psychometric characteristics of the dissociation tension scale. *Journal of Personality Assessment, 92*(3), 269–277. https://doi.org/10.1080/00223891003670232

Stolbach, B. C. (1997). *The Children's Dissociative Experiences Scale and Posttraumatic Symptom Inventory: Rationale, development, and validation of a self-report measure* (Publication No. 9725794) [Doctoral dissertation, University of Colorado at Boulder]. ProQuest.

Stolbach, B. C., Minshew, R., Rompala, V., Dominguez, R. Z., Gazibara, T., & Finke, R. (2013). Complex trauma exposure and symptoms in urban traumatized children: A preliminary test of proposed criteria for developmental trauma disorder. *Journal of Traumatic Stress, 26*(4), 483–491. https://doi.org/10.1002/jts.21826

Struik, A. (2014). *Treating chronically traumatized children: Don't let sleeping dogs lie!* Routledge/Taylor & Francis Group.

Tamar-Gurol, D., Şar, V., Karadag, F., Evren, C., & Karagoz, M. (2008). Childhood emotional abuse, dissociation, and suicidality among patients with drug dependency in Turkey. *Psychiatry and Clinical Neurosciences, 62*(5), 540–547. https://doi.org/10.1111/j.1440-1819.2008.01847.x

Tanner, J., Zeffiro, T., Wyss, D., Perron, N., Rufer, M., & Mueller-Pfeiffer, C. (2019). Psychiatric symptom profiles predict functional impairment. *Frontiers in Psychiatry, 10,* 37. https://doi.org/10.3389/fpsyt.2019.00037

Tarrier, N., Pilgrim, H., Sommerfield, C., Faragher, B., Reynolds, M., Graham, E., & Barrowclough, C. (1999). A randomized trial of cognitive therapy and imaginal exposure in the treatment of chronic posttraumatic stress disorder. *Journal of Consulting and Clinical Psychology, 67*(1), 13–18. https://doi.org/10.1037/0022-006X.67.1.13

Taylor, S. (2003). Outcome predictors for three PTSD treatments: Exposure therapy, EMDR, and relaxation training. *Journal of Cognitive Psychotherapy, 17*(2), 149–161. https://doi.org/10.1891/jcop.17.2.149.57432

Teicher, M. H., Glod, C. A., Surrey, J., & Swett, C., Jr. (1993). Early childhood abuse and limbic system ratings in adult psychiatric outpatients. *The Journal of Neuropsychiatry and Clinical Neurosciences, 5*(3), 301–306. https://doi.org/10.1176/jnp.5.3.301

Teicher, M. H., & Samson, J. A. (2016). Annual research review: Enduring neurobiological effects of childhood abuse and neglect. *Journal of Child Psychology and Psychiatry, and Allied Disciplines, 57*(3), 241–266. https://doi.org/10.1111/jcpp.12507

Teicher, M. H., Samson, J. A., Anderson, C. M., & Ohashi, K. (2016). The effects of childhood maltreatment on brain structure, function and connectivity. *Nature Reviews Neuroscience, 17*(10), 652–666. https://doi.org/10.1038/nrn.2016.111

Teicher, M. H., Samson, J. A., Polcari, A., & McGreenery, C. E. (2006). Sticks, stones, and hurtful words: Relative effects of various forms of childhood maltreatment. *The American Journal of Psychiatry, 163*(6), 993–1000. https://doi.org/10.1176/ajp.2006.163.6.993

Tellegen, A., & Atkinson, G. (1974). Openness to absorbing and self-altering experiences ("absorption"), a trait related to hypnotic susceptibility. *Journal of Abnormal Psychology, 83*(3), 268–277. https://doi.org/10.1037/h0036681

Terence Tramaine Andrus v. Texas, 596 U.S. _____ (2022). https://www.supremecourt.gov/opinions/21pdf/21-6001_3d9g.pdf

Theodor-Katz, N., Somer, E., Hesseg, R. M., & Soffer-Dudek, N. (2022). Could immersive daydreaming underlie a deficit in attention? The prevalence and characteristics of maladaptive daydreaming in individuals with attention-deficit/hyperactivity disorder. *Journal of Clinical Psychology, 78*(11), 2309–2328. https://doi.org/10.1002/jclp.23355

Thomas, S., Höfler, M., Schäfer, I., & Trautmann, S. (2019). Childhood maltreatment and treatment outcome in psychotic disorders: A systematic review and meta-analysis. *Acta Psychiatrica Scandinavica, 140*(4), 295–312. https://doi.org/10.1111/acps.13077

Tichenor, V., Marmar, C. R., Weiss, D. S., Metzler, T. J., & Ronfeldt, H. M. (1996). The relationship of peritraumatic dissociation and posttraumatic stress: Findings in female Vietnam theater veterans. *Journal of Consulting and Clinical Psychology, 64*(5), 1054–1059. https://doi.org/10.1037/0022-006X.64.5.1054

Tombaugh, T. N. (1997). The Test of Memory Malingering (TOMM): Normative data from cognitively intact and cognitively impaired individuals. *Psychological Assessment, 9*(3), 260–268. https://doi.org/10.1037/1040-3590.9.3.260

Tombaugh, T. N. (2003). The Test of Memory Malingering (TOMM) in forensic psychology. *Journal of Forensic Neuropsychology, 2*(3–4), 69–96. https://doi.org/10.1300/J151v02n03_04

Torem, M. S., Egtvedt, B. D., & Curdue, K. J. (1995). The eye-roll sign and the PAS dissociation scale. *The American Journal of Clinical Hypnosis, 38*(2), 122–125. https://doi.org/10.1080/00029157.1995.10403190

Trickett, P. K., Noll, J. G., & Putnam, F. W. (2011). The impact of sexual abuse on female development: Lessons from a multigenerational, longitudinal research study. *Development and Psychopathology, 23*(2), 453–476. https://doi.org/10.1017/S0954579411000174

van der Hart, O., Nijenhuis, E. R. S., & Steele, K. (2006). *The haunted self: Structural dissociation and the treatment of chronic traumatization.* W. W. Norton & Co.

van der Heide, D., & Merckelbach, H. (2016). Validity of symptom reports of asylum seekers in a psychiatric hospital: A descriptive study. *International Journal of Law and Psychiatry, 49*(Pt. A), 40–46. https://doi.org/10.1016/j.ijlp.2016.05.007

van der Kloet, D., Giesbrecht, T., Lynn, S. J., Merckelbach, H., & de Zutter, A. (2012). Sleep normalization and decrease in dissociative experiences: Evaluation in an inpatient sample. *Journal of Abnormal Psychology, 121*(1), 140–150. https://doi.org/10.1037/a0024781

van der Kloet, D., Merckelbach, H., Giesbrecht, T., & Lynn, S. J. (2012). Fragmented sleep, fragmented mind: The role of sleep in dissociative symptoms. *Perspectives on Psychological Science, 7*(2), 159–175. https://doi.org/10.1177/1745691612437597

van der Kolk, B. A. (2014). *The body keeps the score: Brain, mind, and body in the healing of trauma.* Viking.

van der Kolk, B. A., & Ducey, C. P. (1989). The psychological processing of traumatic experience: Rorschach patterns in PTSD. *Journal of Traumatic Stress, 2*(3), 259–274. https://doi.org/10.1002/jts.2490020303

van der Kolk, B. A., Pelcovitz, D., Roth, S., Mandel, F. S., McFarlane, A., & Herman, J. L. (1996). Dissociation, somatization, and affect dysregulation: The complexity of adaptation of trauma. *The American Journal of Psychiatry, 153*(7, Suppl.), 83–93. https://doi.org/10.1176/ajp.153.7.83

van der Kolk, B. A., Roth, S., Pelcovitz, D., Sunday, S., & Spinazzola, J. (2005). Disorders of extreme stress: The empirical foundation of a complex adaptation to trauma. *Journal of Traumatic Stress, 18*(5), 389–399. https://doi.org/10.1002/jts.20047

Vanderlinden, J., Van Dyck, R., Vandereycken, W., & Vertommen, H. (1994). The Dissociation Questionnaire (DIS-G): Development, reliability and validity of a new self-reporting Dissociation Questionnaire. *Acta Psychiatrica Belgica, 94*(1), 53–54.

van IJzendoorn, M. H., & Schuengel, C. (1996). The measurement of dissociation in normal and clinical populations: Meta-analytic validation of the Dissociative Experiences Scale (DES). *Clinical Psychology Review, 16*(5), 365–382. https://doi.org/10.1016/0272-7358(96)00006-2

van Minnen, A., & Tibben, M. (2021). A brief cognitive-behavioural treatment approach for PTSD and dissociative identity disorder, a case report. *Journal of Behavior Therapy and Experimental Psychiatry, 72*(1), Article 101655. https://doi.org/10.1016/j.jbtep.2021.101655

Van Woudenberg, C., Voorendonk, E. M., Bongaerts, H., Zoet, H. A., Verhagen, M., Lee, C. W., van Minnen, A., & De Jongh, A. (2018). Effectiveness of an intensive treatment programme combining prolonged exposure and eye movement desensitization and reprocessing for severe post-traumatic stress disorder. *European Journal of Psychotraumatology, 9*(1), Article 1487225. https://doi.org/10.1080/20008198.2018.1487225

Vielleux, A. R. (2015). *The sociocultural factors in the misdiagnosis of dissociation in children and a proposal for the SID-C* (Publication No. 0419-4217) [Doctoral dissertation, Wisconsin School of Professional Psychology]. ProQuest Dissertations and Theses Global.

Vissia, E. M., Giesen, M. E., Chalavi, S., Nijenhuis, E. R. S., Draijer, N., Brand, B. L., & Reinders, A. A. T. S. (2016). Is it trauma- or fantasy-based? Comparing dissociative identity disorder, post-traumatic stress disorder, simulators, and controls. *Acta Psychiatrica Scandinavica, 134*(2), 111–128. https://doi.org/10.1111/acps.12590

Vonderlin, R., Kleindienst, N., Alpers, G. W., Bohus, M., Lyssenko, L., & Schmahl, C. (2018). Dissociation in victims of childhood abuse or neglect: A meta-analytic review. *Psychological Medicine, 48*(15), 2467–2476. https://doi.org/10.1017/S0033291718000740

Voorendonk, E. M., De Jongh, A., Rozendaal, L., & Van Minnen, A. (2020). Trauma-focused treatment outcome for complex PTSD patients: Results of an intensive treatment programme. *European Journal of Psychotraumatology, 11*(1), Article 1783955. https://doi.org/10.1080/20008198.2020.1783955

Waelde, L. C., Silvern, L., & Fairbank, J. A. (2005). A taxometric investigation of dissociation in Vietnam veterans. *Journal of Traumatic Stress, 18*(4), 359–369.

Walker, E. A., Newman, E., Koss, M., & Bernstein, D. (1997). Does the study of victimization revictimize the victims? *General Hospital Psychiatry, 19*(6), 403–410. https://doi.org/10.1016/S0163-8343(97)00061-3

Waller, N., Putnam, F. W., & Carlson, E. B. (1996). Types of dissociation and dissociative types: A taxometric analysis of dissociative experiences. *Psychological Methods, 1*(3), 300–321. https://doi.org/10.1037/1082-989X.1.3.300

Waters, F. S. (2016). *Healing the fractured child: Diagnosis and treatment of youth with dissociation*. Springer Publishing Co. https://doi.org/10.1891/9780826199645

Watson, D. (2003). Investigating the construct validity of the dissociative taxon: Stability analyses of normal and pathological dissociation. *Journal of Abnormal Psychology, 112*(2), 298–305. https://doi.org/10.1037/0021-843X.112.2.298

Weathers, F. W., Blake, D. D., Schnurr, P. P., Kaloupek, D. G., Marx, B. P., & Keane, T. M. (2013). *The Life Events Checklist for* DSM–5 *(LEC–5)*. National Center for PTSD. https://www.ptsd.va.gov/professional/assessment/te-measures/life_events_checklist.asp

Weathers, F. W., Bovin, M. J., Lee, D. J., Sloan, D. M., Schnurr, P. P., Kaloupek, D. G., Keane, T. M., & Marx, B. P. (2018). The Clinician-Administered PTSD Scale for *DSM-5* (CAPS-5): Development and initial psychometric evaluation in military veterans. *Psychological Assessment, 30*(3), 383–395. https://doi.org/10.1037/pas0000486

Webermann, A. R., & Brand, B. L. (2017). Mental illness and violent behavior: The role of dissociation. *Borderline Personality Disorder and Emotion Dysregulation, 4*(1), 2. https://doi.org/10.1186/s40479-017-0053-9

Webermann, A. R., Brand, B. L., & Chasson, G. S. (2014). Childhood maltreatment and intimate partner violence in dissociative disorder patients. *European Journal of Psychotraumatology, 5*(1), 24568. https://doi.org/10.3402/ejpt.v5.24568

Webermann, A. R., Brand, B. L., & Kumar, S. A. (2021). Intimate partner violence among patients with dissociative disorders. *Journal of Interpersonal Violence, 36*(3/4), NP1441–1462NP.

Webermann, A. R., Myrick, A. C., Taylor, C. L., Chasson, G. S., & Brand, B. L. (2016). Dissociative, depressive, and PTSD symptom severity as correlates of nonsuicidal self-injury and suicidality in dissociative disorder patients. *Journal of Trauma & Dissociation, 17*(1), 67–80. https://doi.org/10.1080/15299732.2015.1067941

Welburn, K. R., Fraser, G. A., Jordan, S. A., Cameron, C., Webb, L. M., & Raine, D. (2003). Discriminating dissociative identity disorder from schizophrenia and feigned dissociation on psychological tests and structured interview. *Journal of Trauma & Dissociation, 4*(2), 109–130. https://doi.org/10.1300/J229v04n02_07

Westen, D., Novotny, C. M., & Thompson-Brenner, H. (2004). The empirical status of empirically supported psychotherapies: Assumptions, findings, and reporting in controlled clinical trials. *Psychological Bulletin, 130*(4), 631–663. https://doi.org/10.1037/0033-2909.130.4.631

White, W. F., Burgess, A., Dalgleish, T., Halligan, S., Hiller, R., Oxley, A., Smith, P., & Meiser-Stedman, R. (2022). Prevalence of the dissociative subtype of post-traumatic stress disorder: A systematic review and meta-analysis. *Psychological Medicine, 52*(9), 1629–1644. https://doi.org/10.1017/S0033291722001647

Widows, M. R., & Smith, G. P. (2005). *Structured Inventory of Malingered Symptomatology manual*. PAR.

Wieder, L., Brown, R. J., & Terhune, D. B. (2023). Revisiting the role of verbal suggestion in dissociative psychopathology. *Acta Psychiatrica Scandinavica*. https://doi.org/10.1111/acps.13597

Wieder, L., Brown, R. J., Thompson, T., & Terhune, D. B. (2022). Hypnotic suggestibility in dissociative and related disorders: A meta-analysis. *Neuroscience and Biobehavioral Reviews, 139*, 104751. https://doi.org/10.1016/j.neubiorev.2022.104751

Wieland, S. (2015). *Dissociation in traumatized children and adolescents: Theory and clinical interventions* (2nd ed.). Routledge. https://doi.org/10.4324/9781315740430

Wiggins v. Smith, 539 U.S. 510 (2003). https://supreme.justia.com/cases/federal/us/539/510/

Wilgus, S. J., Packer, M. M., Lile-King, R., Miller-Perrin, C. L., & Brand, B. L. (2015). Coverage of child maltreatment in abnormal psychology textbooks: Reviewing the adequacy of the content. *Psychological Trauma: Theory, Research, Practice, and Policy, 8*(2), 188–197. https://doi.org/10.1037/tra0000049

Williams, L. M. (1994). Recall of childhood trauma: A prospective study of women's memories of child sexual abuse. *Journal of Consulting and Clinical Psychology, 62*(6), 1167–1176. https://doi.org/10.1037/0022-006X.62.6.1167

Williams, L. M. (1995). Recovered memories of abuse in women with documented child sexual victimization histories. *Journal of Traumatic Stress, 8*(4), 649–673. https://doi.org/10.1002/jts.2490080408

Williams v. Taylor, 529 U.S. 362 (2000). https://supreme.justia.com/cases/federal/us/529/362/

Wilson, J. P., & Lindy, J. D. (1994). *Countertransference in the treatment of PTSD*. Guilford Press.

Wolf, E. J., Lunney, C. A., Miller, M. W., Resick, P. A., Friedman, M. J., & Schnurr, P. P. (2012). The dissociative subtype of PTSD: A replication and extension. *Depression and Anxiety, 29*(8), 679–688. https://doi.org/10.1002/da.21946

Wolf, E. J., Miller, M. W., Reardon, A. F., Ryabchenko, K. A., Castillo, D., & Freund, R. (2012). A latent class analysis of dissociation and posttraumatic stress disorder: Evidence for a dissociative subtype. *Archives of General Psychiatry, 69*(7), 698–705. https://doi.org/10.1001/archgenpsychiatry.2011.1574

Wolf, E. J., Mitchell, K. S., Sadeh, N., Hein, C., Fuhrman, I., Pietrzak, R. H., & Miller, M. W. (2017). The dissociative subtype of PTSD scale: Initial evaluation in a national sample of trauma-exposed veterans. *Assessment, 24*(4), 503–516. https://doi.org/10.1177/1073191115615212

Wolf, G. K., Reinhard, M., Cozolino, L. J., Caldwell, A., & Asamen, J. K. (2009). Neuropsychiatric symptoms of complex posttraumatic stress disorder: A preliminary Minnesota Multiphasic Personality Inventory scale to identify adult survivors of childhood abuse. *Psychological Trauma: Theory, Research, Practice, and Policy, 1*(1), 49–64. https://doi.org/10.1037/a0015162

Woods, S. W., Walsh, B. C., Powers, A. R., III, & McGlashan, T. H. (2019). Reliability, validity, epidemiology, and cultural variation of the Structured Interview for Psychosis-risk Syndromes (SIPS) and the Scale of Psychosis-risk Symptoms (SOPS). In H. Li, D. I. Shapiro, & L. J. Seidman (Eds.), *Handbook of attenuated psychosis syndrome across cultures: International perspectives on early identification and intervention* (pp. 85–113). Springer. https://doi.org/10.1007/978-3-030-17336-4_5

World Health Organization. (2021). *International statistical classification of diseases and related health problems* (11th ed.). https://icd.who.int/

Wright, D. B., & Loftus, E. F. (2000). Measuring dissociation: Comparison of alternative forms of the Dissociative Experiences Scale. *Australian Journal of Clinical & Experimental Hypnosis, 28*(2), 103–126.

Xiao, C. L., Gavrilidis, E., Lee, S., & Kulkarni, J. (2016). Do mental health clinicians elicit a history of previous trauma in female psychiatric inpatients? *Journal of Mental Health, 25*(4), 359–365.

Xiao, Z., Yan, H., Wang, Z., Zou, Z., Xu, Y., Chen, J., Zhang, H., Ross, C. A., & Keyes, B. B. (2006). Trauma and dissociation in China. *The American Journal of Psychiatry, 163*(8), 1388–1391. https://doi.org/10.1176/ajp.2006.163.8.1388

Yeager, C. A., & Lewis, D. O. (1996). The intergenerational transmission of violence and dissociation. *Child and Adolescent Psychiatric Clinics of North America, 5*(2), 393–430. https://doi.org/10.1016/S1056-4993(18)30373-0

Yeater, E., Miller, G., Rinehart, J., & Nason, E. (2012). Trauma and sex surveys meet minimal risk standards: Implications for institutional review boards. *Psychological Science, 23*(7), 780–787. https://doi.org/10.1177/0956797611435131

Yehuda, N. A. (2011). Leroy (7 years old)—"It is almost like he is two children": Working with a dissociative child in a school setting. In S. Wieland (Ed.), *Dissociation in traumatized children and adolescents: Theory and clinical interventions* (pp. 285–341). Routledge/Taylor & Francis Group.

Yen, S., Johnson, J., Costello, E., & Simpson, E. B. (2009). A 5-day dialectical behavior therapy partial hospital program for women with borderline personality disorder: Predictors of outcome from a 3-month follow-up study. *Journal of Psychiatric Practice, 15*(3), 173–182. https://doi.org/10.1097/01.pra.0000351877.45260.70

Young, E. (2022). I didn't know where you were. In V. Sinason & R. P. Marks (Eds.), *Treating children with dissociative disorders: Attachment trauma, theory and practice* (pp. 180–197). Routledge.

Zanarini, M. C., Frankenburg, F. R., Dubo, E. D., Sickel, A. E., Trikha, A., Levin, A., & Reynolds, V. (1998). Axis I comorbidity of borderline personality disorder.

The American Journal of Psychiatry, 155(12), 1733–1739. https://doi.org/10.1176/ajp.155.12.1733

Zatzick, D. F., Marmar, C. R., Weiss, D. S., & Metzler, T. (1994). Does trauma-linked dissociation vary across ethnic groups? *Journal of Nervous and Mental Disease, 182*(10), 576–582. https://doi.org/10.1097/00005053-199410000-00008

Zhang, S., Liu, M., Li, Y., & Chung, J. E. (2021). Teens' social media engagement during the COVID-19 pandemic: A time series examination of posting and emotion on reddit. *International Journal of Environmental Research and Public Health, 18*(19), Article 10079. https://doi.org/10.3390/ijerph181910079

Zimmerman, M., & Mattia, J. I. (1999). Axis I diagnostic comorbidity and borderline personality disorder. *Comprehensive Psychiatry, 40*(4), 245–252. https://doi.org/10.1016/S0010-440X(99)90123-2

Zlotnick, C., Johnson, D. M., Yen, S., Battle, C. L., Sanislow, C. A., Skodol, A. E., Grilo, C. M., McGlashan, T. H., Gunderson, J. G., Bender, D. S., Zanarini, M. C., & Shea, M. T. (2003). Clinical features and impairment in women with borderline personality disorder (BPD) with posttraumatic stress disorder (PTSD), BPD without PTSD, and other personality disorders with PTSD. *Journal of Nervous and Mental Disease, 191*(11), 706–713. https://doi.org/10.1097/01.nmd.0000095122.29476.ff

Zoellner, L. A., Roy-Byrne, P. P., Mavissakalian, M., & Feeny, N. C. (2019). Doubly randomized preference trial of prolonged exposure versus sertraline for treatment of PTSD. *The American Journal of Psychiatry, 176*(4), 287–296. https://doi.org/10.1176/appi.ajp.2018.17090995

Index

About the Author

Bethany L. Brand, PhD, is a psychology professor and the director of the Clinical Focus program at Towson University, near Baltimore, Maryland. She has more than 30 years of experience in researching, assessing, and treating the impact of psychological trauma with a specialization in dissociation. Dr. Brand received her clinical training at Johns Hopkins Hospital, George Washington University Hospital, and at Sheppard Pratt Health System's Trauma Disorders program. She has been honored with the endowed Martha E. Mitten Professorship as well as teaching, research, and clinical awards including the Outstanding Contribution to the Science of Trauma Psychology from the American Psychological Association. She is associate editor of the *Journal of Trauma & Dissociation*. Dr. Brand has served on national and international task forces that developed guidelines for the assessment and treatment of trauma-related disorders. She has published more than 100 peer-reviewed papers and two research-based books about treating dissociation, *Finding Solid Ground: Overcoming Obstacles in Trauma Treatment* and *The Finding Solid Ground Program Workbook*. Dr. Brand is the principal investigator on the largest treatment outcome studies to date of dissociative disorders (the Treatment of Patients With Dissociative Disorders [TOP DD] studies). She has delivered hundreds of clinical and research presentations at national and international conferences. In addition to treating patients in her private practice, Dr. Brand serves as a forensic expert in trauma-related cases including state, federal, and capital cases and an international Supreme Court case.